CLINICAL GYNAECOLOGICAL UROLOGY

Clinical Gynaecological Urology

MOGENS ASMUSSEN
MD (Copenhagen), Dr med (Lund)
Gynaecologist, District and University Hospital, Hvidovre, Copenhagen
Formerly: Gynaecologist, County and University Hospital, Århus and
Gynaecologist and Clinical Research Fellow, Norwegian Radium Hospital, Oslo

ASHTON MILLER
MA, MD (Cambridge), FRCS (England)
Emeritus Consultant Urologist,
United Bristol Hospitals
Formerly: Hunterian Professor and Member of
Court of Examiners, Royal College of Surgeons of
England; Lecturer in Urology, University of Bristol;
Urologist, Norwegian Radium Hospital, Oslo

BLACKWELL SCIENTIFIC PUBLICATIONS
OXFORD LONDON
EDINBURGH BOSTON MELBOURNE

Editorial offices:
Osney Mead, Oxford, OX2 0EL
8 John Street, London, WC1N 2ES
9 Forrest Road, Edinburgh, EH1 2QH
52 Beacon Street, Boston
Massachusetts 02108, USA
99 Barry Street, Carlton
Victoria 3053, Australia

First published 1983

Photoset by Enset Ltd.,
Midsomer Norton, Bath, Avon
and printed and bound in Great Britain by
Camelot Press, Southampton

DISTRIBUTORS

USA
Blackwell Mosby Book Distributors
11830 Westline Industrial Drive
St Louis, Missouri 63141

Canada
Blackwell Mosby Book Distributors
120 Melford Drive, Scarborough
Ontario, M1B 2X4

Australia
Blackwell Scientific Book Distributors
31 Advantage Road, Highett
Victoria 3190

British Library
Cataloguing in Publication Data

Asmussen, Mogens
Clinical gynaecological urology.
1. Genito-urinary organs—Diseases
2. Generative organs, Female—Diseases
I. Title. II. Miller, Ashton
616.6 RG484

ISBN 0-632-00886-5

Contents

Introduction

The complex development of the female genital and urinary tracts from the stage where they shared a common outlet to the development of two adjacent but separate systems makes it inevitable that pathological conditions in one tract may involve the other simply because of close proximity. The two specialities of urology and gynaecology must therefore overlap in several places. This book is a combined effort by a gynaecologist and a urologist to assemble relevant information on the subject under one cover in order to fill a gap in the ordinary training of a gynaecologist.

The recommendations on the terminology of lower urinary tract function which have been produced by the International Continence Society have been used as a guide. For this reason simultaneous observations of vesical and urethral function form the basis of the physiology and patho-physiology which have been described.

A good deal of space has been devoted to gynaecological cancer surgery in spite of the fact that only a minority of gynaecologists are involved in this to any extent. This has been done because it is in this branch of surgery that urological complications are most conspicuous and it is here that the authors have had most experience of them and of urodynamic research in their elucidation.

Acknowledgements

We are grateful to the Norwegian Cancer Society (Landsforeningen mot Kreft) for having given both of us at different times a research fellowship which enabled us to work in the Department of Gynaecological Oncology at the Norwegian Radium Hospital. To Professor Per Kolstad and his colleagues we are grateful for encouragement and help. Much of what is described in this book is the result of experience gained in dealing with the many patients in his department which were entrusted to our care.

Our special thanks go to Dr med Arent B. Huisman of the University of Groningen in Holland, who very generously provided us with the results of his systematic researches into the complicated anatomy of the female urethra. These results are now published as a Thesis for his Doctorate.

Dr Bjørn Klevmark of the Department of Urology, Ullevål Hospital, Oslo, has kindly commented on the subject of neuropathic dysfunction.

Dr Mona Westby of the Department of Radiology, Norwegian Radium Hospital, who developed the technique of video-filming which we describe, kindly helped us with the technical details.

Mrs Liv Støttum, Secretary to the Department of Pathology at the Rikshospital, Oslo, patiently and efficiently converted our dictation into written English.

We thank Miss Claire Little and Miss Debra Neill-Marsei of Oxford Illustrators, who so professionally translated our preliminary drawings to the illustrations used in this book.

Definitions and Classification of Dysfunction

Dysfunction Any activity which is not within physiological limits.

Micturition Voluntary evacuation of urine through the urethra.

Continence The condition in which urine is retained within the urinary tract.

Urethral continence The condition in which urine is voluntarily or involuntarily retained in the bladder. This implies that the maximum urethral pressure is the same or greater than the bladder pressure under all conditions except micturition

Incontinence Any involuntary loss of urine, for example during exercise (*stress incontinence*) or in association with a strong desire to void (*urge incontinence*).

Extra-urethral incontinence Any urinary leakage other than through the urethra.

Urethral incontinence Any involuntary leakage of urine through the urethra caused by bladder pressure exceeding the maximum urethral pressure, so that the urethral closure pressure becomes negative.

Urge The strong desire to micturate. When urge occurs with an unacceptably small volume in the bladder, leading to frequency of micturition, it becomes pathological.

Neuropathic dysfunction Dysfunction caused by an abnormality in the nervous control of the lower urinary tract.

Neuropathic incontinence Involuntary leakage of urine from the urethra due to dysfunction of the micturition reflex arc and/or its cerebral control.

Idiopathic dysfunction Dysfunction for which clinical investigation provides no explanation.

Unstable urethra Oscillating variation of urethral pressure which is not synchronous with the heart beat or respiration and which is not associated with significant variation of bladder pressure.

Unstable bladder or detrusor instability Involuntary rise in bladder pressure greater than 15 cm of water as measured by simple cystometry. Although this term is frequently used, there is no agreement as to its meaning or pathological significance.

Detrusor/urethra dyssynergia Disruption of the normal interplay between the bladder and urethra. The word dyssynergia means lack of cooperation between two groups of muscles.

Retention of urine Sudden inability to micturate so that the bladder becomes distended and painful is known as *acute retention*. A gradual increase in urethral obstruction produces painless retention of urine and incomplete micturition with *residual urine* in the bladder. If the bladder is palpable, it is called *chronic retention*. When this process continues until the bladder reaches the limit of its capacity, a little urine leaks out involuntarily. It is then known as *overflow incontinence*. This form of incontinence is paradoxical in that the bladder is full all the time and the micturition reflex is abolished. It can occur after major pelvic surgery.

Frequency of micturition Normal frequency is decided by the individual patient. Abnormal frequency begins when micturition becomes a recurrent nuisance in daily life. It is important to appreciate the difference between frequency during the day when the patient is awake and during the night when she is asleep. If a patient does not wake up to void during the night, the bladder capacity must be normal. If she wakes up to micturate, there must be urgency sufficient to interfere with sleep. This can, of course, depend on fluid intake.

Dysuria Micturition which has become difficult or painful. In most cases difficulty is inseparable from pain.

Strangury Extreme dysuria.

If a classification of dysfunction is to have any meaning, it is necessary to exclude the following conditions which can produce urinary dysfunction as part of their symptom complex:

lower urinary tract or genital infections
urinary fistula
vesical tumour
abdominal or pelvic tumour
irradiation effects
interstitial cystitis (Hunner's ulcer)
temporary post-operative dysfunction
urethral pathology
vesical or urethral calculus

It is then possible to use the following three groups as a practical guide:

1 stress incontinence (Chapter 5);
2 neuropathic dysfunction (Chapter 6);
3 idiopathic dysfunction (Chapter 7).

REFERENCES

Asmussen M (1980) Aspects of continence, incontinence and micturition in women. Chapter 10 in *Gynecological Urology and Urodynamics*, ed. D. Ostergard. Williams & Wilkins, Baltimore.

Bates P *et al* (1979) Standardisation of terminology of lower Urinary Tract Function. *J. Urol.* **121,** 554.

Chapter 1 Applied Embryology

This chapter contains only what is necessary to understand the role of embryology in gynaecological urology. If the reader needs more information on the subject he is referred to special textbooks on embryology.

Inevitably, the rarer and more bizarre malformations of the urinary tract have crept in because they serve not only to illustrate the processes which cause them but also to make normal development easier to understand. They have very little relevance for the gynaecologist who practically never sees them and in any case will never treat them.

The site of the future genitalia is first recognizable in the 4 mm embryo during the fourth week of existence. It consists of an endodermal tube called the allantois (future bladder) coming in from the umbilical cord, two mesodermal ducts – one on each side of the mid-line – called the mesonephric or Wolffian ducts, which come down from the mesonephric tubules, and the endodermal hind-gut (future rectum) lying posteriorly in the mid-line. All of these channels open into an endodermal cavity (*cloaca*) which is covered by an ectodermal membrane. This lies in a depression between the umbilical cord and the tail known as the proctodeum (Fig. 1.1).

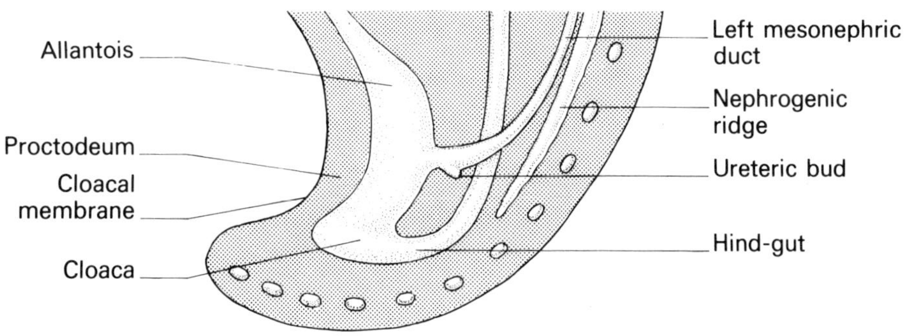

At the lower end of each mesonephric (Wolffian) duct, a *ureteric bud* grows out almost directly backwards on either side of the hind-gut to reach the nephrogenic ridge on the posterior wall at the level of the 2nd sacral vertebra (Fig. 1.2). The *kidney* is formed from the cells of the ridge as a result of the arrival of the ureteric bud. If there is no bud then there will be neither ureter nor kidney (*renal agenesis*), a situation which can be unilateral (about once in 2000 births) or more rarely bilateral (Fig. 1.3). If there are two ureteric buds on one side, then there will be a

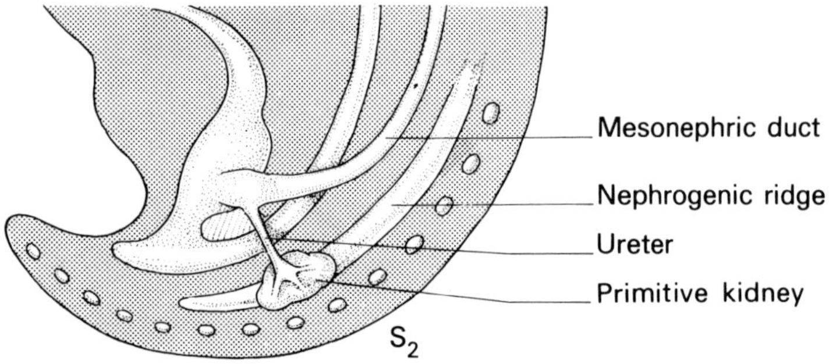

Fig. 1.2. Sixth week. Kidney appears.

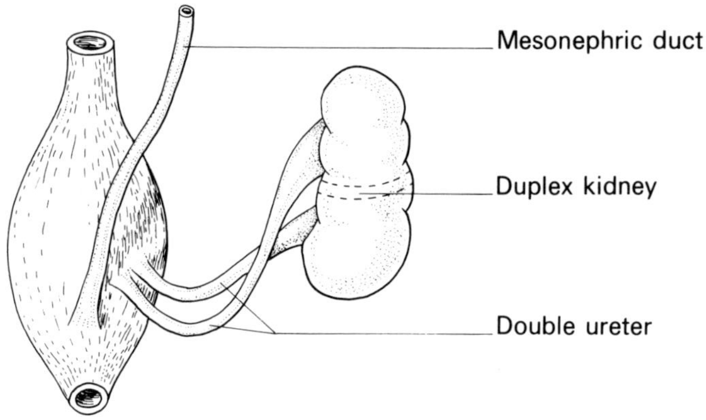

Fig. 1.3. Posterior aspect of primitive bladder. Double right ureter.

kidney in two separate parts, one above the other, a so-called *duplex kidney*, with two ureters (Fig. 1.3). If the original bud divides, the same type of duplex kidney will be formed with the ureter in the form of a Y.

Growth of the cloaca results in the lowest parts of the mesonephric ducts being absorbed into what is to become the bladder, so that the ureters and the mesonephric ducts open into it separately (Fig. 1.4). There is then a considerable period of rapid differential growth in which the relative positions of the orifices of the ureter and mesonephric duct on each side become almost reversed. The posterior part of the primitive bladder grows downwards, carrying the mesonephric duct orifices down with it while the ureteric orifices, now lying more laterally, remain behind (Fig. 1.5). This change of position is not easy to

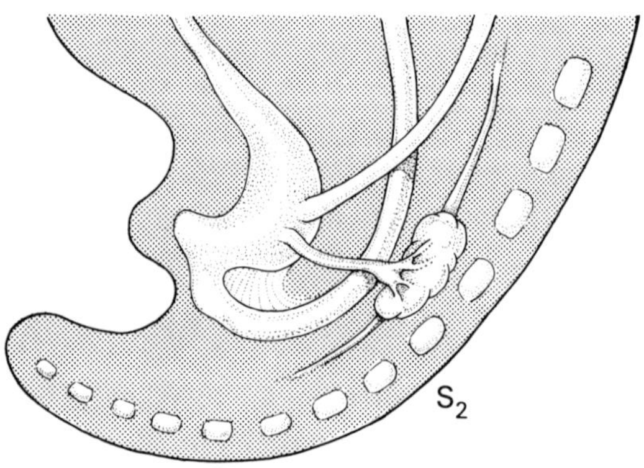

Fig. 1.4. Sixth week. Ureter is separated from mesonephric duct.

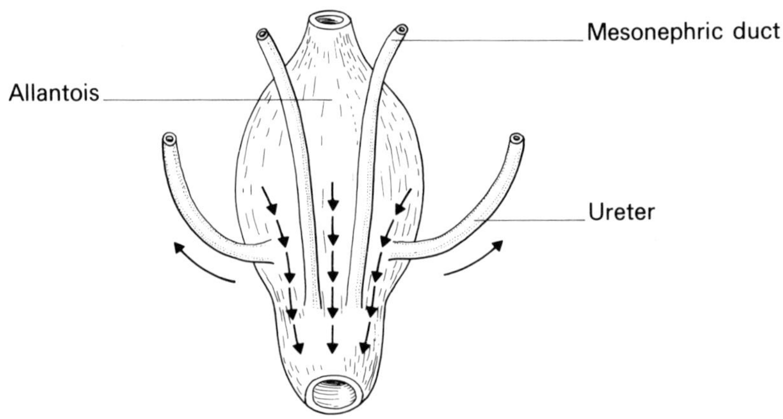

Fig. 1.5. Sixth week. Posterior aspect of primitive bladder.

understand but is the key to the explanation of several anomalies. Occasionally there are two ureteric buds on the same side, as mentioned above; the upper one, which goes to the upper part of the kidney, is moved inwards and downwards in relation to the ureter going to the lower kidney and ends up below it. This explains the otherwise mysterious fact that if one finds two ureteric orifices on one side of the trigone, it is always the lower one that drains the upper part of the kidney. This same ureteric orifice may be carried even further downwards and end up opening into the uterus or vagina, sometimes even adjacent to the external urinary meatus (*ectopic ureter*). These ectopic ureteric orifices leak a little urine almost continuously and are one of the rarer causes of incontinence. It is also understandable why the mesonephric remnants such as Gaertner's ducts can be found further down in the anterior vaginal wall near the urethra.

The primitive kidney is formed at the level of S2 and appears to move upwards to its final position. In reality the embryo straightens itself out at the same time as the whole tail end with the lower limb buds grows downwards past the kidney. Partial or complete failure of this process is not uncommon with the result that a normally functioning kidney can be found anywhere between S2 and the upper lumbar vertebrae. Figure 1.6 shows a posterior view of the two kidneys in the initial stage where their medial and lower poles are very near one another. They can also become fused together to form a *horseshoe kidney*. The inferior mesenteric artery passes forwards directly above the isthmus so that a horseshoe kidney always lies with its junction just above the promontory of the sacrum. The ureters pass downwards over the front of the isthmus and then take an almost normal course to the bladder. So-called *crossed renal ectopia* is really a horseshoe kidney which has slewed round so that it lies on one or other side of the inferior mesenteric artery. This allows the whole complex to lie at a higher level but makes matters complicated for the ureter from the lower renal pelvis must cross over to the other side of the mid-line to reach the bladder in the normal position. Crossed renal ectopia is much rarer than horseshoe kidney.

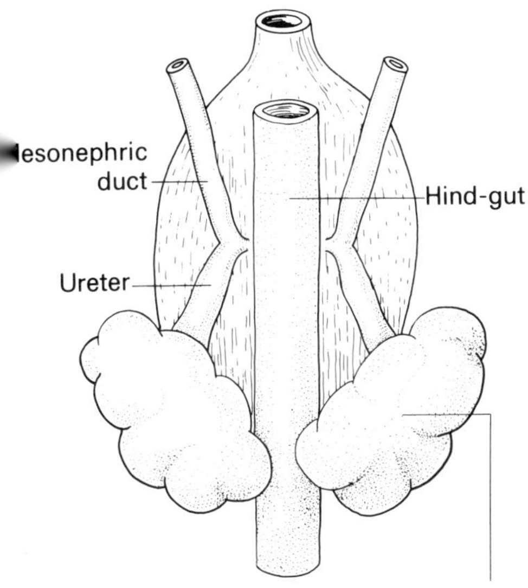

Fig. 1.6. Fifth week. Posterior aspect of primitive kidneys.

A variety of ectopic kidney which can give trouble to the gynaecologist is the *pelvic kidney*. This remains at the S1–S2 level on the posterior abdominal wall in the region of the pelvic brim. It can imitate an ovarian tumour or cause mechnical obstruction during delivery so that caesarian section may be necessary. Furthermore, as in other malformations of the urinary tract, there may be an increased risk of urinary infection. The blood supply comes in the form of a series of arteries from the aorta and common iliac arteries. The renal pelvis tends to lie on the front of the kidney and is therefore an immediate posterior relation of the peritoneum.

The two kidneys may join behind the rectum and stay there, filling the hollow of the sacrum. The condition is then spoken of as *fused pelvic kidney*. The ureters come forward on each side of the rectum.

During the fifth week the cloaca is a large cavity with the allantois entering anteriorly and the hind-gut posteriorly. In between is the urorectal septum, a connective tissue mass which grows downwards until it makes contact with the ectodermal membrane which has up till now closed the cloaca (Fig. 1.7). The region where the septum and the cloacal membrane merge becomes the *perineum* and from this moment, in the sixth week, the hind-gut is completely separated

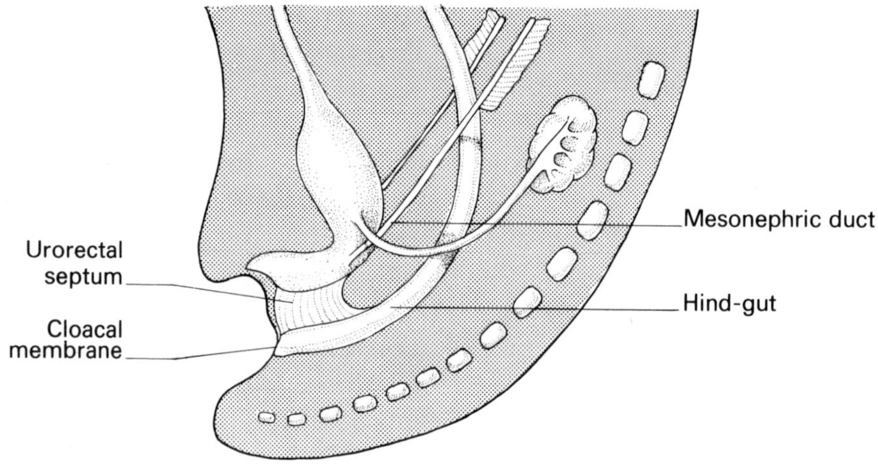

Fig. 1.7. Sixth week. Urorectal septum separates hind gut from primitive bladder.

from the urogenital apparatus. The next step is the disintegration of the cloacal membrane over the hind-gut so that the anal opening is formed. This allows the rectum to open directly into the amniotic cavity. If this process fails, the infant is born with an *imperforate anus*. If the urorectal septum fails to reach the cloacal membrane the rectum will open into the bladder (*persistent cloaca*).

Anterior to the urorectal septum there is considerable activity; the cloacal membrane also disintegrates here, opening this part of the cloaca to the amniotic cavity. This now becomes known as the *urogenital sinus*. Within this sinus can be seen the openings of the mesonephric ducts, symmetrical and near the mid-line, the openings of the ureters further in and farther apart and the channel of the allantois, now beginning to enlarge into the future bladder. It becomes narrower higher up to become the *urachus*. The urachus normally disappears but can occasionally persist as a whole or in part in the form of a tube lined by columnar epithelium. The position at the end of the sixth week is shown in Figure 1.8.

Next, the posterior bladder wall enlarges so that the ureteric orifices are carried laterally away from one another. Fibres from the ureters together with the lower part of the bladder wall forms the bladder base and *trigonal structures*. These

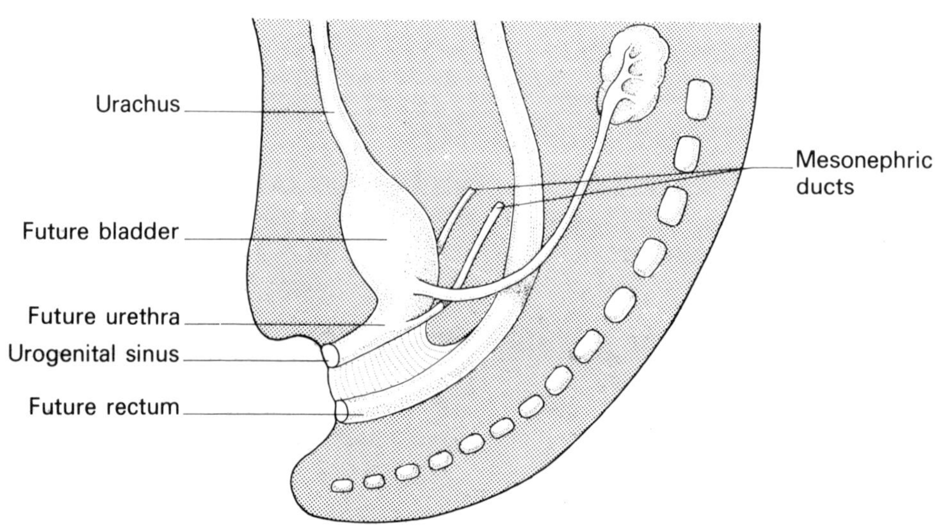

Fig. 1.8. Sixth week. Cloacal membrane disappears.

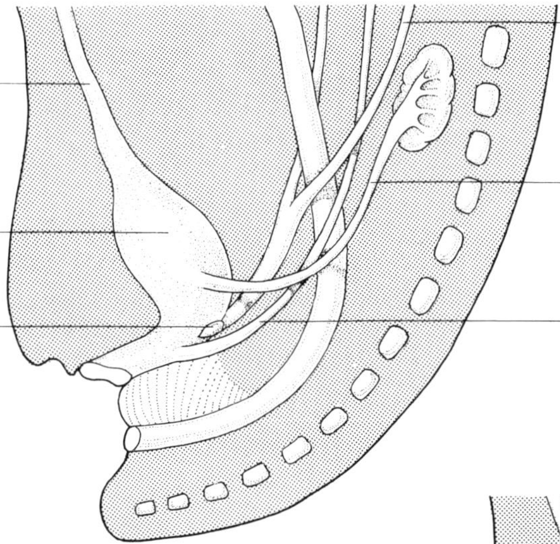

Fig. 1.9. Seventh week. Müllerian duct appears.

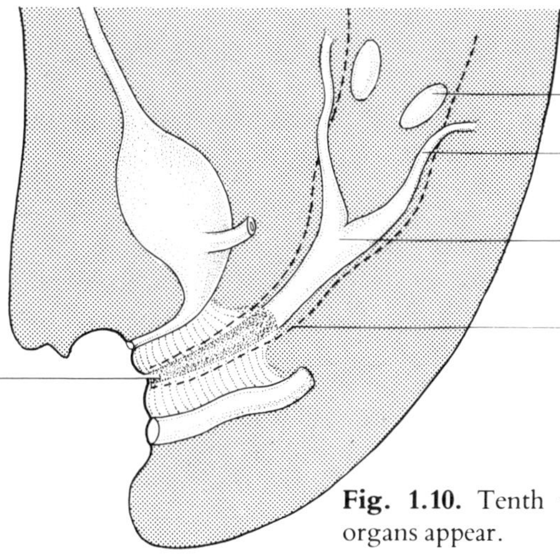

Fig. 1.10. Tenth week. Female genital organs appear.

become narrower to form most of the urethral tube. Failure of this process results in absence of the front wall of the urethra or *epispadias*. This process can be so extensive that it involves the urethra and bladder, with the result that the bladder lies open on the anterior abdominal wall with complete absence of the symphysis pubis. This gross abnormality, *ectopia vesicae,* presents the urologist with one of his most difficult surgical problems.

During the sixth and seventh weeks at about the 12 mm stage, a new duct makes its appearance lateral to and parallel with the upper ends of the mesonephric ducts on the posterior wall of the coelomic (abdominal) cavity. It is called the paramesonephric (Müllerian) duct and its formation extends rapidly downwards until it meets its fellow on the other side. The lower ends of the two ducts blend together and their blind ends form the Müllerian Tubercle in the urogenital sinus between the openings of the mesonephric ducts (Fig. 1.9).

The uppermost vertical portions of the paramesonephric ducts form the *Fallopian tubes,* the mid-portions together with the lower parts form the body of the *uterus,* while the tubercle forms a mass of cells which canalize to form the *vagina*. This canalization is complete with connection to the cavity of the uterus by the twentieth week. The mesonephric ducts largely disappear, remnants sometimes persisting as Gaertner's ducts (Fig. 1.10). The most common anomaly seen by the gynaecologist is a *cyst of Gaertner's duct* which is found on one or both sides of the vagina. The urological relevance of this is that the bladder base and urethra may be direct relations of the cyst and therefore liable to injury during removal.

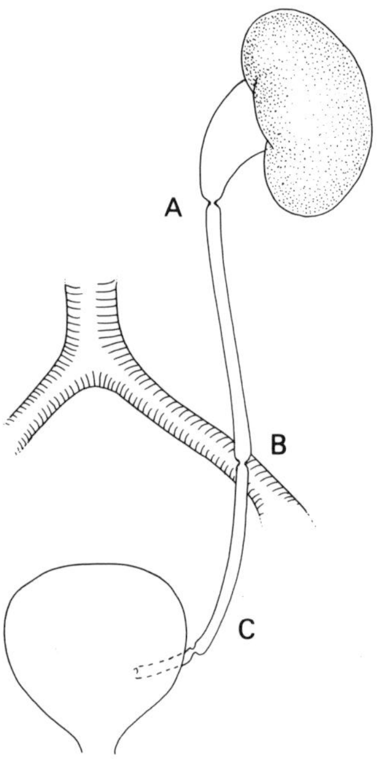

Fig. 1.11. Sites of stenosis in the ureter.

Any of the various tubes can develop a *stenosis*.

The ureter is the site of anatomic or functional stenosis more often than the bladder and urethra. This occurs in 3 places – *A, B* and *C* in Figure 1.11. *A* is the commonest and produces a hydronephrosis. *C* is the next commonest and is situated just outside the bladder wall where the ureter lies in close relation to the uterine artery and passes through the vesico-uterine ligament. Stenosis here produces dilation of the pelvic ureter, sometimes of the whole length of the ureter together with the renal pelvis. Stenosis at *B* is very rare; it is worth noting that the dilatation of the ureters above this point is the same as that which normally occurs in pregnancy. *D* is a stenosis at the junction of the ureteric epithelium with the bladder epithelium which produces a cyst-like dilatation which projects into the bladder. This is known as a *ureterocele* and is therefore easily seen with a cystoscope and shows itself as a typical filling defect on intravenous urography (Fig. 1.12).

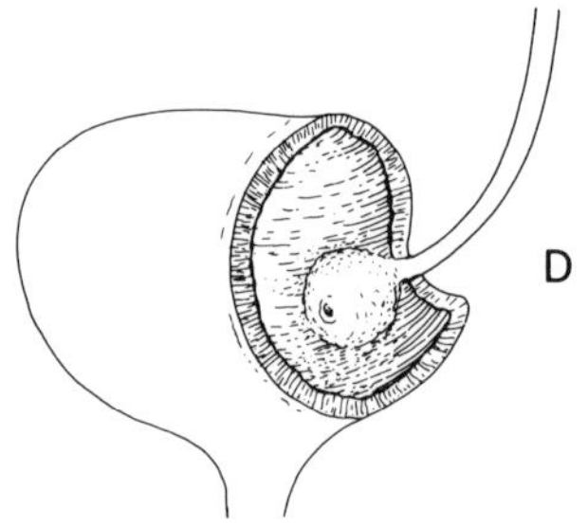

Fig. 1.12. Another stenosis site in the ureter.

The gynaecologist should note that congenital malformations seldom exist singly. Whatever hormonal or other influence has been responsible for one malformation in intrauterine life can also have exerted its effect upon other developing parts. In practice this means that if the gynaecologist finds some congenital anatomical variation in the female genital tract he should look for an abnormality in the nearby urinary tract.

One can sum up development by saying that the bladder, urethra, introitus and outer part of the vagina originate from endoderm, while the rest of the internal female genitalia and the kidneys, ureters and the trigone of the bladder are of mesodermal origin. An exception of course is the germ cells in the ovaries. The epithelial lining does not correspond accurately with these two origins.

REFERENCES

Hamilton WJ, Boyd JD & Mossman H.W. (1972) *Human Embryology*, 4th edn. Williams & Wilkins, Baltimore.

Johnston JH (1969) *Neonatal Surgery*. Butterworths, London.

Williams DI (1968) *Paediatric Urology*. Butterworths, London.

Chapter 2 Applied Anatomy

Recent events in the research world have raised doubts about the accepted views on the mechanism of dysfunction of the bladder and urethra. We will therefore go into considerable anatomical detail in order to explain the basis for these doubts. It reveals that the lower urinary tract in the female is a much more complicated and delicate region than was originally thought.

BLADDER AND URETHRA

The bladder and urethra should be thought of as one anatomical unit. For practical anatomical purposes it is divided into the *dome* or *vault*, the *bladder base* (which includes the trigone) and the *urethra* (Fig. 2.1). The bladder base and the urethra have more muscular layers and a greater nerve supply than the bladder dome. It is not easy to define the exact anatomical boundary between the bladder base and the urethra because this is based more on physiological properties than on a distinct anatomical situation.

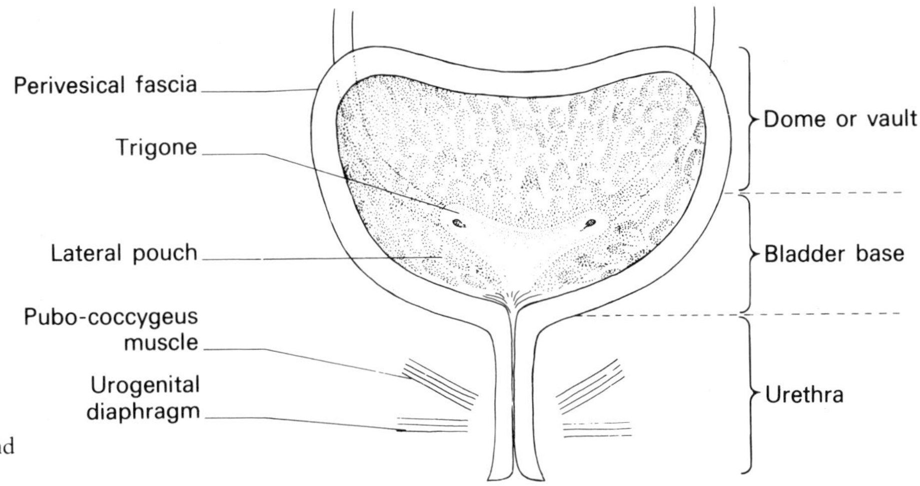

Fig. 2.1. The dome, the bladder base and the urethra.

Epithelial lining

The lining is transitional epithelium, known as the urothelium, resting on a submucosa containing blood vessels and lymphatics which allows considerable mobility of the epithelium everywhere except on the trigone, where it is firmly fixed to the underlying muscle.

There are no true glands in the urothelium except some which open posteriorly into the urethra just above the urogenital diaphragm. Two other small glands, known as Skene's glands, open on either side of the external urinary meatus.

The transitional epithelium in the urethra normally alters to non-keratinizing squamous epithelium in the lower quarter without any sharp line of demarcation. Nearly the whole length of the urethra can be lined by squamous epithelium in the elderly woman while in young women almost the whole length can be transitional. This is probably a metaplasia caused by hormone influences. The squamous epithelium seems to be more susceptible to infection. The urethral epithelium is affected by oestrogen, in the same way as the vaginal mucosa.

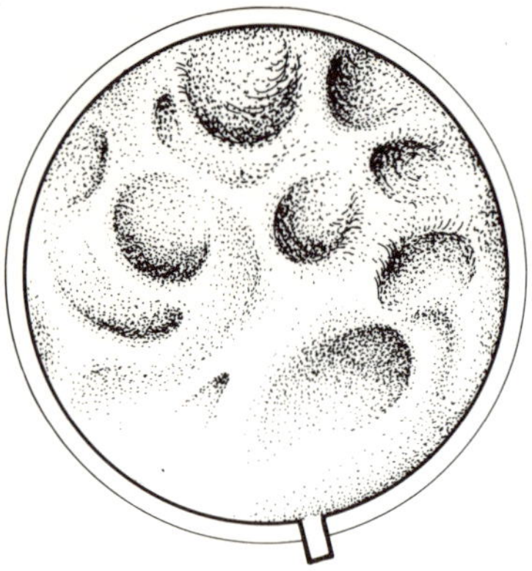

Fig. 2.2. Trabeculation of the bladder.

The dome

In the embryo the musculature consists of three smooth muscle layers, but after birth all layers are merged together. The thickness increases towards the base where the layers are more apparent though they can never be completely separated from one another. The internal coat is much thicker and stronger and is formed like a network of muscle bundles. This layer was originally called the detrusor muscle but this name is now used to mean all three layers. The internal coat can be seen through the cystoscope and produces the appearance known as 'trabeculation' (Fig. 2.2).

The bladder base and urethra

The detailed anatomy here becomes so complex that it is difficult to interpret its function. However, three things are so striking that they must have clinical significance.

1 The blood supply of the urethra far exceeds the needs of nutrition.

2 The circular smooth and striated muscle fibres in the urethra are so thin and so apparently disorganised in the adult woman that a sphincteric effect based on muscular contraction alone seems doubtful.

3 The different structures in the urethra undergo considerable changes with age.

Main blood supply

Besides branches from the inferior vesical arteries, the bladder receives several smaller vessels such as the superior vesical artery. This is not always present because of the enormous vascular variation in the pelvis. When it is present it often comes off the hypogastric (internal iliac) artery where the uterine artery originates. There must be many small vessels which can provide an alternative blood supply to the lower urinary tract for both the superior and inferior vesical arteries on one side can normally be divided without producing necrosis of the bladder wall.

The venous drainage is more complex and even more variable. This becomes obvious if the lower bladder wall is injured during a pelvic operation.

The detailed anatomy of the urethra is illustrated in Figs 2.3, 2.4 and 2.5.

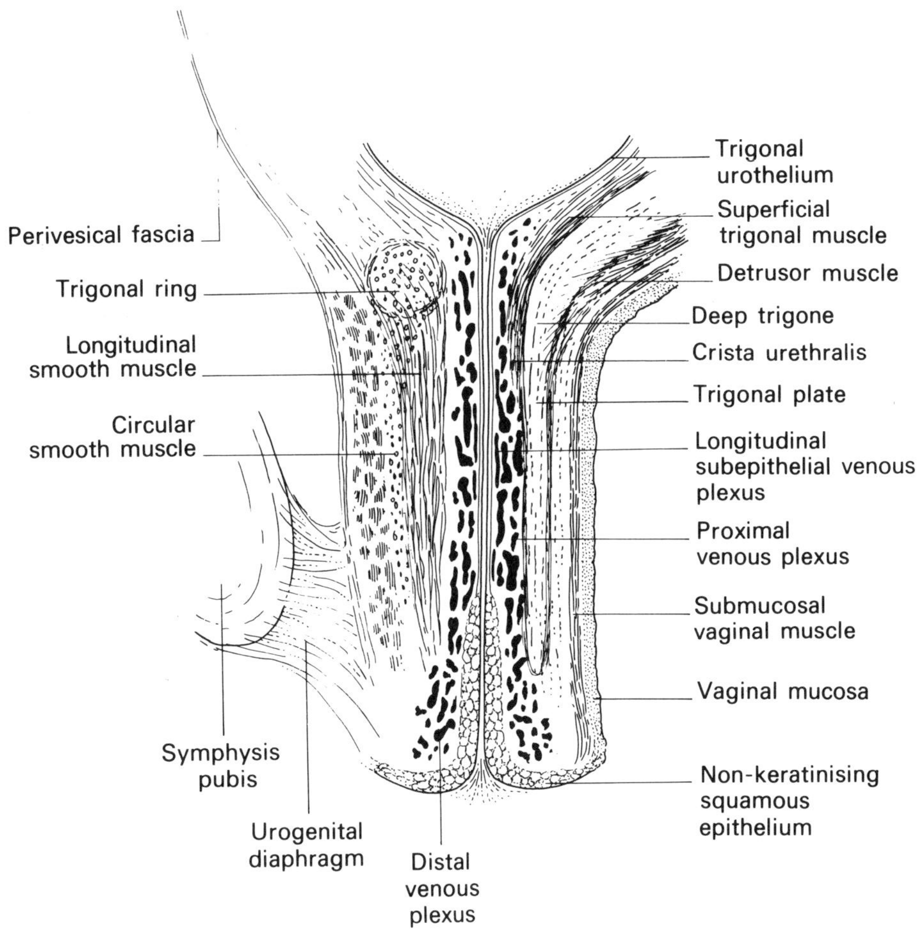

Fig. 2.3. Sagittal section of the urethra.

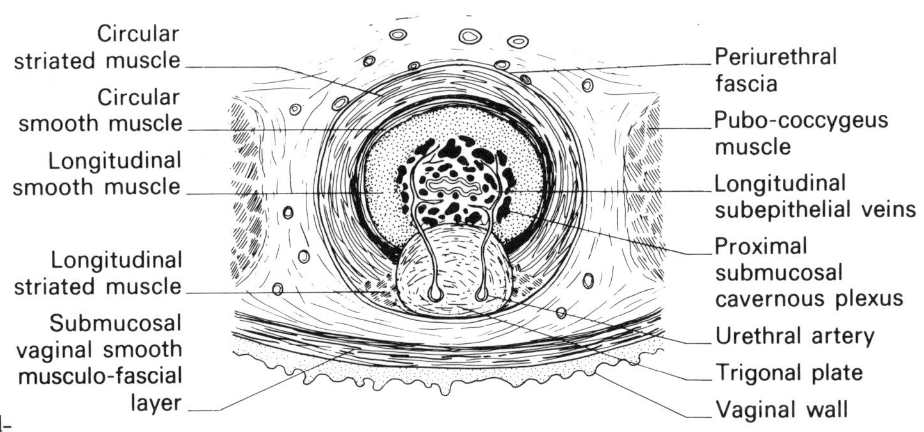

Fig. 2.4. Cross-section through the mid-urethra.

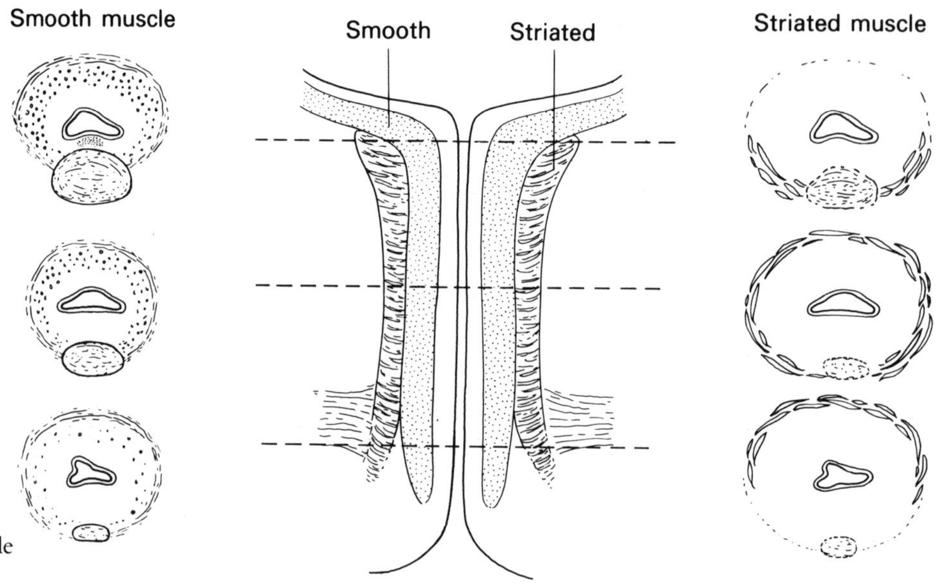

Fig. 2.5. Distribution of smooth muscle fibres.

Submucosa

Many small veins lie directly under the epithelium throughout the whole length of the urethra and on all sides of it. They run longitudinally in the mucosal folds and form two plexuses consisting of wide, thin-walled tortuous vessels. The proximal plexus surrounds the urethra below the vesico-urethral junction with its veins extending among the longitudinal smooth muscle fibres. The other plexus is smaller and lies just above the external meatus. The proximal plexus, with its many arterio-venous anastomoses, and the longitudinal veins lying directly under the epithelium give the submucosa in the upper half of the urethra a cavernous structure. This venous system is closely connected with the arterial system by complex anastomoses without any intervening capillary bed.

The venous plexuses are poorly developed in the new-born, but mature around the menarche so that in the young woman they have marked valve-like folds and are so tortuous that they must contain a large quantity of blood. These valves gradually diminish in size with age and the veins themselves become less flexible and have thicker walls.

The inferior vesical artery sends its terminal branch into the trigonal muscle posteriorly on each side of the mid-line. This divides at the vesico-urethral junction into a muscular branch which continues within the trigonal plate to the level of the urogenital diaphragm and a branch in the submucosa which descends postero-laterally. This latter vessel gives off small arterioles which open into the proximal venous plexus by means of arterio-venous anastomses which are found in the proximal half of the urethra and are distributed all over the mucosa.

Elastic tissue fibres run longitudinally in the submucosa throughout the length of the urethra. The few circular elastic fibres are found at the vesico-urethral junction. There is a great increase with age in the amount of elastic tissue in the urethra.

Nerve supply

The bladder and urethra are innervated by a motor and sensory autonomic nerve supply, both of sympathetic and parasympathetic origin. The sympathetic fibres come from T11–L2 in very thin bundles on each side of the lumbar and sacral vertebrae as the inferior hypogastric nerves (Fig. 2.6). These are not in fact nerves like peripheral nerves but a ribbon-like collection of thin fibres which run to the rectum, uterus and bladder and meet the parasympathetic fibres from S2, 3 and 4 at the pelvic wall. Some of these fibres then condense and continue as the inferior hypogastric plexus together with the inferior vesical artery in the deepest part of the *lateral retinaculum*. They are surrounded by fat and small veins as they run forwards. They connect with the intramural ganglions in the wall of the bladder and urethra. The nerve supply to the uterus runs mainly in the posterior retinaculum.

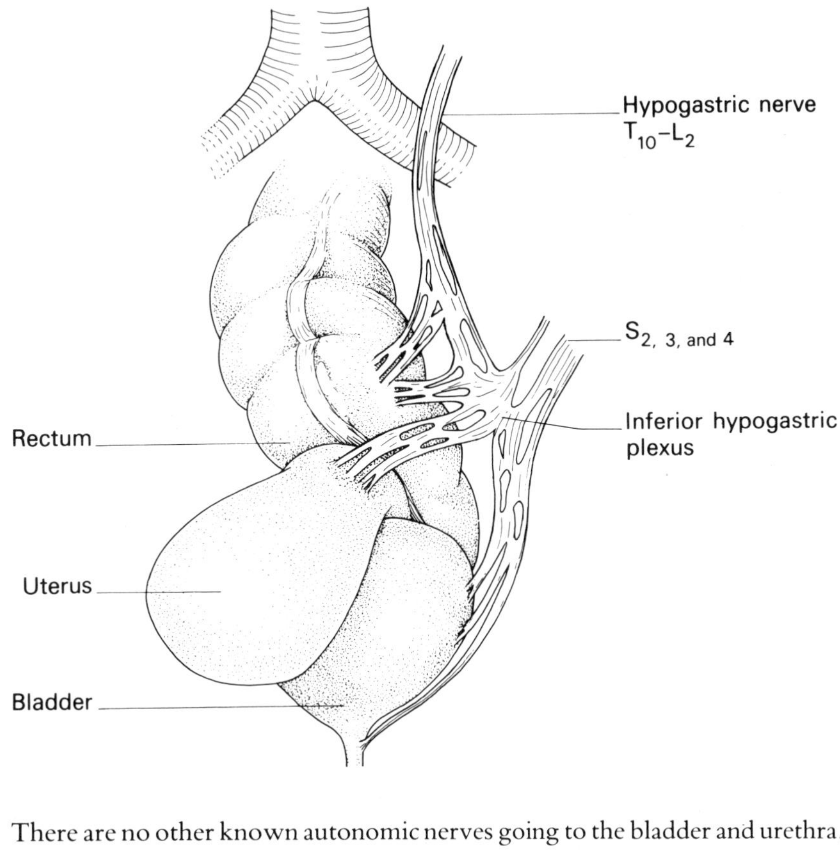

Fig. 2.6. Nerve supply of bladder and urethra.

There are no other known autonomic nerves going to the bladder and urethra, so that if they are cut in an abdominal operation (e.g. radical hysterectomy) the patient will not only lose the ability to micturate normally but also the normal sensations of bladder fullness and urgency.

The nerve supply to the bladder and urethra is also accessible from the vagina, a fact that has led to the use of the vaginal denervation operation for extreme urgency or urge incontinence. In all vaginal operations for prolapse or stress incontinence, the proximity of these nerves makes them liable to injury by stretching or haematoma formation with the possibility of micturition difficulties as a result.

Histo-chemical and pharmacological studies have demonstrated that a complicated mechanism exists for the nervous control of lower urinary tract function. The bladder dome has little nerve supply and detrusor contraction occurs for the most part by intermuscular signal. This explains the slow rise in bladder pressure which is characteristic of detrusor contraction.

The bladder base and urethra have a much richer nerve supply, mostly of sympathetic origin. Both α and β receptors have been demonstrated but, as yet, the picture of the nerve supply is incomplete. The mode of interaction of the sympathetic with the parasympathetic is also little understood. Recent advances

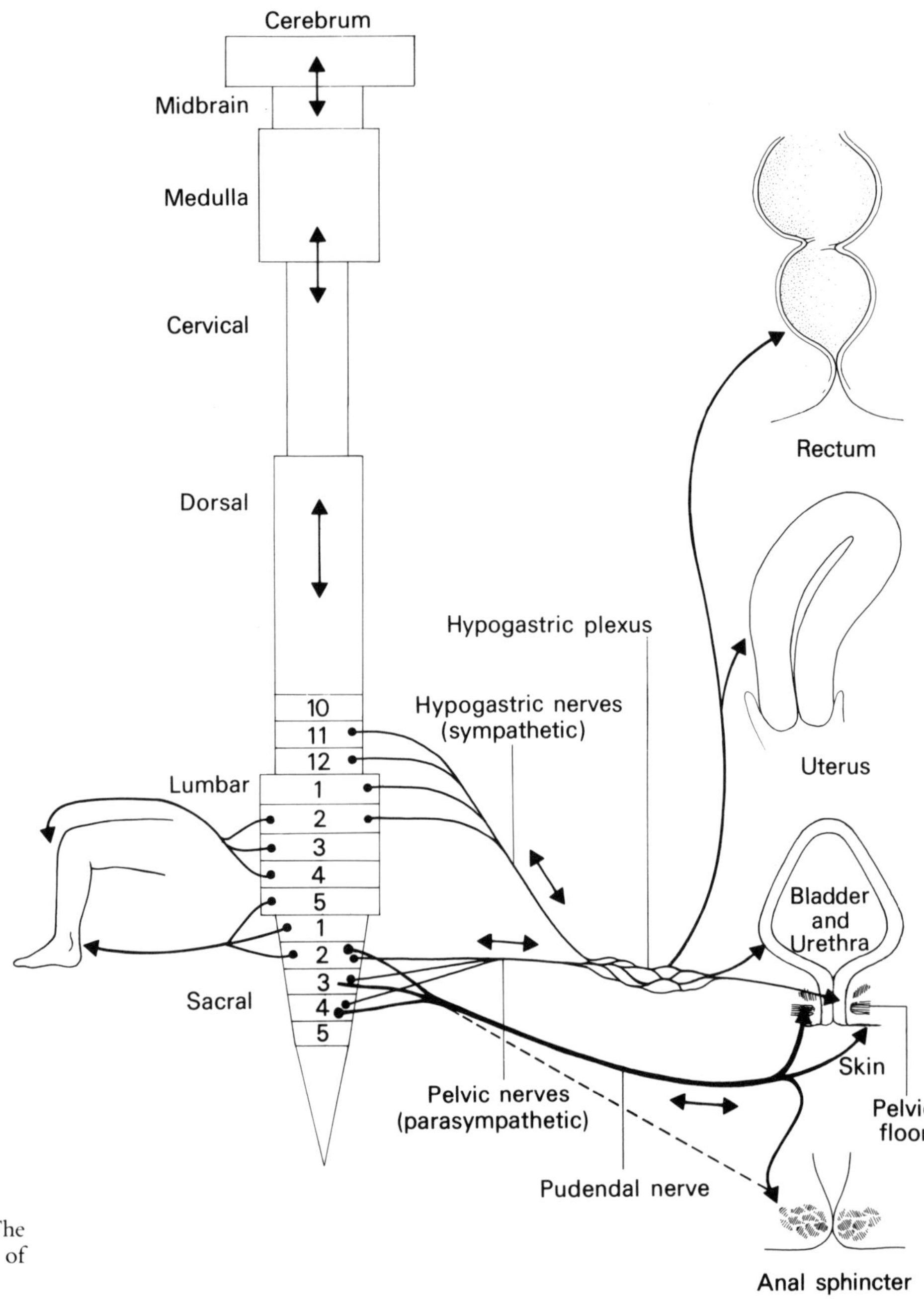

Fig. 2.7. Micturation reflex arc. The dotted line shows the direct innervation of pubo-coccygens from S2, 3 and 4.

show that sympathetic stimulation has an inhibiting effect on the parasympathetic ganglia. Furthermore, there seem to be other receptors such as purinergic and petidergic, which might have a function. Extensive research is in progress in this area with the object of finding drugs which will have a use in the treatment of dysfunction. For further information see de Groat (1981).

The ganglia which contain the synapses of the nerve fibres which supply the detrusor and urethral muscle lie in the bladder and urethral walls and not in the hypogastric plexus. An interesting observation has demonstrated a considerable amount of sympathetic transmitter substance in the mid-urethra. Stretch receptors in the bladder wall are responsible for the proprioceptive sensations which indicate bladder filling. It seems reasonable to think that there may be other kinds of receptors, especially in the urethra.

The pudendal nerve from S2, 3 and 4 supplies the urogenital diaphragm and part of the levator ani muscles with somatic fibres. It is not known whether it contains autonomic fibres which go to the urethra. The pubo-coccygeus part is supplied directly from S2, 3 and 4. All these centres are connected to the various spinal centres, especially S2, 3 and 4. Fig. 2.7 shows the reflex arc which is concerned with continence and micturition. The sacral centres are connected with the sympathetic outflow, T11–L2. These centres are also connected via the afferent fibres in the cord to the brain, where the sensory impulses are analysed.

The spinal centres are, to a certain extent, under the control of efferent impulses from the brain. The micturition reflex is therefore governed by a complicated series of inhibiting and stimulating impulses from the higher centres. This implies that dysfunction can occur not only by direct interference with the lower urinary tract itself but also by interference with any or all of the nervous pathways in the presence of a normal lower urinary tract.

Smooth muscle

The crista urethralis extends downwards from the vesico-urethral junction on the posterior wall, and is very marked in young girls, causing the urethra in its upper half to be shaped like a half moon with concavity backwards. It is a continuation downwards of the *superficial trigone,* which in turn is a continuation of the ureteric muscle (Fig. 2.8). The lumen of the urethra gradually becomes more like a transverse slit in fertile and postmenopausal women because of the flattening of the crista.

The deep trigone, which is a continuation of the fibro-muscular periureteric fascia, together with some detrusor fibres spreads out at the vesico-urethral junction to form the *trigonal ring* around the upper part of the anterior aspect of the urethra and the trigonal plate on the posterior aspect (Figs. 2.9 and 2.10). The trigonal plate extends downwards as far as the urogenital diaphragm. The ring and the plate are made up of a meshwork of short thin fibres in dense connective tissue.

The two smooth muscle coats of the urethra are in close connection with the trigonal ring. Fibres of this ring extend downwards as a firm inner longitudinal

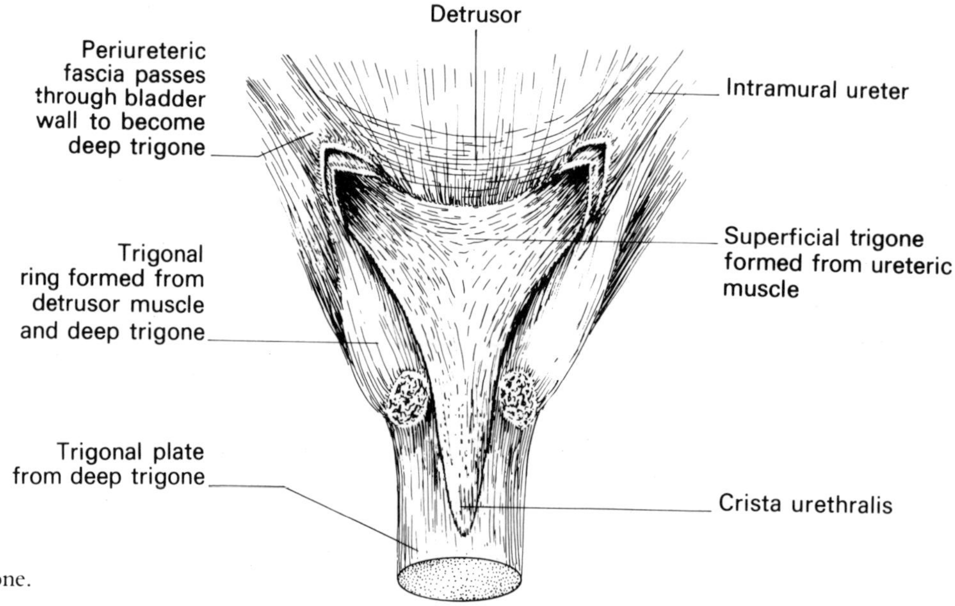

Fig. 2.8. Formation of superficial trigone.

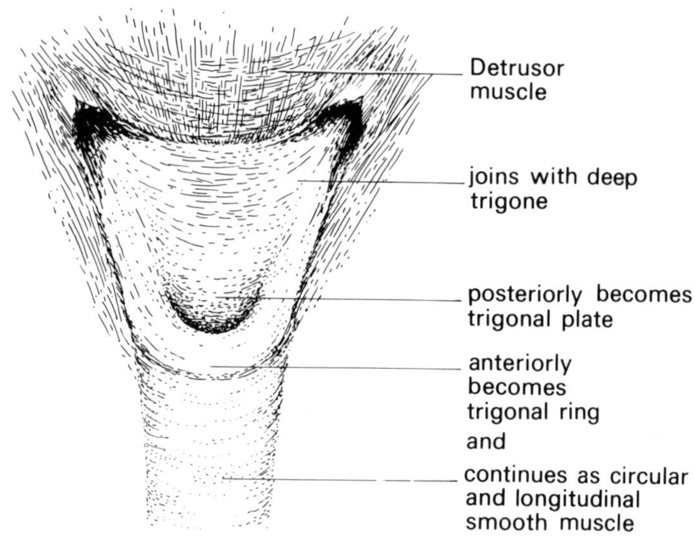

Fig. 2.9. Ureteric muscle and superficial trigone removed.

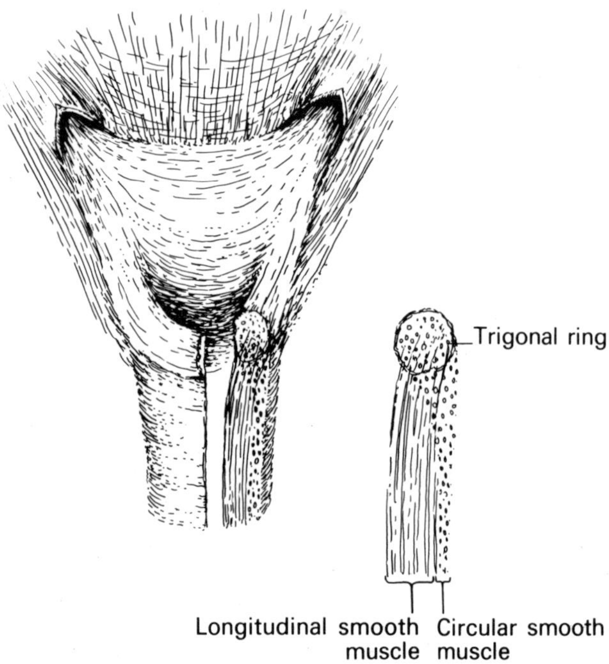

Fig. 2.10. Trigonal ring and urethral smooth muscle.

coat and a thin outer coat. They extend between the trigonal ring and the urogenital diaphragm. Underneath the diaphragm the muscle coats can no longer be identified (Fig. 2.5).

Striated muscle

Fibres in the shape of a horseshoe form the major part of the striated muscle coat and extend from the lower margin of the trigonal ring to the urogenital diaphragm on the outer aspect of the urethra. They are inserted posteriorly into the trigonal plate and below this fan out into the periurethral connective tissue at the level of the urogenital diaphragm. A few fibres reach the antero-lateral wall of the vagina and others join the fibres of the bulbo-cavernous muscle. There is no connection with either the pubo-coccygeus or transversus perinei muscles (Fig. 2.5) and there is no distinct boundary between smooth and striated muscle fibres within the urethral wall.

The individual muscle fibres are only one third to one quarter the size of the fibres in the levator ani muscle group. Their innervation is still unknown. They are most marked in the new-born and gradually diminish in number until they are almost rudimentary in the adult.

THE URETERS AND TRIGONE

The ureter is a muscular tube about 25 cm long and 4 mm in diameter consisting of three very ill-defined layers of smooth muscle with a lining of urothelium. It lies in the retroperitoneal space loosely adherent to the peritoneum all the way from the renal pelvis to a point where it passes through the lateral and anterior retinacula (cardinal and vesico-uterine ligaments) just before it enters the bladder wall. There is a thin layer of connective tissue ensheathing the ureter which is inseparable from the muscle coat but which serves to separate it from other organs and to permit peristalsis. This periureteric fascia is of great value to the surgeon because it protects the ureter from inflammatory and neoplastic processes in its neighbourhood and enables him to dissect it free and unharmed even after it has been surrounded. Injuries to this ensheathing fascia can sometimes lead to stricture and fistula formation, but if the ureter is normal without any obstruction, they heal without difficulty – as is seen, for example, after removal of a calculus.

There are three places where there may be a physiological and sometimes anatomical stenosis: at the pelvi-ureteric junction, near the brim of the pelvis and just before the ureter enters the bladder wall (Fig. 1.11).

Blood supply reaches the ureter in the female at three points: at the pelvi-ureteric junction from the renal artery; near the pelvic brim from the internal iliac and/or the ovarian arteries; and just outside the bladder from the superior and sometimes also the inferior, vesical arteries (Fig. 2.11). The lowest vessel is occasionally absent. There is no blood supply from the peritoneum even though the ureter is loosely attached to it by areolar tissue. Urologists have a rule of

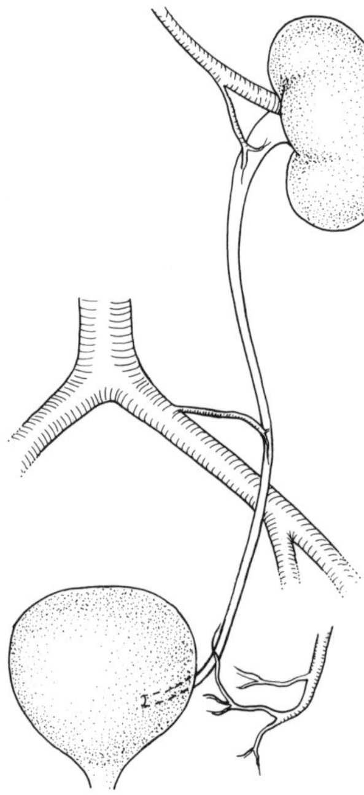

Fig. 2.11. Blood supply of ureter.

thumb that, where the normal ureter is concerned, only one of these three groups of vessels is necessary to supply the whole length with blood.

When the ureter reaches the bladder wall, all the muscle fibres become longitudinally orientated. The roof opens so that the fibres become flattened out to form the *superficial trigonal muscle* together with fibres from the opposite side. This is tightly adherent to the mucosa over the whole area of the trigone and is continued about halfway down the urethra as the *crista urethralis* (Fig. 2.8).

A few centimeters from the bladder wall, as the ureter passes through the lateral and anterior retinacula, the periureteric fascia becomes thicker and more distinct (Waldeyer's fascia). This then continues on the surface of the ureter as it passes through the detrusor muscle and allows separation of the ureter from the bladder muscle. The periureteral fascia opens out in the same way as the muscle fibres and forms the *deep trigone* with fascial fibres from the other side. This passes downwards on the posterior aspect of the urethra as the *trigonal plate*, which is composed of dense fibro-muscular tissue and contains the two arteries, one from each inferior vesical artery, which are the main blood supply of the urethra. The lateral parts of the periureteric fascia merge with detrusor muscle fibres to form the *trigonal ring* around the front of the upper urethra (Fig. 2.9) and continue as circular and longitudinal smooth muscle in the urethral wall (Fig. 2.10).

Both motor and sensory autonomic nerves supply the ureter. This is well demonstrated in ureteric colic.

Lymph drainage of the lower urinary tract

This is described in Chapter 13, under cancer of the urethra.

Perivesical and periurethral fascia

Around the bladder and urethra there is a condensation of fascia which allows these organs to be separated from adjacent structures. It also allows for the movement necessarily associated with bladder filling and micturition. This loose fascial tissue merges with the fascia covering the ureters and also with the tough fascia covering the vagina. It allows separation of the bladder base and urethra from the vagina though this requires careful dissection. Around the urethra it contains a large number of elastic fibres and small veins. Laterally it unites with the fascia covering the pubo-coccygeus muscle.

Suspension apparatus of the bladder and urethra

In the mid-line the lower part of the bladder and the urethra are only loosely attached to the back of the symphysis. On each side there is a condensation of pelvic fascia containing a few smooth muscle fibres which fixes the anterior vaginal wall to the back of the pubic bones and to the pelvic wall near the anterior part of the arcus tendineus. This has the effect of holding the vesico-urethral junction and urethra firmly in position (Fig. 2.12 and 2.13). This fixation may be damaged during delivery so that the fascial condensation becomes stretched. This means that the vesico-urethral junction is allowed freer movement. The fascial bands now become known as the *pubo-vesical ligaments*.

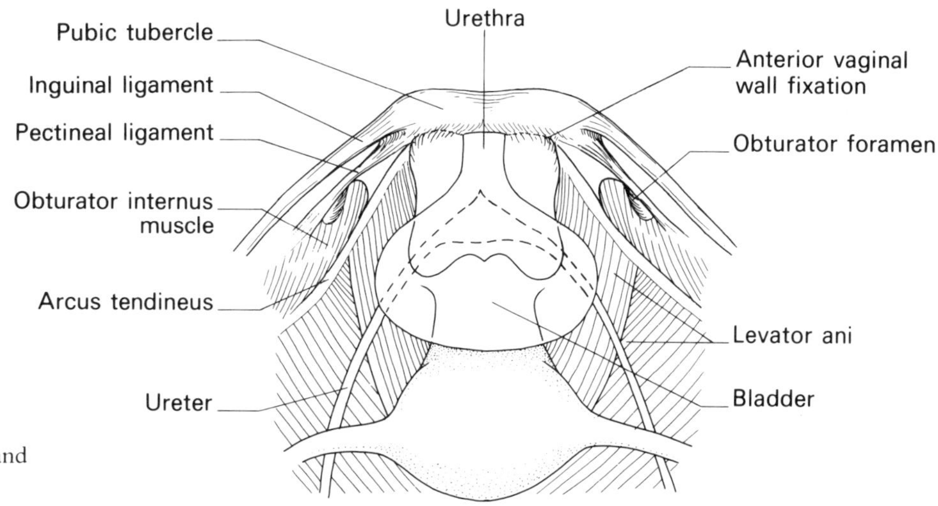

Fig. 2.12. Suspension of bladder and urethra by vaginal fixation.

Relations

The peritoneum covers the dome of the bladder, to which it is loosely attached, and then dips down in front between the bladder and pubis to form the shallow *pre-vesical pouch*. The posterior wall of the bladder lies in front of the lower part of the body of the uterus and the trigone is on the front of the anterior fornix of the vagina. During simple hysterectomy, the bladder can be easily dissected free from the uterus down to the level of the cervix, but here the areolar tissue changes

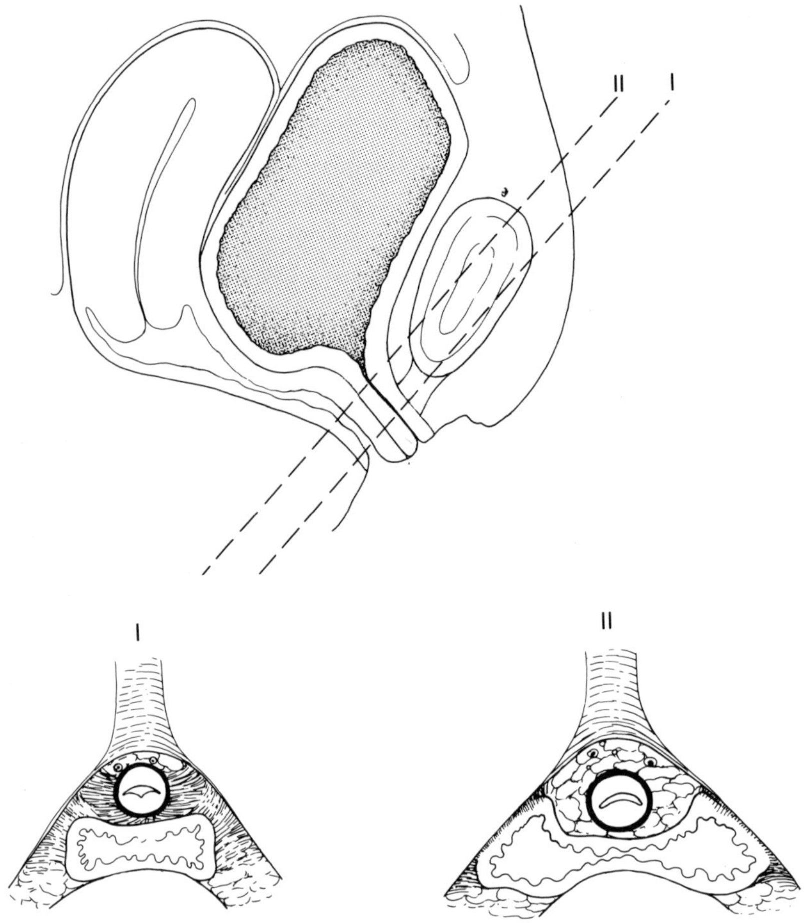

Fig. 2.13. Normal fixation of anterior vaginal wall on each side of the urethra.

so that it is more difficult to separate the bladder base from the anterior vaginal wall. This separation is hazardous for it is here that bladder injury and vesico-vaginal fistula formation most often occurs. Previous surgery in this region of course makes the separation all the more difficult. Lateral to the ureteric orifices in women there is quite a considerable pouch of the bladder wall which when distended reaches outwards over the levator ani muscles nearly to the pelvic wall. This, however, can be very easily separated by blunt dissection from the pelvic wall without bleeding, opening up a space called the *paravesical fossa* which is a landmark in radical hysterectomy. The distended bladder is never spherical because of these pouches and because the anteverted uterus makes a considerable impression on the posterior wall. When the bladder is empty the posterior wall is in contact with the internal urinary meatus and the dome does not reach to the level of the top of the symphysis pubis. It is only when it is distended by at least about 250 ml that the dome rises sufficiently to reach above the top of the symphysis pubis. It is important to remember this when suprabubic bladder puncture is done.

The urethra passes through the urogenital diaphragm, which is really the deep transversus perinei muscle and the fascial layers above and below it. It is only loosely attached to this and can be completely separated from the muscle of the diaphragm.

The bladder base rests on the pelvic floor so that the inner part of the pubo-coccygeus muscle is only 2–3 mm from the lateral aspect of the urethra.

REFERENCES

Curtis AH *et al* (1952] Anatomy of the pelvic autonomic nerves in relation to gynaecology. *Surg. Gynecol. Obstet.* **75,** 743.

Gosling JA, Dixon JS, Lendon FG (1977) The autonomic innervation of the human male and female bladder neck and proximal urethra. *J. Urol.* **118,** 302.

de Groat WC *et al* (1981) Organisation of the sacral parasympathetic reflex pathways to the urinary bladder and large intestine. *J. auton. nerv. syst.* **3,** 135.

Huisman AB (1979) Morfologie van de vrouwelijke urethra. MD Thesis, University of Groningen.

Notley RG (1971) The structural basis for normal and abnormal ureteric motility. *Ann. R. Coll. Surg. Engl.* **49,** 248.

Olsen KP, Gran V (1976) The suspensory apparatus of the female bladder neck. *Urol. Int.* **31,** 33.

Richardson AC, Edmonds PS, Williams NL (1981) Treatment of stress urinary incontinence due to paravaginal fascial defect. *Obstet. & Gynaecol.* **57,** 357.

Tanagho EA, Pugh RCB (1963) Anatomy and function of the uretero-vesical junction. *Brit. J. Urol.* **35,** 151.

Woodburne RT (1968) Anatomy of the bladder and bladder outlet. *J. Urol.* **100,** 474.

Chapter 3 Applied Physiology

BLADDER AND URETHRA

The bladder and urethra should be regarded as a physiological unit in which the bladder is the reservoir and the urethra forms the outlet or biological valve.

When the pressure in any part of the urethra is the same or greater than the pressure in the bladder, no urine can pass through the urethra. This is known as *urethral continence*. To allow urine to pass out, the maximum urethral pressure must be lower than the bladder pressure. This simple statement is the physiological basis of urinary continence and micturition. The simultaneous measurement of bladder and intraurethral pressures at any bladder volume and under any conditions such as coughing, straining or changing position, has provided a more accurate picture of the normal physiology of the lower urinary tract.

The *bladder pressure* depends on:

- the volume of fluid in the bladder;
- that part of the intra-abdominal pressure that is transmitted to the bladder;
- tension in the bladder wall, which is partly passive elasticity and partly activity in the detrusor muscle.

The *intraurethral pressure* is more complex and depends on:

- striated muscle fibres in the urethral wall and around the urethra;
- smooth muscle fibres in the urethral wall;
- the vascular content of the submucosal cavernous plexus;
- passive elasticity in the wall;
- that part of the intra-abdominal pressure that is transmitted to the urethra.

The urethra is a short tube which has a lumen only during micturition, that is for a few minutes each day. The pressure by which the walls are kept together varies considerably, at rest, from the inner to the outer end. The pressures can be drawn as a curve which is known as the *urethral pressure profile* (Fig. 3.1). The *total urethral length* is defined as that part of the urethra between the point at which the pressure exceeds the bladder pressure and the point where atmospheric pressure is reached. That part of the total length where the pressure exceeds the bladder pressure is called the *functional urethral length*. This part can be considered as preventing loss of urine and therefore functions as a sphincter. *Closure pressure* means urethral pressure minus bladder pressure.

The point of maximum urethral pressure normally lies very close to the middle of the functional urethral length. This point is about half a centimetre proximal to the urogenital diaphragm, which means that the urogenital

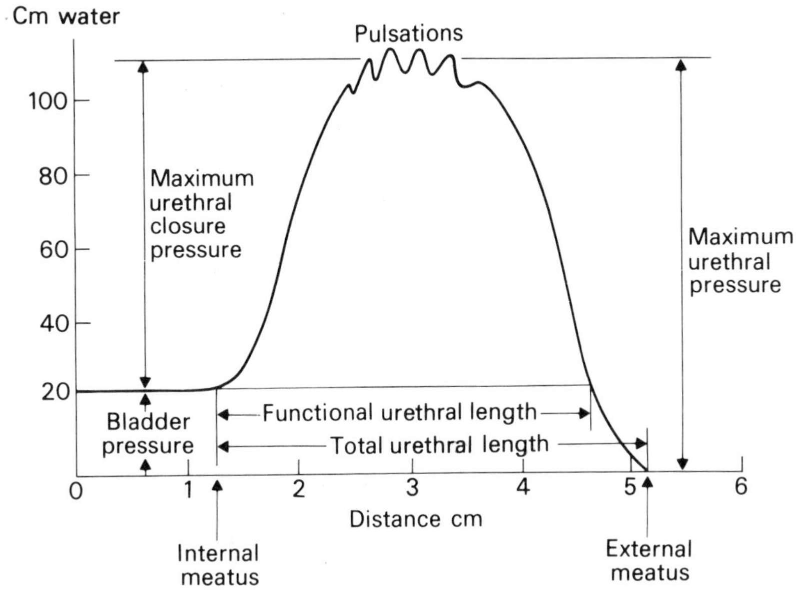

Fig. 3.1. Urethral pressure profile.

diaphragm is not at the point of maximum sphincteric action. This fact is an important contribution of the urethral pressure profile to the explanation of the physiology of continence. Furthermore it corresponds well with the detailed anatomy of the urethra which shows that the urethral tube has no direct connection with the muscle of the urogenital diaphragm and that the submucous cavernous plexus, the bulk of the smooth and striated muscle and the bulk of the autonomic nerve supply are all most obvious at the point of maximum urethral pressure.

Another contribution of the urethral pressure profile is the surprising fact that after surgical resection of the distal half of the urethra for tumour, the point of maximum urethral pressure is still located at about the middle of the functional length of the remaining urethra (see Chapter 13).

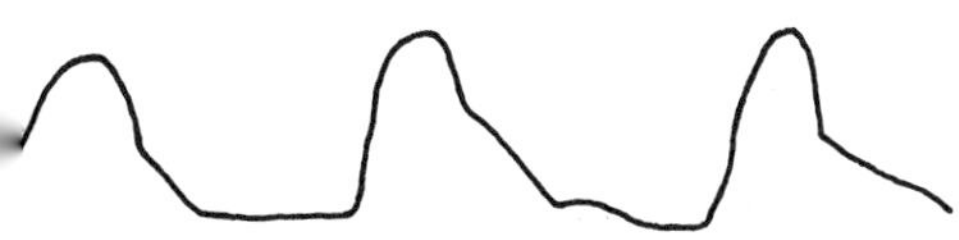

Fig. 3.2. Pulsation at point of maximal urethral pressure.

The urethral pressure profile shows oscillations of pressure which are synchronous with the heart beat and most marked at the point of maximum urethral pressure. This indicates filling of the plexus with blood. In younger women these oscillations have the same shape as an aortic pressure curve; one can even see the place where the aortic valve closes (Fig. 3.2). This confirms the direct connection with aortic pressure which is indicated by the direct arterio-venous anastomoses in the submucosa. In younger women, the oscillations can be as large as 20 cm water. They gradually diminish in size with increasing age until in the post-menopausal stage they are seldom over 5 cm water. There are great variations in each age group. Women with stress incontinence appear to have the same oscillations as the average for their age group.

The functional length as measured on the urethral pressure profile normally varies from 2 to 4 cm, but the relevance of this to the maintenance of continence is unknown; there is no direct relationship between functional and total length, which is about 0.5 cm longer.

The various factors which make up intraurethral pressure appear to work together as an integrated function as shown in Fig. 3.3. It is impossible for this reason to estimate the relative importance of each component as regards continence and micturition. The submucosal plexus can be considered as a cylindrical cushion-like structure which closes the lumen by approximating mucosa to mucosa over a certain distance. This mechanism for the production of a watertight closure can be continued almost indefinately so long as the heart continues to beat and remains connected to the plexus. It is not subject to muscle fatigue.

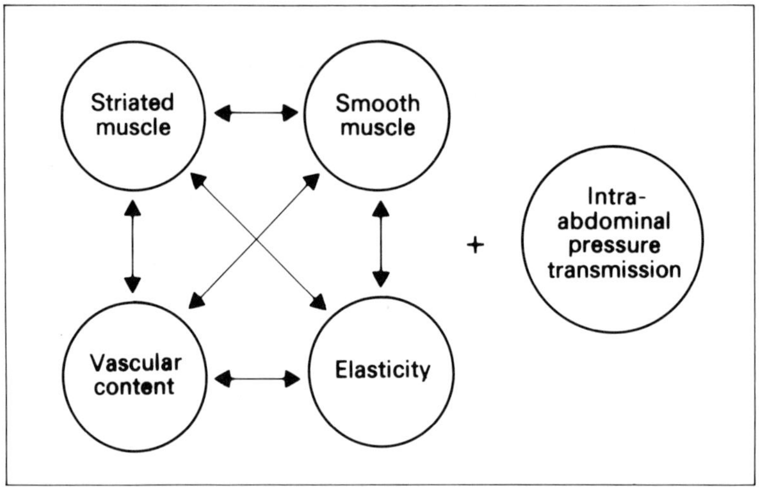

Fig. 3.3. The various elements which make up intraurethral pressure.

Experiments have shown that if both internal iliac arteries are occluded in the human female, the pulsation disappears immediately and the pressure profile is significantly flattened out. When the occlusion is removed, both pulsation and profile quickly return to normal.

The main action of the smooth and striated muscle in the urethra may well be to regulate the amount of blood in the plexus rather than to exert a direct effect on intra-urethral pressure. This hypothesis is supported by the fact that most of the smooth muscle fibres lie parallel to the axis of the urethra. Also, the circular smooth and striated muscle fibres in the adult woman, in whom intra-urethral pressure is at its maximum, have diminished in number and in size compared with the young girl and have become almost rudimentary. That direct muscular activity by itself can be responsible for the major part of intra-urethral pressure seems therefore unlikely. The striated muscle in the urethra appears to have a short-term effect in preventing loss of urine during periods of urgency and straining, while the smooth muscle is in constant activity. This has not been completely elucidated.

It is difficult to imagine that the transversus perinei muscle has any direct sphincteric effect at rest since its fibres lie at right angles to the axis of the urethra. It appears to act by fixing the lower urethra. The levator ani muscles act on the bladder base and urethra in a way which can best be described as holding them in the optimum position for efficient sphincteric action. Direct sphincteric action clearly seems impossible. The gynaecologist will notice a marked effect on the

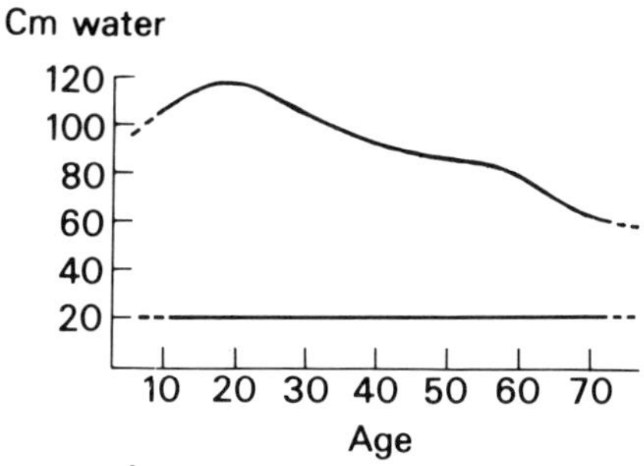

Fig. 3.4. Alteration of average maximum urethral pressure with age. Bladder pressure (lower curve) remains almost the same.

urethra if he asks his patient to contract her perineal muscles during a vaginal examination. The same effect can be seen on a micturating cysto-urethrogram when the patient is asked to perform the same movement.

The urethral pressures alter with age (Fig. 3.4) and this corresponds with the anatomical age changes which have already been described. There is an increase to the age of 20 and then a gradual fall until the menopause. After this there is a steeper fall.

The changes in bladder and intra-urethral pressures during bladder filling

The normal female bladder will hold a certain amount of urine before the *first sensation* is noticeable and then several hundred additional millilitres can be tolerated before the urge to void is so strong that micturition cannot any longer be prevented. This is called the *maximum bladder capacity*. The first sensation of fullness varies from individual to individual and also in the same individual under different conditions, indicating that sensory signals from the lower urinary tract are not always interpreted by the brain in the same way. This is illustrated by the phenomenon which everybody has experienced, that a strong urge to void can suddenly be forgotten if attention is distracted. First sensation is considered normally to occur between 200 and 300 ml and the maximum bladder capacity lies between 400 and 600 ml in most women. In pregnancy these figures increase considerably and in patients with urgency they may be considerably lower. Figure 3.5 shows the bladder and intra-urethral pressures during slow filling of the bladder at a rate of 15 ml/min in a normal woman in a natural sitting position. This rate is probably within the normal physiological limits of urine production

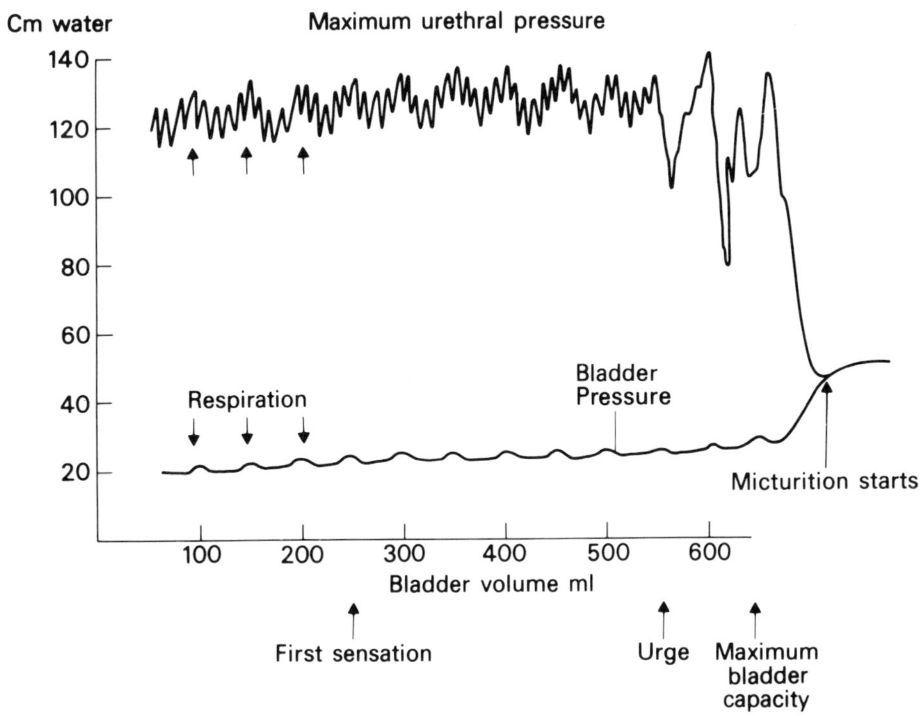

Fig. 3.5. Simultaneous urethro-cystometry during slow bladder filling.

by the kidneys. The bladder adapts to this and the bladder pressure only increases slightly when its contents increase from from 100 to 500 ml of urine, while the maximum urethral pressure remains almost unaltered apart from the variations synchronous with the heart beat and respiration. At 250 ml the patient notices that something is going on and experiences the first sensation but there is no accompanying rise in pressure. This means that impulses have begun to reach consciousness. The pressure within the bladder does not seem to increase more than the weight of the water that is put into it. From about 400 to about 600 ml there is increased activity in the striated muscle in the pelvic floor. The maximum urethral pressure often rises a little more than the bladder pressure as a result of this. When the volume reaches about 600 ml she feels an extremely strong desire to void. If the filling continues she will be unable consciously to prevent the start of micturition.

Urgency just before micturition becomes so unpleasant that the patient tries to suppress it by contraction of the striated pelvic floor muscles. This is a normal voluntary or involuntary mechanism which produces marked variations in intra-urethral pressure without any change in the bladder pressure. It has been called the 'unstable urethra'; its pathological significance has not been proven so it cannot be used as a criterion of underlying abnormality.

Micturition

When urgency becomes so great that micturition cannot be prevented any longer, it is started by a decrease in intra-urethral pressure in association with a relaxation of striated muscle, followed a few seconds later by a moderate and slow increase in bladder pressure. This produces a maximum intra-urethral pressure less than the bladder pressure and urine escapes (Fig. 3.5). The bladder base and the vesico-urethral junction drop at the same moment as the intra-urethral pressure falls (Figs. 3.6, 3.7). This indicates that the pelvic floor muscles cease to support the urethra and by this process facilitate funnelling of the bladder outlet. Figure 3.8 shows the same woman when she is asked to micturate at a lower bladder volume when she has no urge to void. Here again micturition is initiated in the same way by a decrease in intra-urethral pressure followed by a slight bladder contraction.

To sum up, normal micturition occurs as a result of lowering of urethral resistance followed by slight increase in the bladder pressure which occurs a few moments later. The bladder pressure during micturition never exceeds the maximum intra-urethral pressure at rest except when a Valsalva manoeuvre is performed. In fact there is always activity in the urethra during micturition. The view, based on simple cystometry, that urine is expelled as a result of contraction of the detrusor muscle which increases the bladder pressure sufficiently to overcome the resistance in the urethra does not fit in with the above findings. Women explain that all that is necessary when they wish to start micturition is relaxation of pelvic musculature. And indeed simultaneous pressure measurements show that in some women, especially older women, the only change that occurs when they initiate micturition is a decrease in the

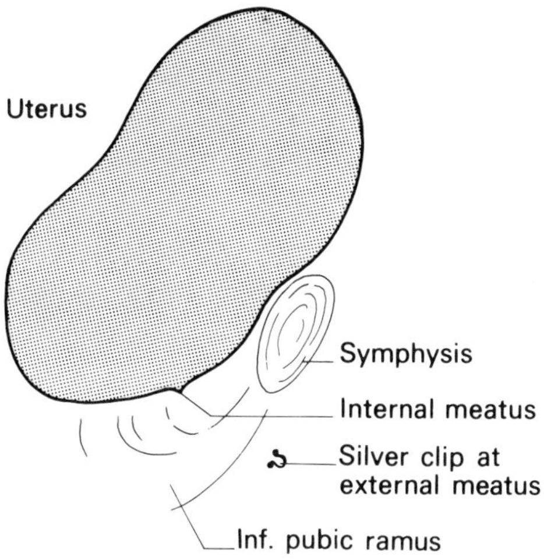

Fig. 3.6.

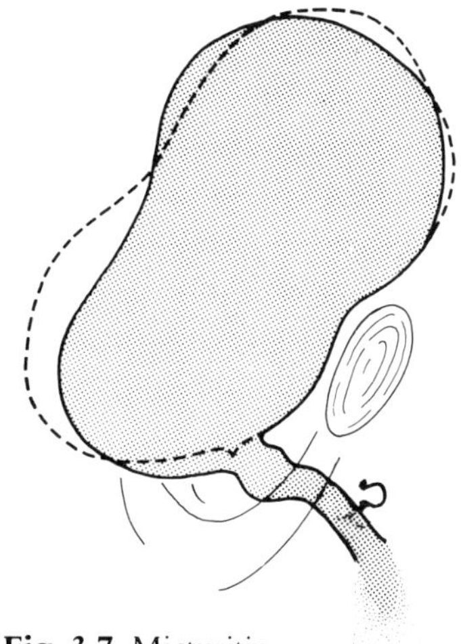

Fig. 3.7. Micturition.

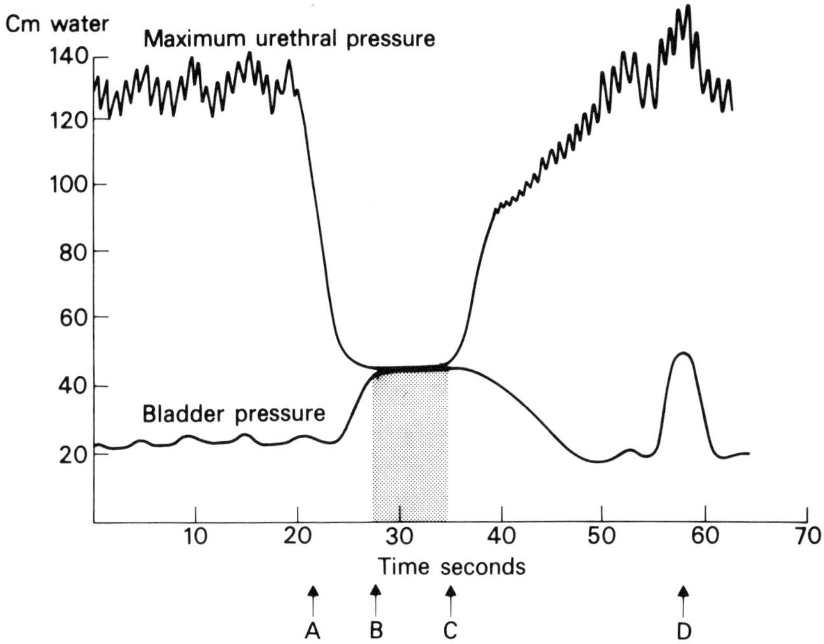

Fig. 3.8. Micturition at a lower bladder volume than maximum capacity.

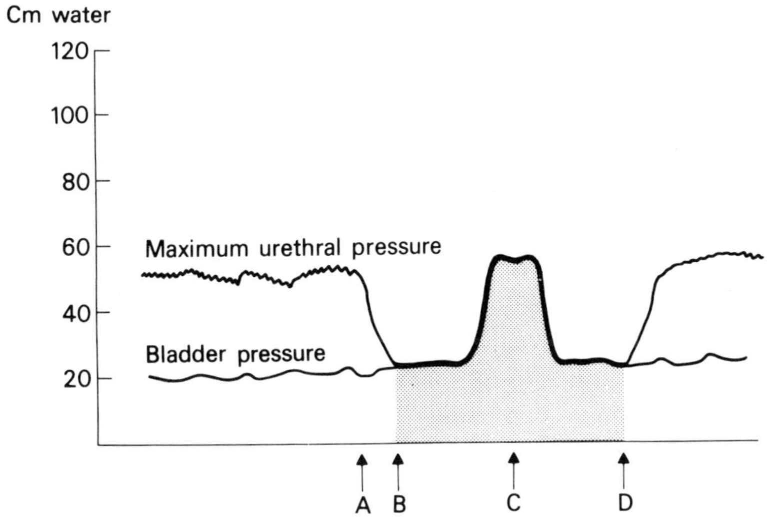

Fig. 3.9. Micturition without detrusor contraction:
A, Urethral pressure falls;
B, micturition starts;
C, flow increased by Valsalva manoeuvre;
D, micturition voluntarily stopped.

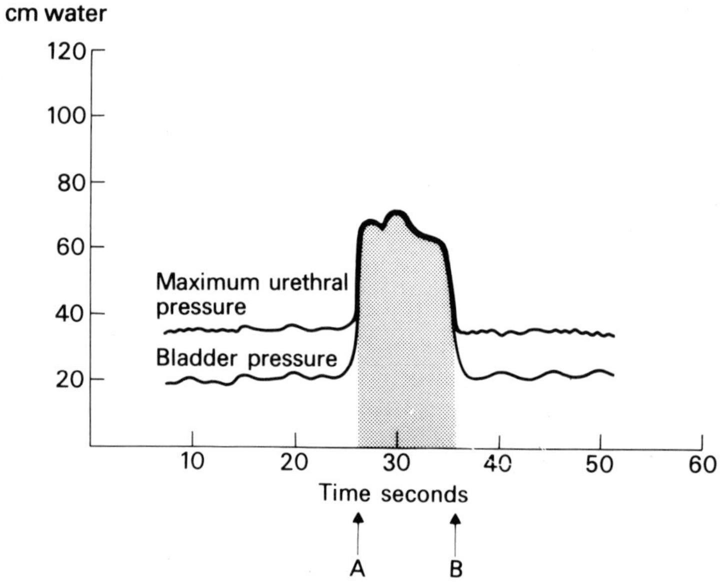

Fig. 3.10. Micturition by Valsalva manoeuvre.

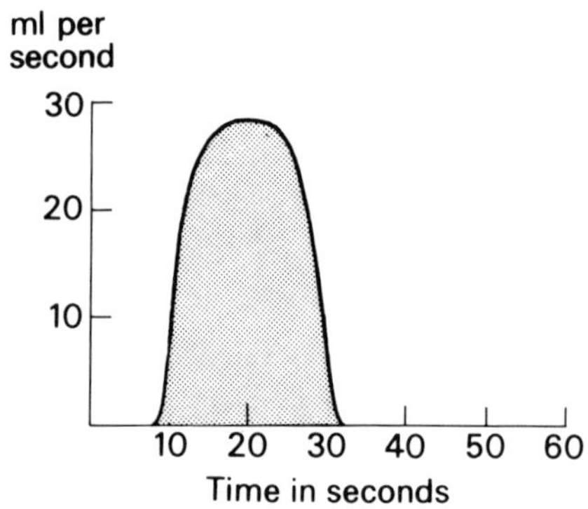

Fig. 3.11. Normal flow rate.

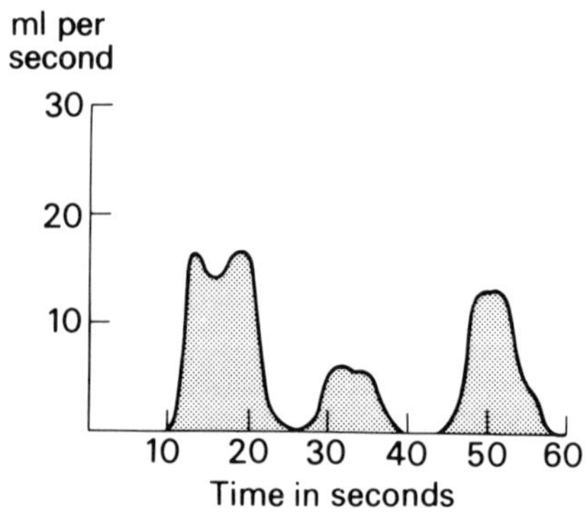

Fig. 3.12. Valsalva flow rate.

intra-urethral pressure. It becomes less than the bladder pressure and urine runs out sufficiently fast to empty the bladder within a short period of time without any detrusor activity which increases bladder pressure (Fig. 3.9).

In some normal women, a Valsalva manoeuvre comes into play when they are asked to initiate micturition (Fig. 3.10). This may be a way of increasing flow-rate or a means of initiating micturition when there is no desire to void. The interpretation of this is difficult for it can to some extent be caused by the strange surroundings and lack of privacy. Figure 3.11 shows a normal flow-rate and Fig. 3.12 shows the flow-rate during a Valsalva manoeuvre.

Women should be able to empty their bladders (about 500 ml) almost completely within about 20 seconds. The definition of *residual urine* is therefore the amount of urine which remains in the bladder after micturition which has been as complete as the subject can manage. Most urologists, however, regard small amounts of residual urine under 100 ml as not significant because under the unfamiliar conditions of investigation and lack of privacy, the bladder may not completely empty itself.

It is often said that the normal woman should be able to interrupt micturition when asked to do so but it is not yet certain if this statement is completely true or whether it can be used to assess dysfunction of the lower urinary tract. The sequence of events when she is asked to stop micturition is shown in Fig. 3.8. The pelvic floor musculature around the urethra contracts and the intra-urethral pressure rapidly increases to a level which is adequate to interrupt the stream; from this point the intra-urethral pressure rises more slowly and its pulsations gradually increase until the maximum urethral pressure is reached in about 10 seconds. This indicates that the submucosal cavernous plexus is being filled with blood by arterial pulsation. The process can be seen on a video film as a narrowing of the distal part of the urethra where it passes through the urogenital diaphragm (Fig. 3.13). This interrupts the stream. At the same time the bladder base and vesico-urethral junction is lifted up by the levator ani muscles. After this, the urine in the part of the urethra above the urogenital diaphragm can be seen to be pushed back into the bladder. This is called the 'milk back'. When this series of events is nearly complete, the situation is as shown in Fig. 3.14 where the bladder base is lifted up by the pelvic muscles.

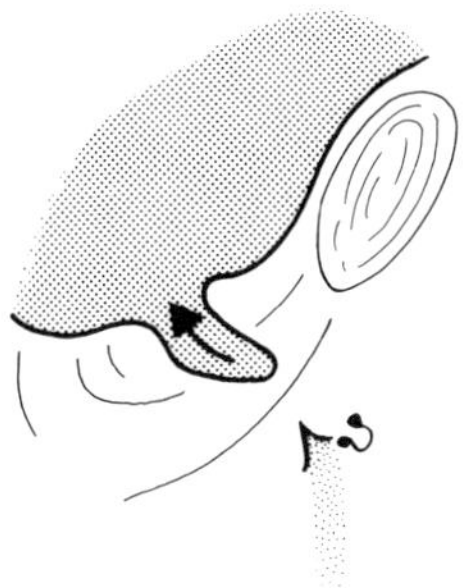

Fig. 3.13. Interruption of micturition—'milk back'.

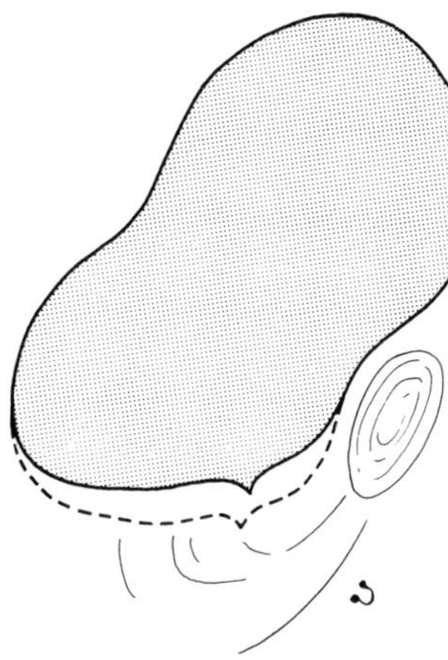

Fig. 3.14. 'Hold back' contraction of pelvic floor muscles.

How the different components interact to reduce intra-urethral pressure at the beginning of micturition is not yet known, but it is assumed that both striated and smooth muscle work together in the same manner as during continence. The mechanism of emptying the submucous cavernous plexus is also still unknown. The conception that continence is partially maintained by the amount of blood in the urethral vessels is both new and fascinating.

Normal micturition is, therefore, the result of conscious and unconscious inhibiting and stimulating efferent cerebral impulses which act on the micturition reflex arc. These impulses are initiated as a result of afferent signals from the lower urinary tract and, perhaps, its surroundings during the bladder filling phase. The main stimulus which initiates micturition seems to be bladder filling. All levels of the nervous system are involved in this process by means of complicated reflex arcs. Proprioception and exteroception in the lower urinary tract are still very little understood. Further information can be found in Fletcher & Bradley (1978).

The bladder and intra-urethral pressures during coughing and straining

The fast and short-lived rise in intra-abdominal pressure caused by a cough, or the more prolonged rise when the woman strains to lift something, would produce leakage of urine simply because the bladder pressure will exceed the maximum intra-urethral pressure. This is prevented by a combination of passive and active events which lead to a sufficient increase of pressure in at least one place in the urethra to prevent loss of urine.

The passive element is provided by the fixation of the urethra behind the pubis and the active part is contributed by the striated muscle fibres in the urethra and in the pelvic floor muscles.

Passive element

Any exertion which results in a short fast rise in intra-abdominal pressure, such as coughing or jumping, leads to the transmission of pressure to the part of the urethra above the urogenital diaphragm to such a degree that the intra-urethral pressure is raised by a sufficient amount to compensate for the rise in bladder pressure (Fig. 3.15). This is dependent upon the fixation of the upper urethra and vesico-urethral junction behind the pubis on each side. At the same time the rise in bladder pressure leads to funnelling of the vesico-urethral junction. In the young woman this funnelling is minimal, but after the birth of children and also in the post-menopausal woman it is much more marked. An extreme degree of funnelling produces stress incontinence. Adequate fixation of the urethra at the vesico-urethral junction resists this effect by preventing expansion of the urethra. If this fixation is inadequate, there is insufficient transmission of pressure and increased funnelling. How much of the intra-abdominal pressure is transmitted to the urethra compared with the bladder is not easy to measure and exactly how the funnelling occurs is still the subject of discussion. The transmission of the rise in intra-abdominal pressure during a cough is most marked in the upper two-thirds of the urethra where the maximum urethral pressure is located. This is above the level of the urogenital diaphragm.

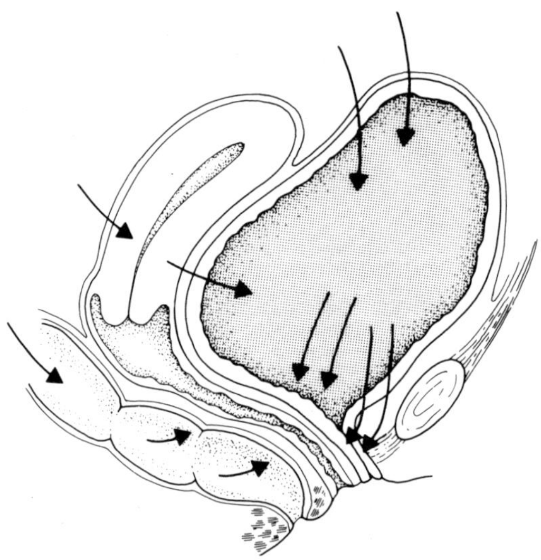

Fig. 3.15. Passive transmission of intra-abdominal pressure to the urethra.

Active element

When the pelvic muscles contract while the subject is 'holding back', there is a rise in intra-urethral pressure throughout almost the whole functional length of the urethra, that is to say nearly down to the external meatus. This corresponds to the region where the striated muscle is located. The amplitude of the rise in pressure in the urethra diminishes with age. For anatomical reasons it seems impossible for the striated muscle in the levator group and in the urogenital diaphragm to exert any direct effect on intra-urethral pressure but there is no doubt that they lift up the whole bladder base.

Simultaneously with any short, sharp rise in intra-abdominal pressure there is normally a reflex contraction of the pelvic floor muscles as with voluntarily interrupted micturition. This leads to a rise in intra-urethral pressure and to a more rigid fixation of the urethra by contraction of the pubo-coccygeus muscles. Normal women who do not or cannot contract the pelvic muscles quickly enough because the increase of intra-abdominal pressure occurs so suddenly and unexpectedly can experience leakage of urine, though they may be completely continent otherwise.

During a longer strain, there is a slower rise of intra-abdominal pressure which is then continued over a period of time. The pressure changes in the urethra are somewhat different. The funnelling of the vesico-urethral junction and movement of the bladder base are more marked than during short-acting stress, but the contraction of the pelvic floor musculature occurs in the same way and prevents leakage (Figs 3.16, 3.17).

Figure 3.18 shows the maximum urethral pressure and the bladder pressure during a cough.

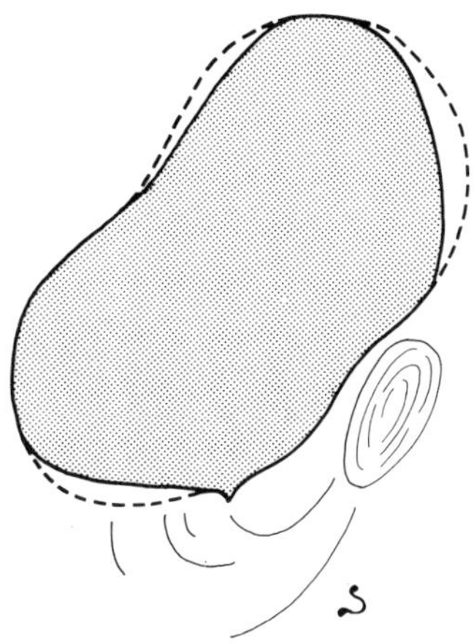

Fig. 3.16. Voluntary stress condition—cough. Note very little movement in a young woman.

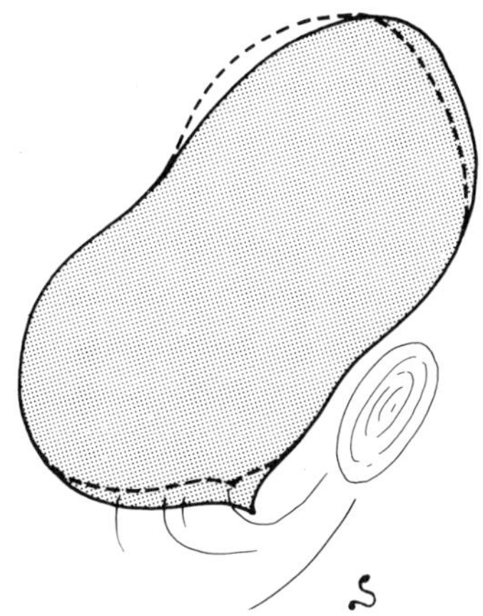

Fig. 3.17. Strain.

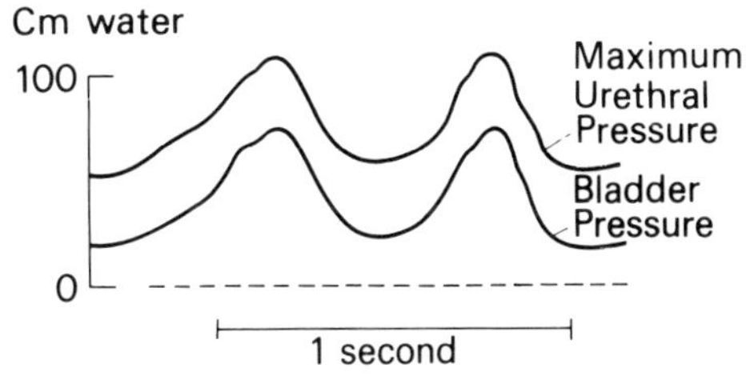

Fig. 3.18. Maximum urethral pressure and bladder pressure during a cough.

THE URETERS

There is normally no lumen except when urine is passed from the kidney to the bladder. Urine is secreted by the kidney almost continuously in amounts which vary up to a maximum of about 15 ml per minute, and is collected in the renal pelvis which serves as a reservoir. Distension of the muscular wall of the renal pelvis initiates a contraction which pushes 1 to 3 ml of urine into the upper ureter causing the ureteric wall to contract and pushing the bolus further down at a rate of 3 to 5 cm per second. There may be a short pause outside the bladder. There is no evidence that autonomic innervation plays any part in the 'peristalsis' because the ureter can be completely removed from the body and contraction be seen to proceed unaltered for a time. Also, no ganglia have been demonstrated in or on the ureteric wall.

It seems certain now that the contraction wave passes by direct intercellular signal, as is predominantly the case in the bladder wall. Contraction can be stimulated by pinching the ureter gently between the blades of a pair of forceps anywhere in its length; the resulting contraction may pass upwards or downwards. This is known to surgeons as 'vermiculation' and is much used as a means of identifying the ureter. Another method depends upon the fact that the ureter is a firm smooth cord when felt between the finger and thumb, so firm that it can be 'snapped' by the fingers.

The pressure within the renal pelvis at rest is normally equivalent to less than 5 cm water but it can rise a little during a diuresis and to more than 30 cm of water in the presence of obstruction.

REFERENCES

Asmussen M (1975) Urethro-cystometry in women. MD Thesis, University of Lund.

Asmussen M, Ulmsten U (1976) Simultaneous urethro-cystometry by a new technique. *Scand. J. Urol. Nephrol.* **10,** 7.

Asmussen M (1980) Aspects of continence, incontinence and micturition in women. Chapter 10 in *Gynecologic Urology and Urodynamics,* ed. D Ostergard. Williams & Wilkins, Baltimore.

Bates P *et al* (1979) Standardisation of terminology of lower urinary tract function. *J. Urol.* **121,** 554.

Enhørning G (1961) Simultaneous recording of intravestical and intraurethral pressure. *Acta Chir. Scand.,* Suppl. 276.

Fletcher TF, Bradley WE (1978) Review article: Neuro-anatomy of the bladder/urethra. *J. Urol.* **119,** 153.

Kiil F (1967) *The Function of the Ureter and Renal Pelvis.* WB Saunders, Philadelphia.

Quinn EL, Kass EH (1960) *The Biology of Pyelonephritis.* Little, Brown, Boston.

Rud T, Ulmsten U, Vestby M (1979) Initiation of micturition. *Scand. J. Urol. Nephrol.* **13,** 259.

Rud T *et al* (1980) Factors maintaining the intraurethral pressure in women. *Invest. Urol.* **17,** 343.

Rud T (1980) Urethral pressure profile in continent women. *Acta obstet. gynecol. Scand.* **59,** 331.

Tanagho EA, Miller ER (1970) Initiation of voiding. *Brit. J. Urol.* **42,** 175.

Ulmsten U (1974) Studies on urethral function in women. MD Thesis, University of Lund.

Westby M, Asmussen M (1981) The site of maximum urethral pressure and the location of the urogenital diaphragm in the female urethra as studied by simultaneous urethro-cystometry and voiding urethro-cystography. *Proc. International Continence Society,* 11th Annual Meeting.

Chapter 4

Examination of the Urinary Tract

It is possible to learn a great deal by the use of simple methods. A good history which includes the patient's own notes on micturition, urine examination, clinical examination, measurement of residual urine, the stress test, a limited neurological examination, cysto-urethroscopy and simple cystometry with roughly estimated flow measurement are often all that is necessary. All these methods can and should be used by any gynaecologist. As in other branches of modern medicine, a lot of complicated and expensive equipment which goes with highly specialized methods of investigation has been developed in urology. Most gynaecologists will never need to perform these investigations, but it can nevertheless be an advantage for them to have heard of them and to understand the indications for their use.

MICTURITION CHART

If there is any question of lower urinary tract dysfunction, it is often a great help to have the patient note down on a piece of paper how much she drinks, the times she passes urine and the amounts passed during a period of about a week before the examination.

CLINICAL EXAMINATION

It is convenient to make *examination of the urine* the first step in the clinical examination. Before the patient is placed on the examination couch she should be asked to micturate and try to empty her bladder. The technique of a *mid-stream specimen* is explained to her. It is recommended that a mid-stream urine specimen should be taken from all patients. It can be used for investigation of the cellular content, culture of organisms, chemical examination and cytological examination for malignant cells.

Details of the various methods of taking urine specimens, the significance of culture results and methods of examination of the urine in the consulting room or office will be found in Appendix A. Guidance on the clinical interpretation of 'urinary infection' will be found in Appendix B.

Inspection of the external genitalia includes examination of the external urinary meatus where one notes any variation in size or site; any suggestion of urethral mucosal prolapse, polyp or caruncle formation is investigated by cytological smear and colposcopy. A swab is taken for bacteriological examination if there is any sign of infection; any suspicion of tumour formation in the urethra indicates a cytological examination and may make admission to hospital necessary for more detailed investigation by biopsy and examination under anaesthetic.

After *vaginal examination* with the speculum, one should *palpate the urethra* and estimate the quality of the supporting tissues around the bladder neck and urethra which are of such importance in stress incontinence. The young gynaecologist should take every opportunity to palpate the bladder neck and urethra in women who have not had a child and who have no urinary symptoms in order to learn the normal anatomical position both in the resting state and when the patient is straining and coughing. The whole length of the urethra and the vesico-urethral junction above it will be found to be quite firmly fixed behind the symphysis and movement when the patient strains and coughs is limited, though some movement is possible from side to side. At the vesico-urethral junction the fixation ceases so that the bladder base above it is quite mobile. The bladder base and urethra are easily palpable against the pubis by a finger in the vagina, but if it is necessary to feel something in the urethral wall, for example a tumour or inflammatory process, it is an advantage to have a hard instrument such as a cystoscope in the urethra.

The next step is a *bimanual gynaecological examination*. Apart from the bladder no structure is normally palpable between the uterus and the pubis. It is quite essential that the patient is relaxed and avoids any form of straining or resistance. If the examiner cannot achieve this by gentleness and reassurance, there should be no hesitation in using some form of intravenous or intramuscular medication to produce relaxation. If this is not done the information obtained will be inadequate. The whole bladder can be felt with the vaginal fingers in front of the cervix against the hand on the abdominal wall. It is possible in a slim woman to feel any amount of residual urine in excess of about 100 ml, but this becomes uncertain in the obese patient. Urine in the bladder prevents adequate bimanual examination of the bladder wall and of the paravesical tissues on either side. It can conceal small pelvic tumours or intravesical calculi and can cause errors in the estimation of the size of the uterus. Significant residual urine is an important clinical sign which indicates that the emptying mechanism is at fault. If therefore there is any question of this the bladder should be emptied under sterile conditions. For those who have the necessary facilities and competence, a cystoscope can be used. With it one can exclude or measure residual urine, exclude a primary lesion in the bladder or urethra and do a simple cystometry. If residual urine is found the bimanual examination should be repeated. While the gynaecologist is examining the vagina he should palpate the levator ani muscles both at rest and when the subject actively contracts her pelvic floor.

In the normal state, the ureter is not palpable through the abdominal wall. A hydroureter, like a hydronephrosis, is also not palpable in the abdomen or in the flank.

In the pelvis the situation is quite different, for here the normal ureter can be felt through the vaginal wall and through the rectal wall. As it runs adjacent to the cervix in its course to the bladder wall it lies very near the lateral fornix of the vagina, so near in fact, that ureteric calculi have been removed through an incision in the vaginal wall (Figs 4.1 and 4.2). In this situation, especially when the patient is thin, a finger in the vagina can palpate a mobile cord between it and a hand on the abdominal wall. More laterally, where the ureter passes from the pelvic wall to the side of the cervix, it is too far from the vaginal wall to be reached. From the rectum, however, it is palpable against the side wall of the pelvis. It is mobile and can be 'rolled' when the finger is passed across its axis.

Detailed urodynamic measurements, whether simple or advanced, should not be performed at the first session because reliable results will not be obtained until the patient is accustomed to her surroundings and fully informed about instrumentation. When she has once experienced urethral instrumentation she will no longer be apprehensive and can behave as normally as possible. This is of extreme importance if a true picture of lower urinary tract function is to be obtained.

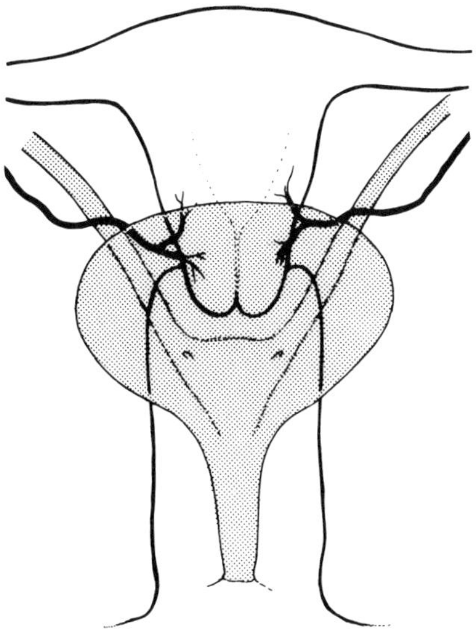

Fig. 4.1. Transverse section through pelvis showing normal relationship between ureters, vaginal wall and cervix.

Stress test

This is done to assess urine leakage during coughing and straining (see p. 53).

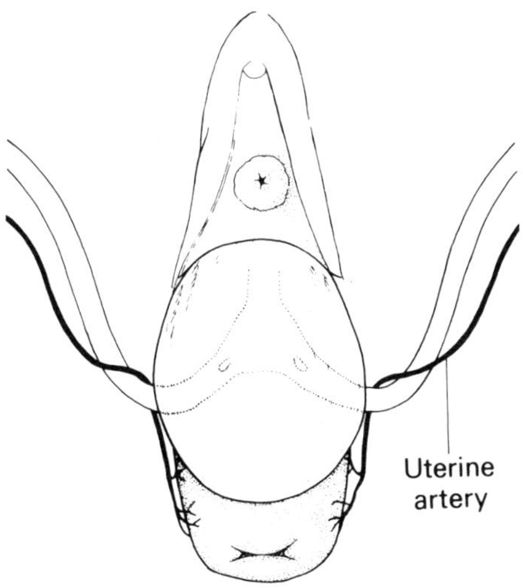

Fig. 4.2. Ureters and trigone in uterine prolapse seen from below.

Cystoscopy

A combined lubricant, antiseptic and anaesthetic gel is squeezed into the urethra. It is wise to remember that this produces only mucosal anaesthesia and that therefore dilatation can be painful. The normal female urethra can, however, be gradually dilated to take an instrument 9–10 mm in diameter without pain (9 Hegar) so it is only in the presence of a stricture that dilatation is necessary to allow passage of the cystoscope. A standard cystoscope is illustrated in Fig. 4.3). When the patient is lying on the couch the urethra is approximately horizontal so the instrument needs to be introduced with the movement illustrated in Fig.

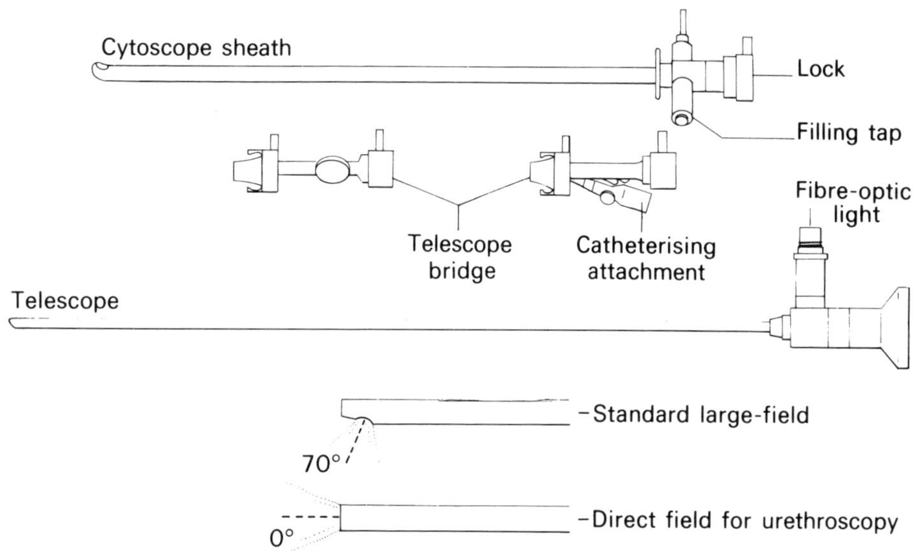

Fig. 4.3. Standard irrigating cystoscope.

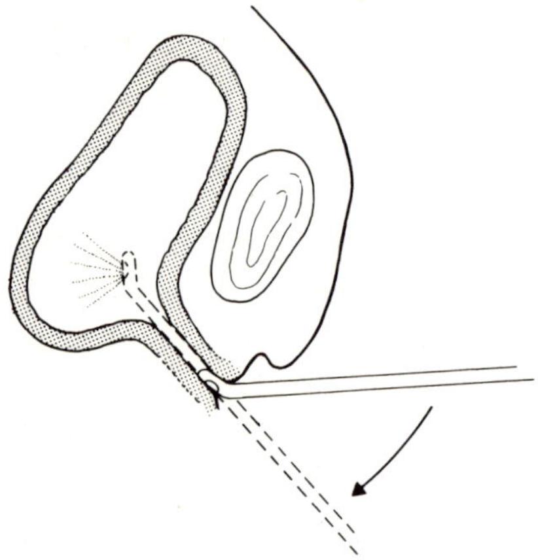

Fig. 4.4. Method of introduction of cystoscope.

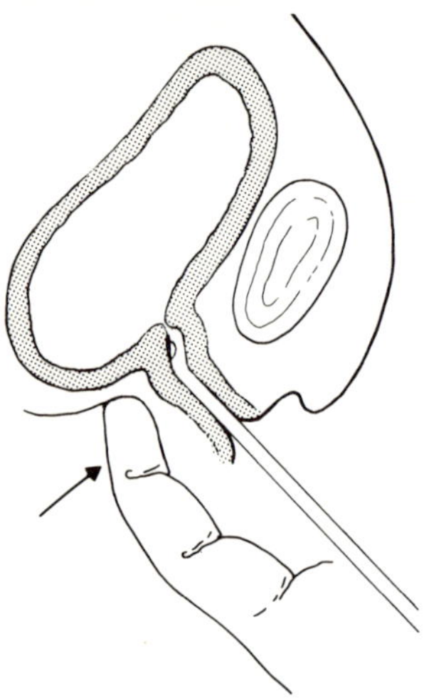

Fig. 4.5. Guidance of cystoscope by finger in vagina.

4.4. In occasional cases it may be difficult to enter the bladder although the instrument passes easily through the outer urethra. The difficulty occurs at the vesico-urethral junction which forms a mucosal ring which catches the beak either anteriorly or posteriorly. If an index finger is introduced into the vagina, the beak of the instrument can be felt through the anterior wall and guided into the bladder (Fig. 4.5). The same method can be used with advantage if there is distortion by tumour growth in or adjacent to the urethra.

When the cystoscope is in the bladder, the telescope is removed so that any urine can run out. This is measured as an estimate of residual urine and also used as a specimen for bacteriological or other examination if necessary. The presence of antiseptic which is picked up by the cytoscope on the way can discourage growth on the culture medium but has no effect on the cellular content of the urine. It is easier and more practical to remove the telescope in order to empty the bladder rather than to use the second tap on the instrument. One tap is used for the in-flowing fluid and the second can be attached to a manometer if a roughly estimated cystogram is required (Fig. 4.6).

The telescope is then re-introduced and locked in place, the light and the fluid switched on and the examination begins as the bladder fills. Filling must not be so quick that it becomes unpleasant for the patient. The field of vision is a cone with an apex of nearly 90° whose axis is about 70° to the axis of the cystoscope. The gynaecologist must accustom himself to the optical distortion and take it into consideration when estimating the position of things he sees in the bladder. It is unnecessary to wait until the bladder is full before beginning inspection, for much information can be deduced from the way the bladder

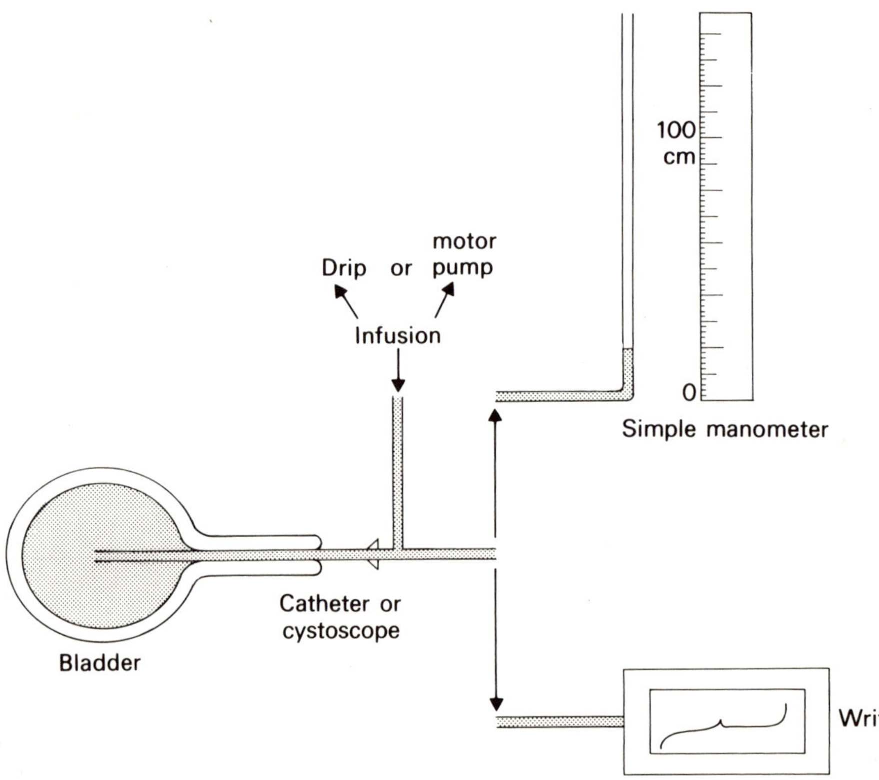

Fig. 4.6. Principles of simple water cystometry.

walls move outwards. When all walls are visible, the water is turned off. This is a better method than to put in a certain amount, say 300 ml, in every patient because the capacity is very variable. Sterile water or normal saline can be used. The patient's first sensation that the bladder is getting full often comes when 200 to 300 ml has run in, and this amount should be noted. When filling is done slowly, the information obtained in this way is reliable.

The view through the cystoscope is extremely good, so that the various parts of the mucosa, the ureteric orifices and the internal meatus can be examined with ease. Even in the presence of a long-standing inflammatory condition, for example when there is a vesico-colic fistula, the stream of clear fluid ensures that the visual field is clear enough; it may be necessary to remove the telescope and empty the bladder once or twice so as to produce a clearer field. Under these conditions the whole examination is conducted with the water turned on. The same procedure is used in haematuria, when there is a source of bleeding in the bladder. It is possible in this way to identify small bleeding arterioles. The gynaecologist should always try to find the source of bleeding and not be afraid that bleeding will make vision impossible – this is almost never the case. The only thing that makes vision quite impossible is the presence of blood clots in the bladder.

With the cystoscope in the moderately filled bladder, the objective is to inspect the whole interior. There are two landmarks which can aid orientation, the internal urinary meatus and the air bubble. If the cystoscope is drawn outwards while the bladder wall is under observation in any direction the ring of the internal meatus will come into view and obscure vision completely. Further out the lens lies in the urethra where one must have the irrigation fluid running to be able to see anything. As soon as the internal meatus comes into view with the operator looking at the trigone it is then rotated 20 or 30 degrees to each side and passed slowly inwards along the same axis. The ureteric orifice normally comes into view about 3 cm from the internal meatus.

If one fails to find an orifice by this method, there is another way which is worth a trial. With the cystoscope lens pointing directly anteriorly or at the ceiling in the lithotomy position, the highest point of the bladder comes into view and here is to be found 'the air bubble'. There is always an air bubble in the highest point of the bladder due to the air that is in the cystoscope when it is introduced. The cystoscope is then rotated through a little less than 180 degrees without altering its axis or moving it in or out and a ureteric orifice should come into view. In some bladders the interureteric bar is prominent and will lead the observer to an orifice if followed in a lateral direction. There is much to be said for learning both these methods of finding ureteric orifices for it is not always easy; there is a natural tendency to a little variation in position, the orifice may be absent or duplicated and also, in just those cases where it is necessary to find and catheterize an orifice, it is obscured by inflammation, oedema or perhaps tumour. Furthermore, the bladder base can sometimes be so grossly distorted by tumour formation in the pelvis that, for example, both ureteric orifices may lie on the same side of the mid-line.

The bladder mucosa is next inspected in all directions always referring to either the air bubble or the internal meatus if one becomes disorientated. The bladder is never spherical, not even during micturition. The posterior wall is pushed forwards by the uterus and two comparatively large lateral pouches are normal findings. The mucosa is a light yellow colour with small blood vessels visible superficially. It forms small folds which flatten out as the bladder fills. On the trigone the mucosa is fixed to the underlying muscle and always flat. It may also be a little more pink and granular here. This is not pathological but something which varies with the menstrual cycle and with age. It is a normal condition that has often been described as 'trigonitis'. Real infection produces redness and oedema, sometimes to the extent that there is bleeding on distension. In-dwelling catheters produce gross local irritative changes in the bladder mucosa on the posterior wall because of contact between the tip of the catheter and the mucosa over a limited area. This can be mistaken for a tumour.

Urethroscopy

This is best done after completion of the examination of the bladder and, because it must be done with fluid running into the bladder all the time, one must remember to begin by emptying the bladder. The vesico-urethral junction is first identified at 12 o'clock and the instrument drawn slowly out until the lens of the telescope reaches the external meatus. The urethral walls will be moved outwards by the stream of water so that they come into focus and folds will be smoothed out. The instrument is then passed in and the examination repeated in the 3 o'clock direction and so on until one has seen the whole urethra. It is easy to recognize parts which do not expand and move outwards and to identify their position by means of a finger in the vagina. The opening of a diverticulum or a fistula can usually be seen without difficulty. If there is infection in the urethral glands, the openings can be seen in the distal part surrounded by small red areas. The patient will certainly remind the surgeon that her bladder is nearly bursting, but he should avoid the necessity for this by emptying out the water that runs in during the examination from time to time.

An additional direct field telescope can be obtained which allows vision in its own axis like a nautical telescope (Fig. 4.3). The advantage of this is that it gives the operator a view of the whole urethra from the lower end so that he can better observe the movement of the vesico-urethral junction during coughing and straining.

CO_2 urethroscopy

CO_2 urethroscopy employs a special instrument which uses gas as a means of distending the urethra. It can also be used to perform cystometry. The urethral mucosa can be beautifully demonstrated and the urethral resistance to gas distension can be observed at rest, during coughing, straining and squeezing with the pelvic floor muscles. The instrument is really a urethroscope and gives a poor view of the bladder because the visual field is in the axis of the telescope and it is therefore difficult to see round the corner at the internal meatus.

Water cystometry

Simple cystometry, which only measures the pressure in the bladder during filling, gives limited information because it reveals nothing of the interplay between activity in the bladder and urethra. However, if cystometry is done as shown in Fig. 4.6 it gives the volume and pressure at first sensation, the maximum subjective bladder capacity and its pressure and the pressure when micturition starts, but nothing more.

The surgeon must appreciate the limitations of the examination. Classical water cystometry was performed with a large balloon catheter and a high filling rate which produced many artefacts. Ideally, the urethral instrument should not be more than the diameter of the urethra during micturition, which is less than 5 mm, and the filling rate should be within physiological limits, which is not more than 15 ml per minute. This means that the examination can take a long time. A filling rate which is greater than that which is produced by the ureters when they carry urine down from the kidneys must produce unphysiological effects because the receptors in the bladder wall are stimulated abnormally.

If an abnormal cystogram is obtained by using a higher filling rate than normal, it should be repeated using a slow rate before any valid conclusions can be drawn from it. Another source of error is the fact that a rise in intra-abdominal pressure produces exactly the same effect on intra-vesical pressure as a detrusor contraction. In fact, if any abnormality is found on simple cystometry, it is an indication for a more detailed examination.

CO_2 cystometry

Gas can also be used to fill the bladder to obtain a cystometrogram. It is very easy to use but provides no advantages over water or saline and introduces a new factor so that the results cannot be directly correlated with water cystometry.

Urinary flow measurement

This has less relevance in women as distinct from men, for obstruction of the female urethra is very uncommon. If a woman complains of a slow urinary stream, it can be measured using a watch and noting the volume passed in a certain time. A normal woman should be able to pass 400 ml within 20 seconds, which gives a mean flow rate of 20 ml/sec. If the rate is 10 ml/second or less and there is a constant flow, this indicates some form of obstruction. Fractionated micturition—small amounts produced by repeated straining—can be seen after peripheral bladder denervation but also frequently appears in a normal subject simply because she is nervous. It can occur, for example, if a flow measurement is done at the first attendance. It is very important to be aware of this artefact.

The combination of flow-rate measurement and measurement of intravesical pressures in order to assess urethral resistance has little place in urodynamics in the female.

Urethral pressure profile measurements

See Fig. 3.1 and p. 43.

RADIOLOGY OF THE URINARY TRACT

In the vast majority of cases, simple radiological investigations which are in daily use in most general hospitals are sufficient. The choice and the interpretation of these is best organized as a cooperative effort by the clinician and the radiologist.

Intravenous urography

The preliminary straight X-ray shows outlines of the kidneys, urinary calculi and calcification. It will also often show large tumour masses and a distended bladder as soft tissue shadows. After the injection of contrast, pictures taken at 5, 15 and 30 minutes will show the progress of contrast through the urinary tract and the outlines of the calyces, renal pelvis, ureters and bladder. Tubular concentration must be considerably reduced before it is obvious on the urograph so it is unwise to put much weight on the examination as a renal function test. At the end the patient can be asked to visit the toilet and try to empty her bladder. A picture of the pelvis after this will give a rough estimate of any residual urine.

Before starting the examination, enquiries should be made about allergic reactions because severe sensitivity to halogen compounds can sometimes be encountered. If it is not essential it should not be done because it can be replaced to some extent by isotope renography. The situation should be discussed with the radiologist and, if the examination is considered essential, everything should be prepared beforehand in expectation of a severe reaction. Premedication with an antihistamine tablet or injection is advisable and an anaesthetist equipped to intubate the larynx should be standing by. Hydrocortisine and antihistamine injections should be drawn up into syringes ready for use and a canula placed in a vein. It can be a fatal mistake to underestimate the need for safety.

If the patient has not drunk or eaten anything for several hours before the investigation, the contrast will appear in the urine in the calyces and renal pelvis within 5 minutes of the injection. Delay in excretion can have many causes; heart failure, renal failure and obstruction to the ureter are the commonest.

The normal ureter is never demonstrated throughout its length because peristalsis empties short lengths periodically, but different parts of the same ureter are usually visible in the different pictures. Abdominal compression will hold up the contrast in the lumbar ureter above the pelvic brim but does nothing to demonstrate the pelvic portion. If the whole length is shown in a film taken about 30 minutes after injection, it suggests that there may be obstruction in the neighbourhood of the bladder. This is a frequent finding after pelvic operations.

Urine leakage from the ureter can also be demonstrated.

Intravenous urography is by far the most useful radiological investigation of the urinary tract, and is of great importance in gynaecological surgery because of its ability to demonstrate ureteric anatomy and function.

Sometimes a kidney is shown on intravenous urography to have two renal pelves and two ureters. It is often impossible for the radiologist to determine if the two ureters join on their way to the bladder because of normal peristalsis. Usually one ureter is seen but seldom two side by side. The gynaecologist wants to know if he will meet one or two ureters in the pelvis and whether they will be together or separate. Cystoscopy will show whether there are two ureteric orifices or only one. If there are two, then the ureter is double all the way from the kidney to the bladder and the two ureters lie together all the way in a common thin fascial sheath. This is an inflexible rule. If there is only one orifice, then the ureters join in the form of a Y somewhere on the way to the bladder. At first sight it might seem desirable to demonstrate the exact point of union, which has to be done by injection of contrast through a ureteric catheter, but in fact it is unnecessary. As the ureters always lie together the finding of one ureter in the pelvis means that the junction must be above this point.

Pyelography and ureterography

For this investigation the solution is introduced through a catheter which can be inserted into the renal pelvis percutaneously (*antigrade pyelography*) or injected into the renal pelvis via a ureteric catheter (*retrograde pyelography*). These methods are useful when renal function is so poor that intravenous urography gives an inadequate shadow; either method can be used to demonstrate the lower ureter. Retrograde catheterization is used for ureterography; the catheter should be withdrawn until only 5 cm remains in the ureter (as seen through the cystoscope) and 3 ml of contrast solution (the same solution as is used intravenously) injected while an exposure is made. Much of the contrast will normally be expelled into the bladder by peristaltic contraction of the ureter but enough will remain to give a good picture. It should be remembered that the ureteric catheter sometimes alters the position of the ureter a little so that it is not always easy to demonstrate its relationship to shadows in the neighbourhood.

Cystography

Normally, there is enough contrast in the bladder urine at the end of urography to give a fair picture of the bladder but it is inadequate to show details.

Radiological demonstration of the bladder can really only be done adequately by emptying the bladder of urine and refilling with a suitable contrast solution.

The cystogram is very rarely used in urological practice because cystoscopy gives sufficient information. It can however be of value in the demonstration of fistulous tracks from the bladder.

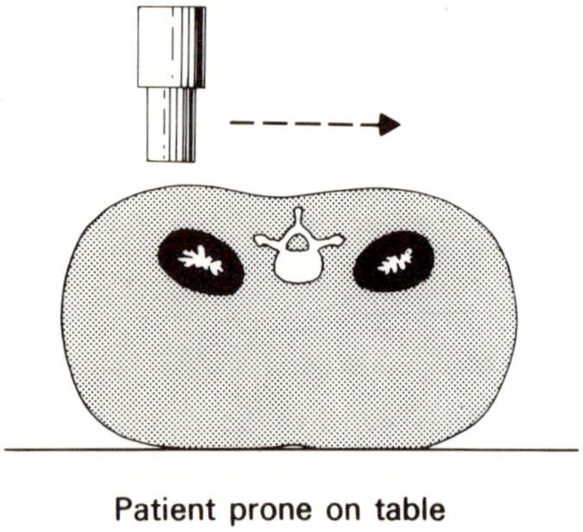

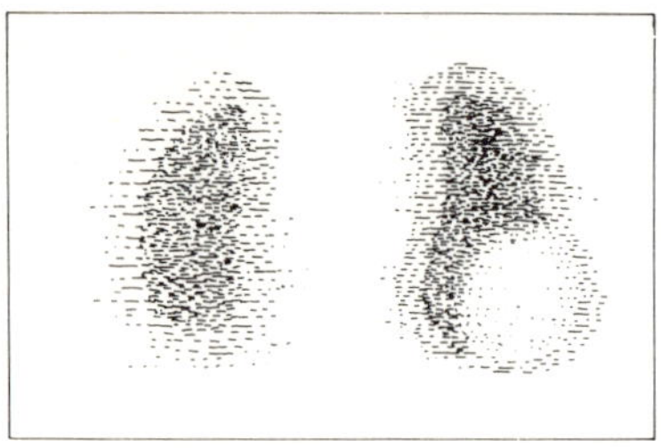

Fig. 4.7. Scintigraphy.

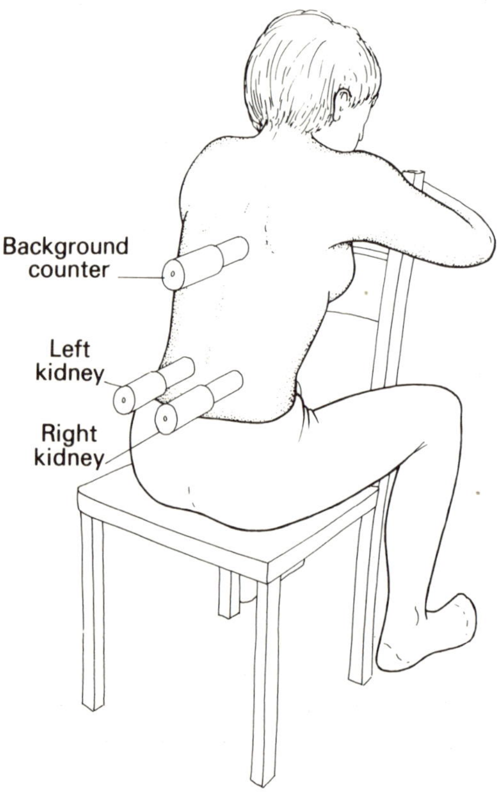

Fig. 4.8. Renography: patient with counters in position.

Urethrography

This is sometimes useful in demonstrating a urethral diverticulum (Fig. 13.4). It must be remembered that it is necessary first to empty the diverticulum by pressure from the vagina otherwise it may not be filled at all.

Micturating cysto-urethrography

Still pictures are first taken while the patient performs a Valsalva manoeuvre with and without contraction of the pelvic floor so as to demonstrate the mobility and shape of the vesico-urethral junction. A bead-chain can be used to show the shape and mobility of the urethra during this manoeuvre. It also shows the outline of the urethra. Still pictures give no information about dynamic events such as coughing, so this examination has been replaced by video filming in centres where the equipment is available.

Isotope investigations

Radioactive isotopes are used to demonstrate the kidneys, ureters and bladder by virtue of their gamma rays which are picked up and measured by gamma cameras placed posteriorly over the kidneys. Some isotopes are almost entirely absorbed by epithelial cells in the kidneys whilst others pass through the nephrons and proceed further in the urine.

Scintigraphy (renal scan, Fig. 4.7)

Scintigraphy is used to demonstrate the size, situation and outline of the kidneys and the presence of space-occupying lesions, that is parts of the kidneys which do not take up isotopes, such as tumours or cysts. The irradiation dose to the kidney is about 10 mGy (1 rad).

Renography (Fig. 4.8)

An isotope which is excreted in the urine can be used to measure renal function by noting its excretion in relation to the passage of time and can also demonstrate ureteric function, especially ureteric obstruction. Some of these isotopes are passed out in the urine by simple filtration. This gives an even smaller radiation dose to the kidneys, about 5 mGy (0.5 rad).

Standard intravenous urography should never be done in pregnancy; a modified examination involving one exposure 20 minutes after injection of contrast can occasionally be permitted if it seems absolutely essential.

If intravenous urography is inadvisable or contraindicated because of pregnancy or iodine sensitivity, isotope investigation can be a very valuable substitute. It gives, of course, a very diffuse outline picture of the kidneys and ureters which is inferior to urography but as a renal function test it is much better. The irradiation dose to each kidney using, for example, ^{131}I-hippuran which is

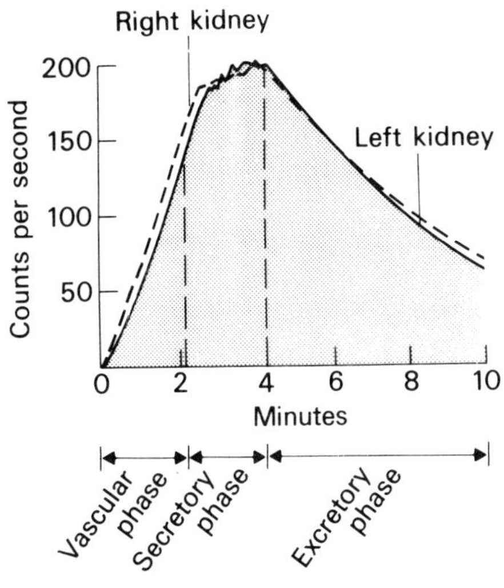

Fig. 4.9. Phases of excretion in normal isotope renography.

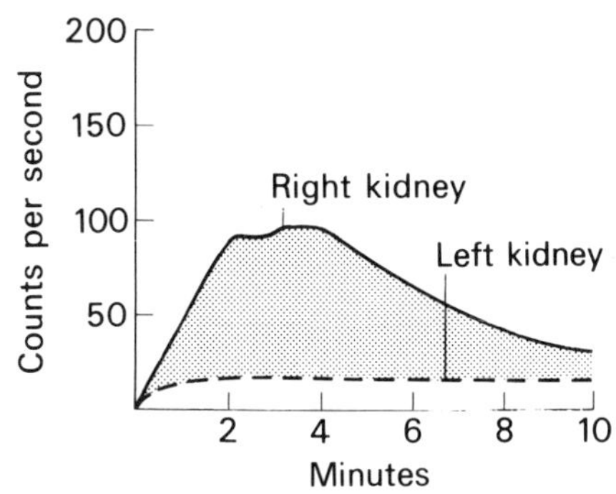

Fig. 4.10. Left kidney shows complete renal failure; right kidney shows partial renal failure due to obstruction.

both filtered and secreted by the kidneys, is only about 2 mGy (0.2 rad), so it is not contraindicated in pregnancy as the dose to the fetus is much less than this.

The isotope is injected intravenously after the patient has drunk enough water to ensure a diuresis (Fig. 4.8). There are three phases of excretion (Fig. 4.9):

1 the vascular phase during which the isotope reaches the renal blood vessels;

2 the secretory phase, during which the isotope is filtered through the glomeruli and passes into the renal tubules; and

3 the excretory phase, during which the isotope passes from the collecting tubules to the calyces, renal pelves and ureters.

Abnormalities which can be demonstrated are:

1 Complete renal failure (Fig. 4.10). There is no increase of density of isotope in the kidneys so that the counter only registers the amount in the blood flowing through the renal circulation.

2 Partial renal failure (Fig. 4.10). Inadequate concentration compared with a normal kidney. The excretory phase is normal.

3 Delay in excretion due to ureteric obstruction which has produced hydronephrosis (Fig. 4.11). In the acute phase of obstruction, the first two excretory phases are normal and only the third phase is affected. The hydronephrosis and hydroureter are shown by accumulation of the isotope in the renal pelvis and upper ureter. If the obstruction continues, the first two phases will be increasingly affected, leading eventually to the picture seen in complete renal failure.

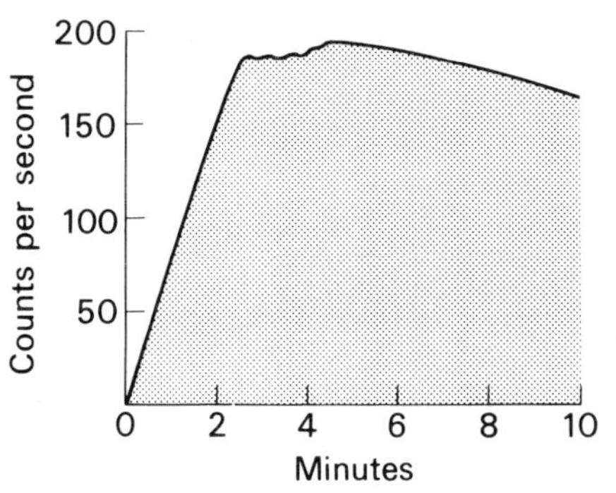

Fig. 4.11. Delay in excretion due to renal obstruction.

Isotope renography as a renal function test

If renography using hippuran is combined with a series of measurements of the blood concentration of the isotope, it is possible to work out the so-called 'effective renal plasma flow' and estimate the amount of functioning tissue in each kidney. This is being increasingly used and may come to play a major part in the pre- and post-operative assessment of renal function where either the disease process or the treatment has resulted in renal damage.

A LOOK AT MODERN URODYNAMICS

Pressure-flow measurements, simple urethral pressure profile studies and electromyography of the pelvic floor muscles give at the present time little relevant clinical information; they are more useful as research instruments. Additional methods of investigation should not be so complicated that they are difficult to perform without a mass of technical equipment with its concomitant technicians and, above all, they should not be so unpleasant for the patient that her reactions become abnormal.

Pressure measurements in the bladder and urethra can be combined with flow measurements, videofilming and electromyography to provide a fascinating total picture of bladder and urethral function in one examination. This, however, is difficult to carry out successfully and, at present, is experimental. It has surprisingly little clinical application. Normal micturition is difficult for the patient: either she cannot start or she attempts to initiate micturition by the Valsalva manoeuvre. The results may therefore easily be misinterpreted.

There is no doubt that the two most important considerations where modern urodynamics is concerned are that *the investigation must be easy to perform* and that *it must not be unpleasant for the patient*. Furthermore, it should be possible, if necessary, to leave her alone so that she can micturate normally. She must be informed in detail about the whole procedure and an informal and relaxed relationship with the examiner must be encouraged.

At the present time two techniques fulfil these criteria. They are simultaneous urethro-cystometry and video-urethro-cystography. They demonstrate simultaneously both static and dynamic events in the bladder and urethra in two completely different ways, the first by pressure measurement, the second by visualization.

Simultaneous urethro-cystometry and urethral pressure profile measurement

This means *measurement of the pressure in the bladder and the urethra simultaneously* under various conditions, such as filling with different amounts in the bladder at rest, while straining as in the Valsalva manoeuvre, when coughing, while contracting the pelvic muscles and during micturition.

Urethral pressure profile measurement means *recording the urethral pressure at all points from the internal to the external urinary meatus.* At present there are three ways of performing this examination:

1 open-end catheters,
2 balloon catheters,
3 micro-transducers built into a catheter.

Open-end catheters and balloon catheters are not as satisfactory as micro-transducers, because their physical properties do not allow measurement of rapid changes of pressure and they often do not react in a linear manner. There are problems with calibration. Both open-end catheter and balloon catheter measurements are difficult to standardize. All this adds up to the fact that neither method can ever have a universal clinical application and it also serves to remind us that the quality and quantity of the results must be adequate to ensure that additional useful information is forthcoming. Micro-transducers are much easier to use and are not subject to the problems described above. A suitable instrument can be made with 2 micro-transducers with surface membranes a few cm apart (so-called tip-transducers) which will measure the pressures in the bladder and at a point in the urethra at the same instant. It can then be moved to another point or moved slowly in or out while pressures are recorded. Alternatively, several mini-transducers can be mounted at intervals along the instrument.

The double micro-transducer catheter which is commonly used is semi-flexible, smooth, radio-opaque and size 7–8 Fr. The area of each of the transducers is 0.75 mm^2 which means that pressure is measured over a very small area. The physical properties such as linearity, stability and measurement of fast pressure variations far exceed what is necessary in the lower urinary tract. The

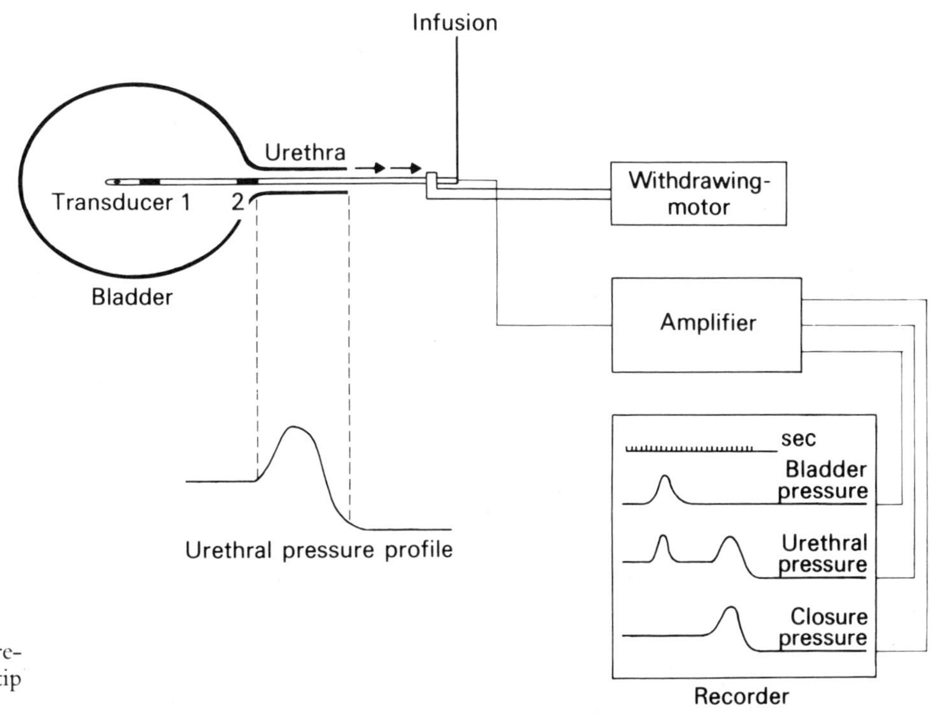

Fig. 4.12. Simultaneous pressure measurement in bladder and urethra using microtip catheter.

catheters are so reliable that electronic calibration is the only thing that is necessary in routine daily use. They are easy to clean and disinfect.

The transducers are connected to a differential amplifier which not only records the pressures but also subtracts the bladder pressure from the intra-urethral pressure to give the closure pressure (Fig. 4.12). This equipment is expensive and delicate, but can provide a lot of reliable information in a short time, so that the cost per examination becomes low in the long run.

Measurement procedure

The patient can be in any desired position, sitting, lying, standing, semi-sitting, etc. The bladder is slowly filled through a thin female catheter to the desired volume (usually 100 ml), then the special catheter is inserted so that both transducers are in the bladder. This special catheter is connected to a withdrawal motor which pulls it out through the urethra at a constant speed. Transducer 2 moves slowly out through the urethra producing a pressure profile while transducer 1 records the bladder pressure. It is usually withdrawn at a speed of 2.5 mm/s which is adjusted to be the same as the speed of the paper on which the pressures are recorded. It therefore also records directly the length of the urethra.

The withdrawal motor can move the catheter in both directions and can be stopped at any point so that a particular place in the urethra can be examined, for example, during coughing.

The urethral pressure profile measurement has been much used in recent years. It has by itself little clinical relevance. The maximum urethral pressure has been the most used parameter. This point is, however, not stable or well defined because it may alter its position in the profile if repeated measurements are made. The length of the urethra varies greatly from one individual to another so that comparison of treatment groups is difficult. In the same individual, quite considerable variation can occur from one examination to another for reasons which are not yet understood.

The most important clinical data are often obtained during bladder filling when transducer 2 is placed at the point of maximum urethral pressure. This is the most interesting point in the urethra particularly where neurogenic lesions are concerned because it represents maximum sphincter activity and is the place where the greatest variations of pressure occur. Contraction of pelvic floor muscles as seen in the unstable urethra or when micturition is voluntarily stopped can also be demonstrated.

The bladder is filled at a constant physiological rate. Micro-transducer 2 can be placed at any point in the urethra while the patient is asked to cough and resulting alterations in bladder pressure, maximum urethral pressure and closure pressure are observed. This is of special interest in patients with stress incontinence because the function of the sphincter can be observed and the appearance of leakage noted and compared with variations in closure pressure. Leakage directly associated with a cough can be differentiated from the leakage which occurs in some neurogenic bladders, due to micturition which is induced by a cough.

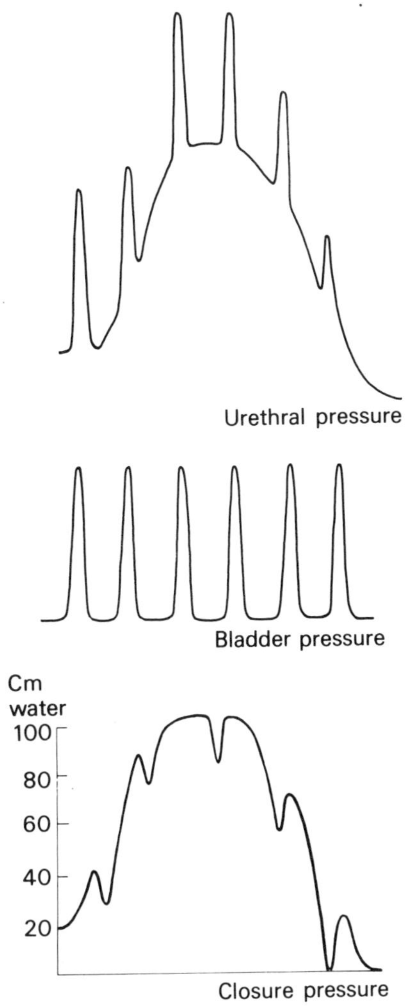

Fig. 4.13. Coughing profile.

The patient can be asked to initiate micturition with a small amount in the bladder. If she cannot do this when requested, it is always possible to continue filling until the urge to micturate becomes so strong that she cannot prevent it. This is often facilitated if the investigator leaves the room. Micturition will be brought into action by the bladder distension. If there is no reflex action, overflow incontinence will occur. This is called *controlled provoked micturition*.

This is really the most important use for simultaneous pressure measurement and an important contribution to urodynamics in recent years. As a result the focus of interest has been shifted from the bladder to the bladder and urethra as the functional unit.

If transducer 2 is withdrawn through the urethra while the patient repeatedly coughs, a so-called '*coughing profile*' is produced (Fig. 4.13). This can be done with different amounts of fluid in the bladder. The closure efficiency during stress throughout the length of the urethra can be demonstrated in this way. Examples of other recordings which are produced have been given in Chapter 3.

The intra-rectal catheter to record rectal pressure, which reflects changes in intra-abdominal pressure, is not usually necessary because a rise in intra-abdominal pressure is transmitted to both the bladder and urethra. A rise in intra-abdominal pressure can more easily be misinterpreted as a detrusor contraction if simple cystometry is used because only the bladder pressure is recorded.

Video recording

Video-urethro-cystography is the simultaneous recording of static and dynamic events in the bladder and urethra in a visual form on tape. The image is produced by the use of contrast medium and X-rays and is demonstrated on a television screen.

The method allows the outlines of the bladder and urethra to be visualized radiologically at the same time so that the changes which occur during straining, contraction of the pelvic floor muscles, coughing and micturition can be recorded. Its advantages are that it gives additional information on the shape and mobility of the bladder neck and the action of the urethra. It also gives incidental information about abnormalities such as diverticulum of the bladder or urethra, ureteric reflux and residual urine. It is also possible to see leakage of urine from the urethra or from a fistula and observe exactly when and how it occurs. Most of these things cannot be demonstrated by simultaneous urethro-cystometry. This means that in order to obtain a fully descriptive picture of the lower urinary tract, both urethro-cystometry and video-filming should be used because they demonstrate different things. The combination of these two examinations so that they can be done at the same time becomes too complicated and bewildering for the patient. Artefacts become too common to be acceptable. A video-tape recorder is easier to use and involves a smaller radiation dose than a cine-camera. Cassette tapes are very convenient and much cheaper than film; they can be played over and over again, reversed and stopped. If documentation is required, a short exposure on 100 mm film can be made and this allows more detailed anatomical measurements to be taken if they are needed. Any modern X-ray equipment with fluoroscope such as is used for angiography or lymphangiography can be used. It is connected to a video-tape recorder which is the same as is commercially available for use with a home TV set (Fig. 4.14). The examiner should be alone with the patient. The bladder is slowly filled with body-warm contrast medium until the patient begins to feel a strong desire to void. A 40% aqueous solution of contrast medium gives a better picture of the urethra than, for example, a 25% solution, especially if the flow is slow. It does not seem to interfere in any significant way with micturition. The bladder should not to be overfilled so that the patient feels discomfort. A little silver clip (as used in neurosurgery) can be placed on the external urinary meatus to act as a marker. A microphone is connected so that instructions to the patient are recorded on the tape. This facilitates subsequent analysis. The patient sits comfortably on a sponge plastic toilet seat which does not give a shadow on the X-ray screen. The bladder is first viewed antero-posteriorly and then laterally. The lateral view is the more useful. The instrument is now focussed and the examination starts. It is possible to see the position and shape of the bladder and vesico-urethral junction and the length of the urethra can be estimated from the internal meatus to the silver clip. The patient is then asked to perform a Valsalva manoeuvre, to cough and then to contract the pelvic floor muscles so that the mobility and shape of the vesico-urethral junction and possible leakage of urine can be observed. She is then asked to micturate so that one can see:

the action of the bladder base,
the funnelling of the vesico-urethral junction and urethra,
the shape and course of the urethra, and
if there is a diverticulum, stricture or fistula.

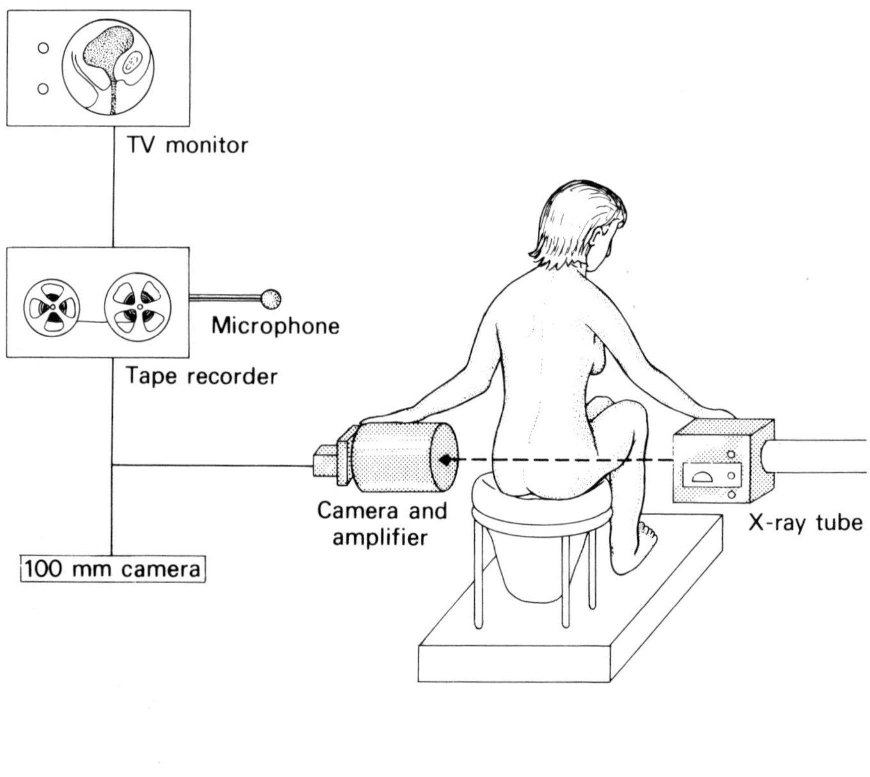

Fig. 4.14. Diagram showing principles of video-urethro-cystography.

When micturition has started, she is asked to stop it voluntarily so that the point in the urethra where 'cut off' occurs can be seen and the 'milk back' can be observed. She is then asked to continue micturition until the bladder is as empty as possible so that residual urine can be observed. A detrusor contraction can be recognized when the bladder shadow alters and becomes rounder ('spherification').

The examination is now complete and the silver clip can be removed. The irradiation dose is low, not more than 2 mGy (200 m rads) per min + 0.1 mGy (10 m rads) per 100 mm still picture as measured in the centre of the bladder. The dosage to the gonads is less than this because of shielding so that an average examination which takes 2 min with ten 100 mm pictures gives a gonad dose which is not more than a straight X-ray of the lower abdomen.

The main use of this examination is in recurrent stress incontinence after exclusion of neurogenic abnormality. It demonstrates very effectively the mechanism of the leakage, so much so that, ideally, it could be used both before and after operation to see the reasons for successful and unsuccessful surgery. This, of course, is a counsel for perfection and not always possible in practice.

REFERENCES

Asmussen M (1976) Intraurethral pressure recording. *Scand. J. Urol. Nephrol.* **10,** 1.

Asmussen M, Ulmsten U (1976) New technique for measurement of urethral pressure profile. *Acta Obstet. Gynecol. Scand.* **55,** 167.

Asmussen M, Ulmsten U (1976) Simultaneous urethrocystometry by a new technique. *Scand. J. Urol. Nephrol.* **10,** 7.

Asmussen M (1980) Aspects of continence, incontinence & micturition in women based on simultaneous urethro-cystometry. In *Gynecologic Urology and Urodynamics,* ed. D. Ostergard. Williams & Wilkins, Baltimore.

Bates P *et al* (1979) Standardisation of terminology of lower urinary tract function. *J. Urol.* **121,** 551.

Britton KE, Brown NJG (1971) *Clinical Renography*. Lloyd-Luke, London.

Davis IH, Cain LG (1956) Positive pressure urethrography. *J. Urol.* **75,** 753.

Drutz HP, Shapiro BJ, Mandel F (1978) Do static urethrograms have a role in the investigation of female incontinence? *Am. J. Obstet. Gynecol.* **130,** 516.

Hodgkinson CP (1978) Metallic bead-chain urethrocystography. *Clinical Obstetrics and Gynecology* **21,** no 3. Harper & Row, New York.

Klevmark B (1981) Hyperactive neurogenic bladder studied with physiological filling rates. *Scand. J. Urol. Nephrol.* Suppl. 60, 55.

Robertson JR (1973) Gynecologic urethroscopy. *Am. J. Obstet. Gynecol.* **115,** 986.

Robertson JR (1974) Gas cysto-metrogram with urethral pressure profile. *Obstet. Gynecol.* **44,** 72.

Vestby M (1982) Video–urethro–cystography in women. In press.

Chapter 5 Stress Incontinence

Mild stress incontinence is common in women. It is unknown in animals so it is presumably part of the price that women pay for the privilege of walking in an upright position. It is only when stress incontinence becomes so severe that it causes the individual to be uncomfortable or interferes with her social activities that it becomes a condition which needs treatment. The surgeon who is called upon to deal with it should remind himself frequently that it is a form of dysfunction and not a disease and, though it may sometimes make life very unpleasant for the patient, nobody has ever died of it.

Such terms as 'genuine stress incontinence' and 'sphincter incontinence' have been avoided because they give no clearly defined information. Stress incontinence occurs most frequently in older women and in multipara, but most women experience it at some time in their lives. It is more frequent in obese women. The history often reveals that it started after delivery of an extra large child, after a rapid delivery or after a forceps delivery. Women who have not borne children seldom complain of it. Mild symptoms are often aggravated at the menopause.

Relationship of cystocele to stress incontinence

Small cystoceles are of two types.

1 *Distension cystocele* is caused by stretching of the vagina from within so that the wall becomes thinner with flattened rugae. The anterior wall descends, bringing with it the attached bladder wall without altering the position of the vesico-urethral junction. Stress incontinence is not a feature of this type.

2 *Displacement cystocele* results from stretching or destruction of the tissues which support the vagina and cervix against the pelvic wall. The vaginal wall is intact with normal rugae. The whole bladder base descends by the mechanism which is described below. Stress incontinence frequently results.

Larger cystoceles lead to over-distension of the bladder with residual urine and overflow incontinence. Ureteric obstruction may even occur.

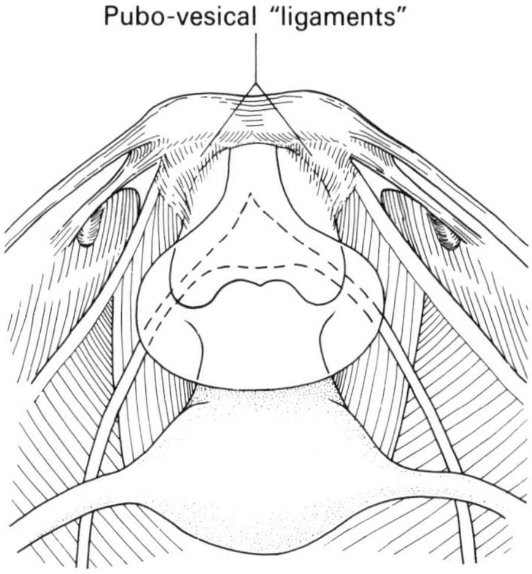

Fig. 5.1. Damage to the fixation of the anterior vaginal wall produces the so-called pubo-vesical ligaments (see also Fig. 2.20).

AETIOLOGY

Passive elements

Vesico-urethral fixation

The attachment of the anterior vaginal wall on either side of the urethra to the back of the pubis and to the pelvic wall becomes damaged so that the vesico-urethral junction and the urethra become more mobile (Figs 5.1 and 5.2). The angle which the trigone makes with the urethra becomes flattened out (Fig. 5.3). This angle is, however, not pathognomonic of stress incontinence, but is one of the results of damage to the fixation. It has been shown that if a group of normal women is compared with a group who have stress incontinence, measurement of this angle at rest and during straining shows considerable overlap between the two groups.

One reason for leakage during a cough is that most of the transmitted energy is lost in producing movement of the urethra instead of being absorbed by a

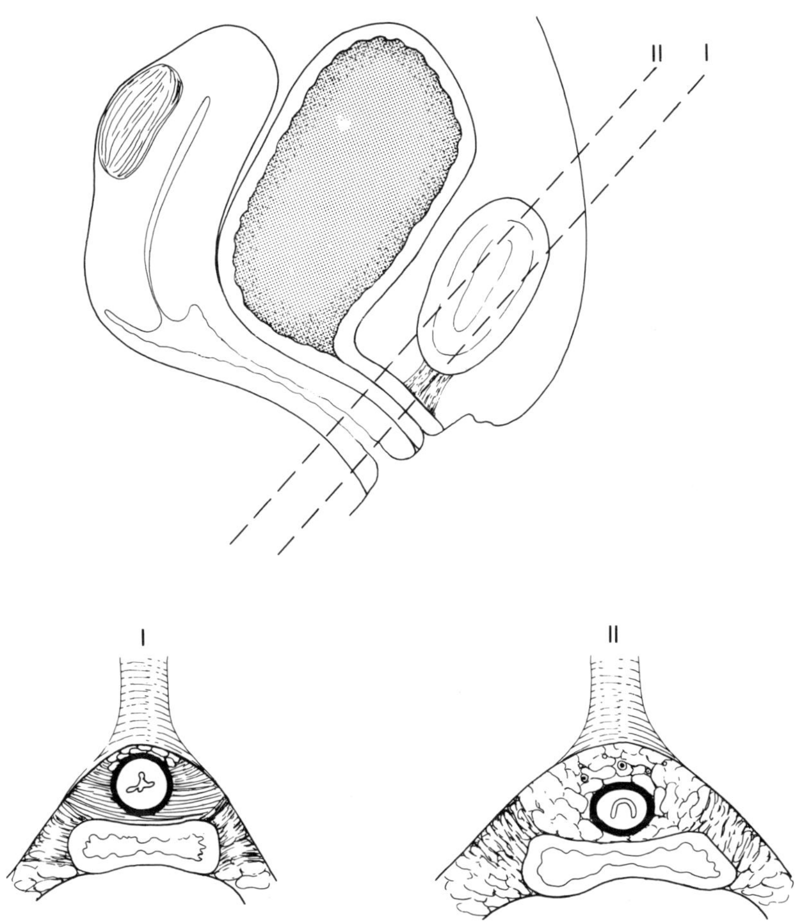

Fig. 5.2. Urethral fixation at the urogenital diaphragm is normal (I). Above this (II) the fixation of the anterior vaginal wall on each side has become loose.

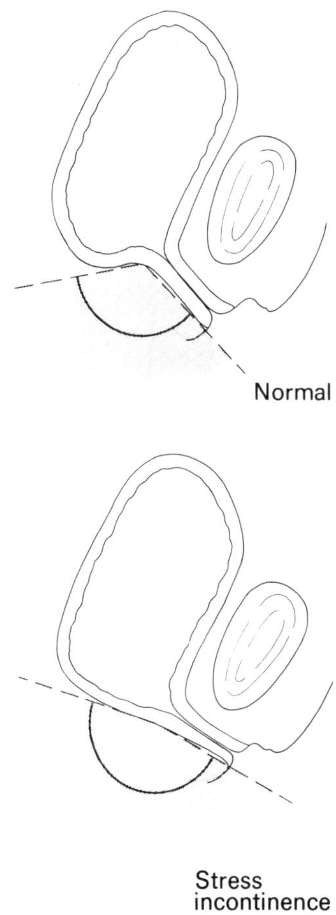

Fig. 5.3. The angle between the trigone and the urethra becomes flatter.

well-suspended urethra so that it increases the intra-urethral pressure sufficiently to prevent loss of urine (see Normal Physiology, Chapter 2). The movement of the upper urethra in both normal and stress-incontinent women is in a downward direction and not in the direction of the urethral axis through the urogenital diaphragm. The upper part of the urethra always remains an intrapelvic organ.

Another equally important reason for leakage is that the poor fixation of the anterior vaginal wall on either side of the vesico-urethral junction allows the upper urethra to open more easily so that it becomes funnel-shaped and therefore contains urine (Fig. 5.4). The bladder base including the trigone, together with the floor of the upper urethra, is pushed directly downwards because of the pressure.

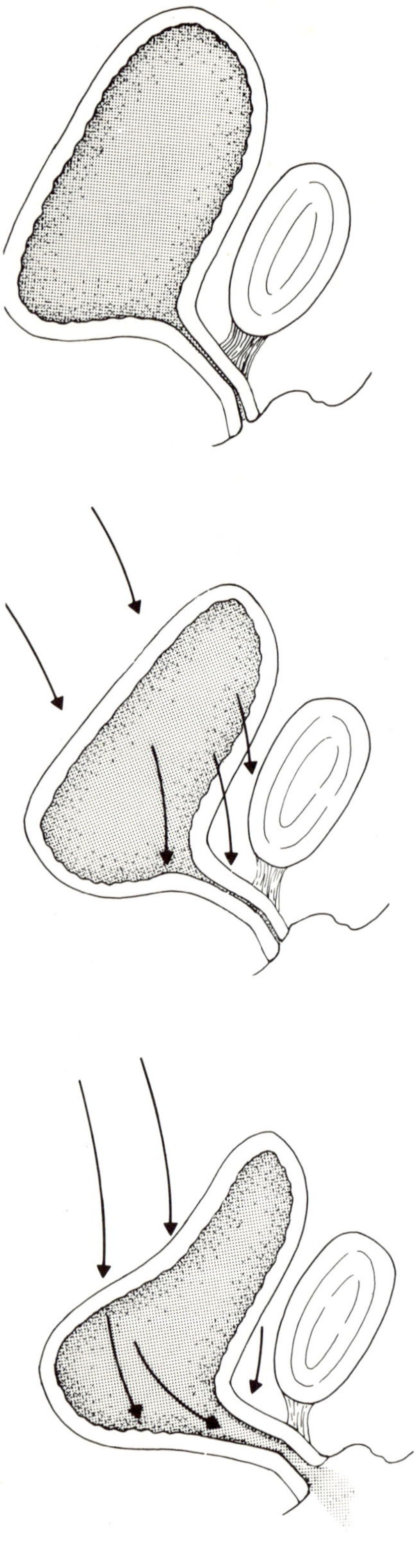

Fig. 5.4. Direction of action of increased intra-abdominal pressure in stress incontinence. This produces funnelling of the urethra with leakage.

Urethral pressure profile

Patients with stress incontinence generally have a somewhat lower urethral pressure profile than continent patients of the same age who have had the same number of children. The reason for this is not clearly understood. However, the difference is not so great that there is no overlap. This means that the lower pressure profile does not necessarily by itself cause the incontinence but helps to produce it by combination with damage to the fixation of the vesico-urethral junction. The margin of safety becomes less because the difference between the bladder pressure and the maximum urethral pressure is reduced. Theoretically, all women can become incontinent as a result of stress if the intra-abdominal pressure is raised to a sufficiently high level.

Urethral length

It has been suggested that a short urethra can produce a low urethral pressure so attempts have been made to treat this by lengthening the urethra. This hypothesis does not fit in with the present knowledge of anatomy and physiology. Moreover, after successful surgery directed at the suspension of the anterior vaginal wall, there is normally no alteration of either the total or the functional length of the urethra.

Urethral scarring and periurethral fibrosis

This results from traumatic deliveries, irradiation therapy, recurrent urethritis, vaginal operations for prolapse – not to mention unsuccessful operations for stress incontinence and internal urethrotomy. In all these conditions, the urethra may be transformed into a rigid tube which is a poor transmitter of rapid variations of intra-abdominal pressure (the so-called 'frozen urethra'). The resting urethral profile may show reduced pressure compared with the normal urethra. The closing pressure becomes inadequate.

Mild degrees of scarring might, perhaps, be the reason for the lower pressure profile in many cases of stress incontinence.

Active elements

The pelvic floor muscles normally provide extra security during a rise of intra-abdominal pressure. Any weakening of these muscles reduces the margin of safety.

As described in Chapter 2, the innervation of the pubo-coccygeus muscle comes directly from S2, 3 and 4 and not via the pudendal nerve. The fibres probably pass on to supply part of the urethra. They are liable to damage during delivery and during major pelvic surgery with resulting degeneration and atrophy of this part of the levator ani muscle.

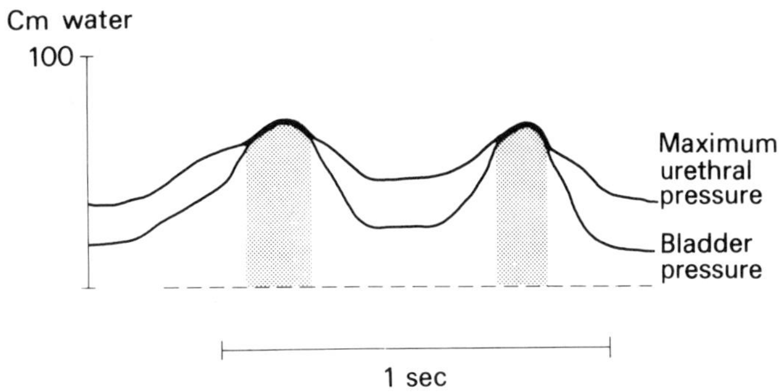

Fig. 5.5. Simultaneous urethrocystometry in a patient with stress incontinence while coughing. The shaded area shows leakage of urine because bladder pressure exceeds maximum urethral pressure.

The relative importance of the active and passive factors is impossible to estimate in the individual patient but in combination they produce a situation where the bladder pressure exceeds the maximum urethral pressure during any sudden rise of intra-abdominal pressure (Fig. 5.5).

PROPHYLAXIS

The obstetrician should do everything to avoid birth complications which can damage the urethra and its suspensory apparatus during delivery. The need for Caesarian section in disproportion is obvious, but other situations exist where there may be too rapid dilatation of the vagina and perineum. Episiotomy can help to a certain extent and it is wise to remember to empty the bladder by catheter before forceps are put on. Generally speaking the patient should always empty her bladder before the head is on the pelvic floor. If she cannot do this herself, a catheter should be used. Huge rises in intra-vesical pressure occur in deliveries in the presence of a distended bladder and this can lead to over-stretching of the bladder and urethral walls with injury to the periurethral tissues. Many women go through a short period of micturition dysfunction, including stress incontinence, immediately after a normal delivery. This indicates that the lower urinary tract has been traumatized to a limited extent. Certain patients may need intermittent catheterization for a few days. Pelvic floor exercises may be useful under these conditions but it is uncertain if they can prevent either stress incontinence or uterine prolapse.

The avoidance of heavy lifting immediately after delivery is self-evident.

INVESTIGATION OF A PATIENT WITH STRESS INCONTINENCE

History

When a patient tells her doctor she has a problem holding her urine during situations such as coughing, jumping, dancing, etc., he must be quite sure that her symptoms correspond with the definition given previously. All these activities lead to sudden increases in intra-abdominal pressure and are included in the term 'stress'. He must go into details so as to exclude other conditions which can imitate stress incontinence. It is often difficult for the patient to describe her symptoms exactly. He must find out when she leaks and how much, and if it occurs during standing, walking, sitting or lying down. The relationship of the leakage to micturition is also important, whether micturition prevents leakage for a time, and also whether urgency is present when she leaks, whether the leakage comes a little while after the cough and whether the bladder is ever involuntarily emptied completely. It is important to note whether she has nocturia or not and whether there is frequency during the day. These factors can indicate that organic lower urinary tract disease is producing urgency or urge incontinence. All details of her micturition pattern should be asked about: does she have to strain, is the urinary stream poor and is it difficult for her to empty the bladder?

It has often been suggested that the differential diagnosis from urge incontinence can be difficult and that lack of proper preoperative evaluation is a more frequent cause of surgical failure than shortcomings of surgical technique. Misdiagnosis can be avoided if a detailed history is taken and then all the simple investigations described here are systematically undertaken.

The number of children and the circumstances of their births should be noted as well as any previous operations or any question of neurological disease. It is useful to remember that when a patient uses anti-hypertensive drugs, the intra-urethral pressure may be lowered to such an extent that the patient complains of stress incontinence. Other drugs, such as ergotamine, can have the same effect.

It is not unusual to encounter patients who have been operated on several times for what has erroneously been thought to be stress incontinence. An example of this was a woman with a large urethral diverticulum who had undergone six operations, some vaginal and some suprapubic, without any improvement. The diverticulum was still there and became filled with urine every time she passed urine. A little urine was then squeezed out of it every time she coughed or strained. The opening could easily be seen with the cysto-urethroscope and the pouch was demonstrated by video-filming. It was removed, but the urethra had now after all these operations been converted into a rigid tube with a very low pressure profile and poor pressure transmission. Little could be done to improve the situation for she had now developed real stress incontinence because of the rigid urethra.

Clinical examination

The patient should be asked to empty her bladder and to take a mid-stream specimen at the same time. She is then put on the examination couch in the lithotomy position and a gynaecological examination carried out in order to exclude pathological conditions in the vagina, uterus and ovaries. Next, the urethra is inspected and palpated through the anterior vaginal wall. If the gynaecologist has learnt to estimate the normal degree of fixation of the urethra and the vesico-urethral junction and the amount of movement caused by coughing and straining in a young healthy woman, he will get some idea of how much he needs to correct any displacement. It is logical to believe that optimum results are obtained by restoration of a normal degree of fixation and not by over-correction.

The next step is to insert a small female catheter (12 F) and measure the amount of residual urine. Two hundred ml sterile saline is then put in, the catheter is removed and the mobility of the vesico-urethral junction is again assessed. The stress test is then performed.

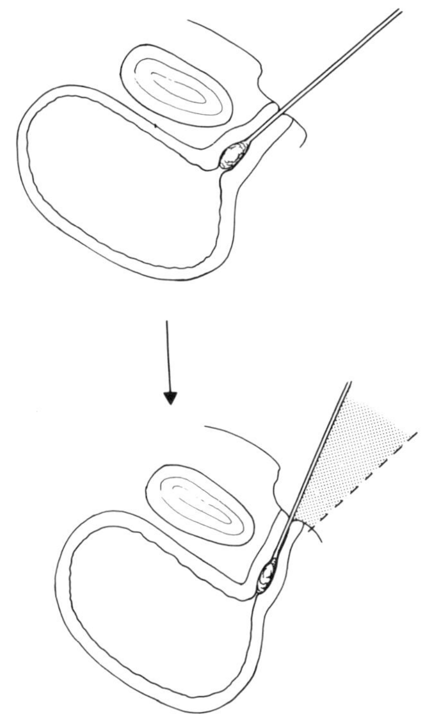

Fig. 5.6. Q-tip test, at rest and while straining.

Stress test

The patient is asked to cough gently. If there is any leakage with 200 ml in the bladder there must be an extreme degree of stress incontinence. If there is no leakage she is asked to cough more forcibly or the amount of fluid in the bladder can be increased. Any leakage associated directly with coughing may not start until there is a much larger amount in the bladder. One must take into account that the test is being carried out in an unusual position for the patient; she has usually been standing when she has noticed leakage of urine. If there is any doubt about leakage, the bladder can be filled with, say, 400 ml saline coloured with a little methylene blue and the patient asked to stand up, cough and walk around while wearing an ordinary sanitary pad. This can give a good indication of the leakage under various conditions of stress and with different amounts in the bladder. The pad can also be weighed before and after exertion. The so-called 'Q-Tip' Test, shown in Fig. 5.6, gives no special indication that surgery would be helpful.

By measuring the pressure profile in the urethra while performing this test it has been conclusively demonstrated that it has no value. When the fingers lift the vesico-urethral junction, it is impossible to avoid compression of the urethral lumen and elongation of the urethra (Fig. 5.7). It is also difficult to apply the fingers to the right place and, even if an instrument is used instead, the effect is the same. The test is therefore liable to be misleading.

Fig. 5.7. Bladder neck elevation test. The action of the fingers is either to compress the urethra and raise the intra-urethral pressure or to elongate it and reduce the pressure.

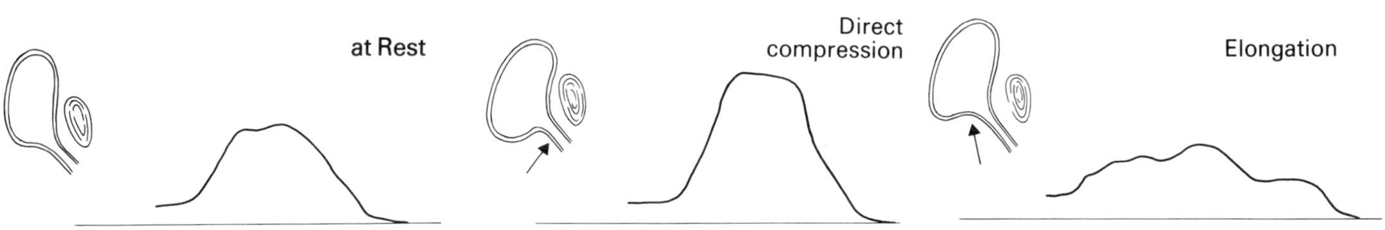

Simple cystometry

The information that simple cystometry gives is limited because it tells us nothing about the activity in the urethra. However, if its limitations are taken into account, the rough relationship between pressure, sensation and volume can be used to recognize a normal curve. This is usual in stress incontinence and excludes such abnormalities as a very large or very small capacity and extreme variations in sensation and control that can indicate neurological disease. Only very simple inexpensive equipment is necessary for this and it can with advantage be done at the same time as the cystoscopy.

Urethro-cystoscopy

This should be done to exclude intrinsic pathology in the bladder and urethra. Palpation of the urethra against the shaft of the cystoscope should not be forgotten in order to eliminate the possibility of a diverticulum.

All the above investigations can and should be performed by any gynaecologist dealing with patients with stress incontinence. They will certainly lead to a correct diagnosis in most cases. If the following more advanced methods are available, they can of course be used, but in the majority of cases they are not necessary. If, however, there is still uncertainty or if it is a case of recurrent stress incontinence after operation, there is every reason to refer the patient to a special urodynamic department.

X-ray investigations

Urography is not usually necessary; most urologists will use it to exclude renal and ureteric abnormalities, but in the absence of indications in the history or clinical examination which point to renal or ureteric problems, it can be regarded as an extra investigation which may be justified in special circumstances.

Micturating cysto-urethrography in its original form with still pictures taken at rest, when straining and during micturition, gives little extra information that is not available from simple clinical examination. The main reason for doing it is to obtain a visual record of the mobility of the vesico-urethral junction before and after operation. This can be very instructive to the surgeon who has operated on the patient and it only requires simple equipment; he must himself decide whether it is worth doing in every case. Occasionally gross pathology such as diverticulum or vesico-vaginal fistula can be revealed.

Video films can be a very useful help both before and after operation in difficult cases but it is obvious that they can only be available in larger radiological departments.

INDICATIONS FOR OPERATION

It is impossible to give definite advice on when and if a patient should be treated by surgery because of the large number of variables. Patients vary greatly in how clever they are to avoid situations which produce leakage; some find out that if they empty the bladder before any activity which involves physical stress they can keep themselves dry enough. There is no doubt that a large number of women do this and never consult their doctors about it. Other women with the same degree of leakage cannot be bothered or cannot remember to do this and go in search of a surgeon who will operate on them. The patient's social background plays a large part in deciding whether or not she goes to a doctor and, for example, a desire to take part in sport, which almost always produces situations where abdominal pressure is raised, will also make her think about treatment. Many similar external factors can influence what the patient desires as regards improvement of symptoms.

On the part of the surgeon there are other criteria which play their part; he must always remember that surgical treatment carries a risk, not only the risk which is inherent in all operations but also a risk that the resultant improvement will be inadequate. In addition, he cannot get away from the fact that treatment consists in performing a cosmetic operation, so he must persuade himself that an operation is really necessary. Surgeons in different situations will obviously vary in the ease with which they can persuade themselves, or perhaps it will be the patient who will persuade them. Experience in general has shown that surgeons have difficulty in getting good results in fat women: it can be done, but it is technically difficult to remove all the fat which seems to prevent good fixation of the vesico-urethral junction. The operation must be done at the bottom of a deep hole without the advantage of the wider opening which is available, for example, when doing a hysterectomy in an obese patient. A warning finger can also be raised where young women who have not had children are concerned; it is all too easy to jump to the conclusion that stress incontinence is the cause of the leakage of which they complain when, in reality, there is another cause – urge incontinence or a diverticulum, for example.

Most gynaecologists in the end reach a compromise between how much they think a patient needs operation, how much the patient herself thinks she needs operation and how much he thinks he can improve her symptoms.

CHOICE OF OPERATION

Over 100 different procedures have been advocated for the treatment of stress incontinence. They include approaches from the suprapubic region or the vagina or a combination of these two, the use of various kinds of sling – either fascial, absorbable or unabsorbable, the use of the round ligament, anteversion of the uterus, vaginal hysterectomy and vaginal repair operations. This multiplicity alone suggests that there must be something wrong with the basic principles underlying most of these operations. Perhaps the most significant advance in the treatment of stress incontinence has been agreement on what we are trying to do, namely *to re-establish normal fixation of the vesico-urethral junction and urethra*, thus lessening mobility and funnelling and at the same time ensuring effective transmission of abdominal pressure. The moral is: restoration of function comes with restoration of anatomy.

The retropubic approach gives a better view of the situation and allows a more accurate operation than when operating from the vagina, where one tries to push the urethra into position without being able to see how much the position has been altered and without being able to be certain that the normal periurethral tissue containing blood and nerve supply is preserved intact. The retropubic approach also allows correction of mild and moderate degrees of displacement cystocele. Vaginal operations for stress incontinence generally speaking, are, not recommended. A possible exception to this is the very obese patient in whom any retropubic operation is difficult.

The retropubic operation

COLPO-SUSPENSION OR VAGINOPEXY

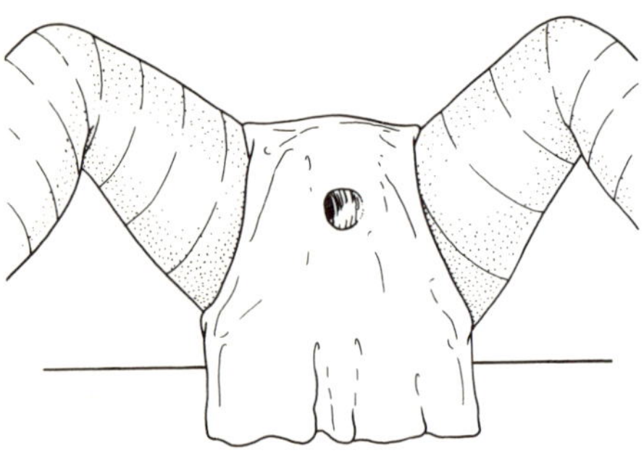

The patient is placed in the lithotomy position, preferably that version of the position which is used by urologists where the thighs are moderately abducted and flexed. This allows the surgeon and his assistant good access to the suprapubic region and at the same time permits the necessary access to the vagina. The vagina should be prepared for operation and it is a good plan to make use of the sterile finger stall combined with drape that is used by urologists in transurethral resection of the prostate (Fig. 5.8). After the usual preparation of the urethra, a large balloon catheter, size 24 F, is passed into the bladder. All urine is drained out and the balloon inflated; this allows easy identification of the vesico-urethral junction and the urethra. The catheter is immediately connected to a closed drainage system.

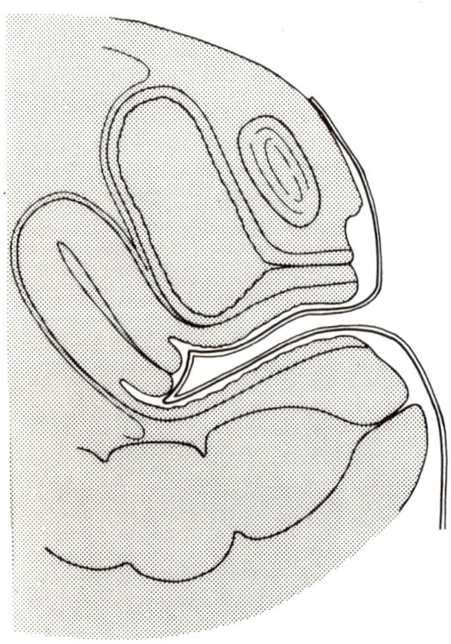

Fig. 5.8. Sterile finger stall combined with drape.

Incision

A transverse incision a little concave upwards is adequate, but some prefer a mid-line incision; there is little difference as far as access is concerned.

If the transverse incision is used, it should cross the mid-line just above the symphysis and then the upper skin edge and the anterior rectus sheath should be undercut upwards so as to expose the rectus muscles for at least 10 cm. They are then separated by retractors. Behind them lies the thin transversalis fascia, fastened to the symphysis at the lower end of the wound and covering the peritoneum at the upper end. This fascia should be divided with scissors immediately adjacent to the pubis and the incision extended laterally on each side behind the rectus muscles. The two index fingers are then inserted to open up the retropubic space on each side. This space is easily opened and the fingers pass deeper behind the pubis to reach the bladder base and vagina, and can palpate the catheter lying in the mid-line. Now, blunt dissection is carried laterally to open the paravaginal and paravesical spaces on each side until the obturator canal with its nerve and blood vessels, the arcus tendineus and the levater ani muscles are visible. The dissection avoids the region near the mid-line but goes down behind each pubic bone until the anterior vaginal wall is exposed on each side. It is important to have enough room so that stitches can be accurately placed and sutures tied.

The next step is to remove all the fatty tissue on both sides and divide defective pubo-vaginal fixation, avoiding the mid-line region (Figs 5.9 and 5.10). The object of this is to arrange for fixation of the vaginal wall to the back of the pubis and pelvic wall by solid growth of fibrous tissue. Any fatty tissue remaining will impede this fixation and permit the same movement of the vesico-urethral junction which gave rise to the stress incontinence. The fatty tissue sometimes contains thin-walled veins which are best divided between ligatures without traction. If the cut ends are pulled up to the slightest degree the veins tend to rupture under the symphysis or in the obturator fossa and the resultant bleeding is difficult to stop. Diathermy coagulation is often unreliable because of the fatty tissue adherent to the veins. Continuous swab pressure can be effective or the site of bleeding can be under-run with a stitch on a small curved needle. After previous retropubic operations the bladder and upper urethra is often stuck to the pubis and the dissection can be difficult. This is not where the fixation should be, so this part of the bladder wall must be freed as a first step when opening the retropubic space. The secret of avoiding injury to the bladder is to do the dissection as near the bone as possible either with a knife or scissors and not to pull on the bladder wall. If the surgeon is tempted to pull he will find that the adhesions to the pubis are stronger than the muscle of the bladder wall and the

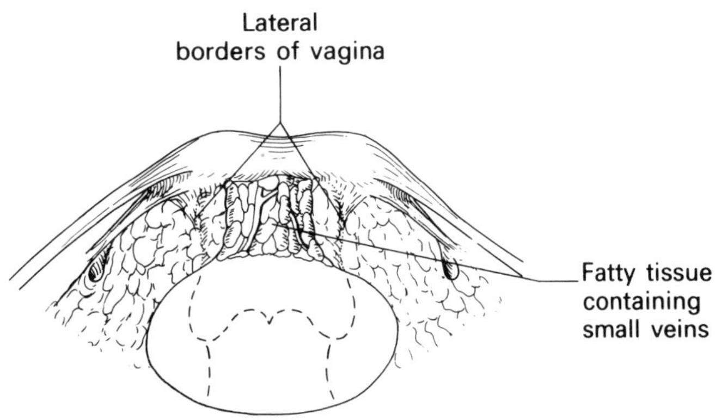

Fig. 5.9. Retropubic space.

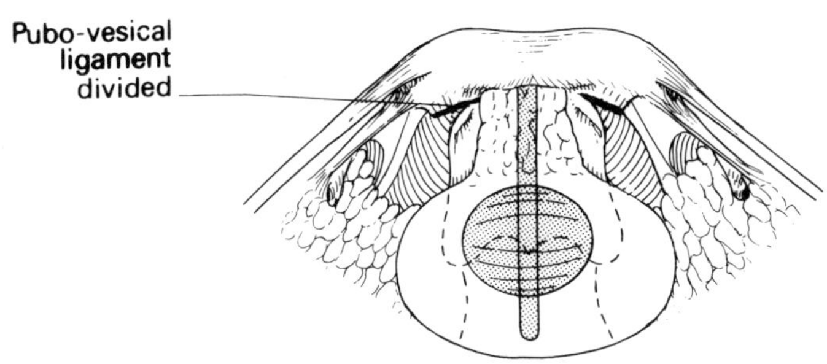

Fig. 5.10. Steps in the clearance of the anterior vaginal wall and the paravaginal space on each side.

inevitable result will be a hole. Where there is a hole in the bladder, there is always a danger of fistula formation, so it pays to be extra careful here. It is usually easy to see when the bladder wall has been damaged. Some surgeons put methylene blue or sterile milk in the bladder to make injury obvious. When one comes nearer the urethra in these patients who have been operated on before, the balloon catheter in the bladder and urethra is of great help.

If it is found that previous operation has fixed the urethra to the symphysis by sutures which pass through or lie very close to the urethral wall, these should be removed so that the urethra and anterior vaginal wall are freed down to the pelvic floor. This sometimes requires sharp dissection close to the symphysis in order to mobilize the 'frozen urethra'. It is not the urethra which must be fixed, it is the vaginal wall on each side.

Suture material

Long-lasting absorbable sutures size 1 or 0 should always be used. There is a danger that unabsorbable sutures placed in or even adjacent to the bladder wall or urethra will migrate into these organs and give trouble by causing recurrent infection, inflammation or stone formation. Another reason for using absorbable material is that fibrous tissue formation is to be encouraged and this is exactly what absorbable sutures do. After the formation of fibrous tissue the sutures play no further part in the fixation of the vesico-urethral junction.

Putting in the sutures

The periosteum on the pubic bone is liable to tear and give way if it must support the vaginal wall. The stitch to the pelvic wall should therefore pick up the fascia covering the obturator internus muscle or even include some fibres of the muscle itself in order to get a good grip. Two or three sutures should be used on each side and should be put in as shown in Fig. 5.11. The uppermost suture should lie at the vesico-urethral junction, so it is best to begin – as always in pelvic surgery – with the deepest and most difficult stitch. The vaginal wall should be pushed upwards by the assistant's or the surgeon's finger so that it can be picked up by a stitch about 2 cm lateral to the urethra (Fig. 5.12); the bites in the tough vaginal wall must be adequate to obtain a good grip. In his anxiety to achieve this the surgeon may go right through into the vaginal lumen but this seems to do little harm. Atraumatic cutting needles often have too big a curve and bend or break very easily. Halfcircle, 1.5 to 2.0 cm round-bodied needles or J-shaped needles of the type used in femoral hernia operations are to be preferred. In most cases two to three sutures on each side of the urethra are enough, but sometimes more support is necessary, especially when there is a minor degree of prolapse. Here one can make use of the pectineal (Cooper's) ligament or the attachment of the obturator internus, which provides a solid anchorage for the uppermost stitch which must take up the lateral fornix of the vagina just above the level of the vesico-urethral junction as far laterally as possible. A warning is apt at this point. It is not difficult to over-correct and fix the vaginal wall so that the urethra is compressed. This is where the region directly anterior to the

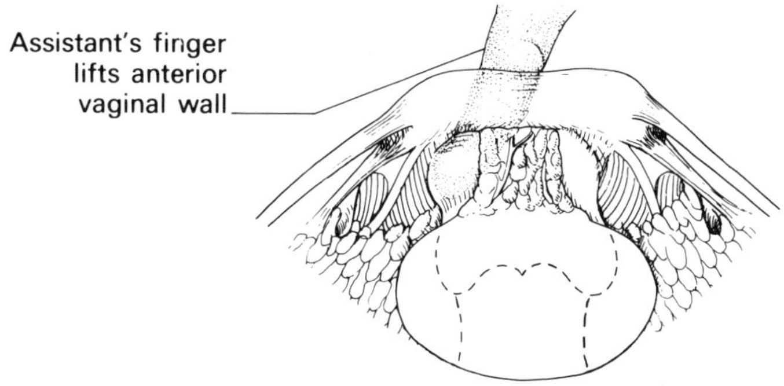

Fig. 5.11. Anterior vaginal wall lifted forwards.

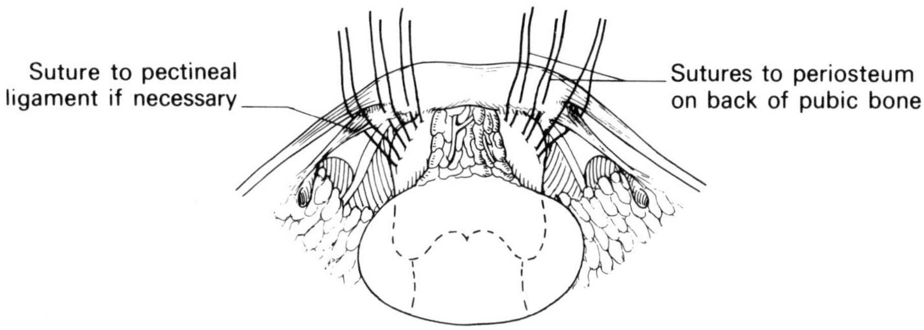

Fig. 5.12. Site of sutures which fix anterior vaginal wall.

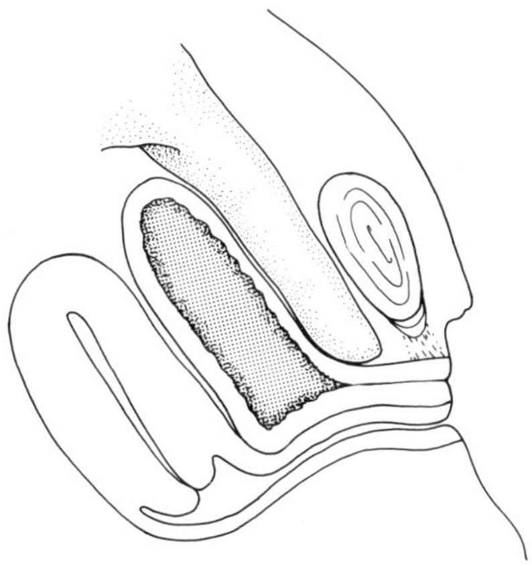

Fig. 5.13. Finger tip passed down between urethra and symphysis pubis.

urethra which has been avoided until now comes into use. It should be possible at the end of the operation to put a finger down between the symphysis and the upper urethra (Fig. 5.13). The penalty for urethral compression is post-operative micturition difficulty and residual urine.

When the sutures are tied the assistant should put a finger in the vagina to lift the anterior fornix forwards. The knots can then be tied without tension. One must bear in mind that there is great individual variation in anatomy and that the flexibility of the vaginal wall can vary from patient to patient. Flexibility is, of course, greatly reduced by previous vaginal operations.

It is an advantage to drain the bladder by a suprapubic catheter to avoid the inflammation and infection which always occurs when a urethral catheter is used.

Another advantage of this which appears later is that the patient can make her first attempts at micturition while the suprapubic catheter is still in position. A small balloon catheter (for example 14 F) or a special suprapubic drainage catheter is used. The wound is then closed leaving a small retropubic drain in the mid-line for 48 hours. This can be a suction drain if preferred. The urethral catheter is then removed. A light pack in the vagina lessens the chance of haematoma formation and assists fixation (Fig. 5.14). The suprapubic catheter is connected to a closed drainage system.

If a urethral catheter is used post-operatively, a small (about 14 F–18 F) balloon catheter should be substituted for the large one. This ensures that the bladder is empty all the time and this assists fixation by minimizing tension in the region of the operative field. The patient should be up and about from the first post-operative day and should be encouraged to drink large quantities of fluid. This helps to keep the catheter draining and to prevent infection. Her first attempts at micturition can be made by simply placing a clip on the catheter and

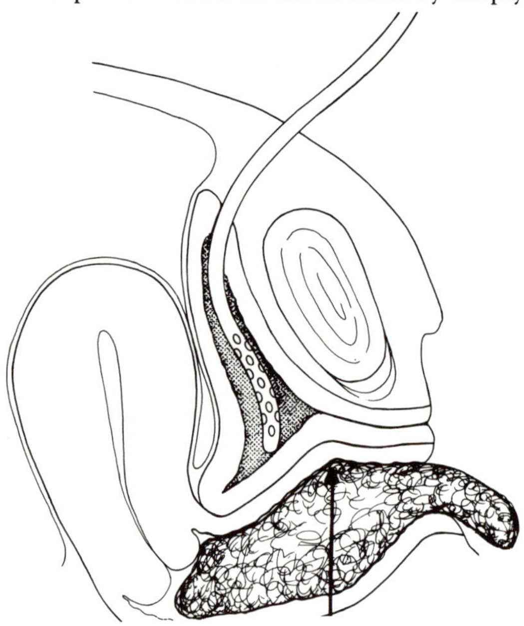

Fig. 5.14. Light pack in vagina provides pressure at site shown by arrow.

waiting until she feels the desire to empty the bladder. If she has difficulty to begin with, it is better to keep the catheter in place a little longer until convincing micturition is possible. It is essential after the catheter is removed to avoid anything in the nature of bladder distension because this will interfere with the fixing of the vaginal wall that is the key to success. The patient also should be advised to void as soon as she feels any urge for the first weeks.

Post-operative residual urine is seldom more than a temporary problem after this operation but it cannot be avoided in every case. Every patient should be followed up carefully in the days and weeks after removal of the catheter by measuring the residual urine and examining mid-stream specimens. If the patient has a slow stream and residual urine, outflow obstruction is probably the cause. Ideally, all patients should have normal urine during the whole of the post-operative period, but nobody attains this ideal in all cases. Infection must first be treated and the site and degree of obstruction should then be investigated by urethral instrumentation. A 20 F (6 mm dia.) instrument should pass easily into the bladder. A cysto-urethroscope can well be used for this purpose. This rules out any serious mechanical obstruction. If the 20 F instrument will not pass, the outflow obstruction must be considered to be serious and then the only rational treatment is to re-open the wound and relieve this by dissection. This may certainly interfere with the intended result and might well have been avoided if the surgeon had assured himself that the urethra had been left intact in the mid-line and that there was room for a finger to pass down behind the symphysis. The use of urethrotomy to reduce urethral resistance and to produce a better urinary stream has been advocated but is liable to produce additional scar formation and lower intra-urethral pressure.

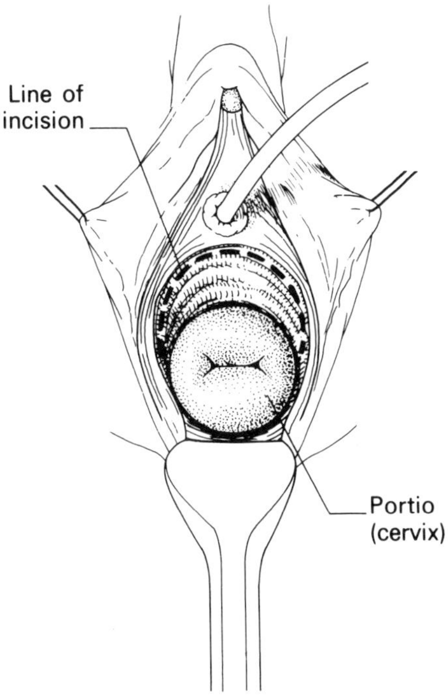

Fig. 5.15. Incision for vaginal operation for stress incontinence.

The vaginal operation

If a vaginal approach is decided upon, the following type of operation is suggested. The patient is placed in the lithotomy position and the vagina cleansed. Antiseptic gel is placed in the urethra and a size 24 F balloon catheter passed into the bladder which is emptied. A transverse incision is made through the vaginal mucosa just behind the external urinary meatus and continued 3 cm on each side of the mid-line (Fig. 5.15). The anterior vaginal wall is dissected free from the urethra and bladder base, keeping carefully in the right layer, and exposing about 2 cm above the vesico-urethral junction and as far laterally as the limits of the vagina (Fig. 5.16). Next, the upper 2 cm of the urethra and the vesico-urethral junction are mobilized on the lateral sides. The pelvic fascia on either side of the urethra is incised so that the pubo-coccygeus muscles come into view. Both muscles are then dissected free so that they can be divided (Fig. 5.17).

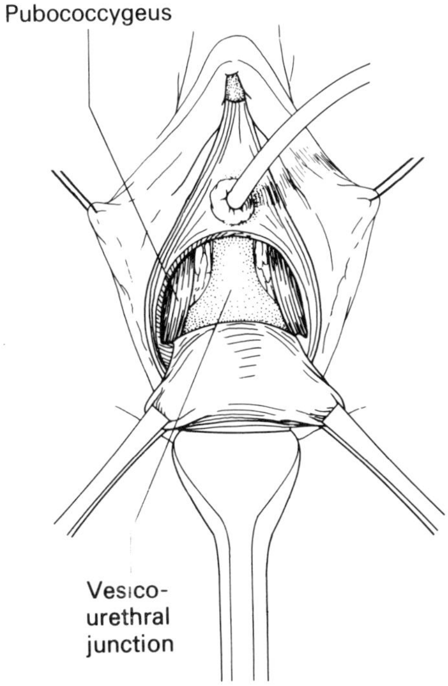

Fig. 5.16. Exposure of the vesico-urethral junction and the pubo-coccygeus muscles.

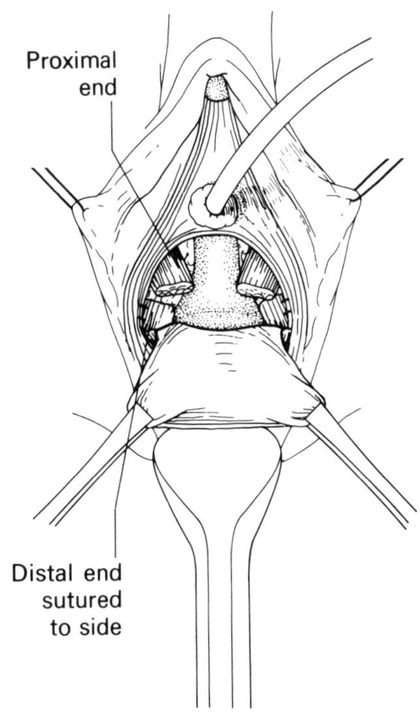

Fig. 5.17. Division of pubo-coccygeus muscle.

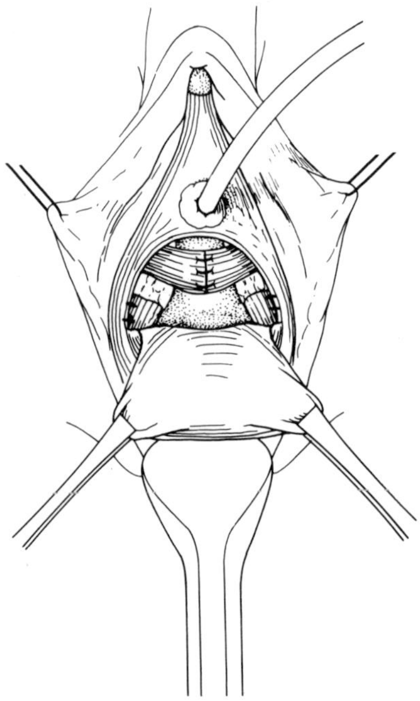

Fig. 5.18. Pubo-coccygeus muscles sewn together under urethra.

This allows the anterior ends to be brought together and sutured so that they hold the vesico-urethral junction in a better position behind the symphysis (Fig. 5.18). The anterior vaginal wall is then loosely sutured back in position. A light pack soaked in chlorhexidine is placed in the vagina and is kept there for a day. A 14 F catheter is connected to a closed drainage system for 5–7 days.

The main indication for this operation is obesity, so urethral catheter drainage is used and the patient is up and about from the first day. The long term effect is that the muscles become converted to a fibrous plate which supports the vesico-urethral junction. It gives good long-lasting results compared with the simpler plication of the anterior vaginal wall.

TREATMENT OF RECURRENT STRESS INCONTINENCE

The object of any operation for stress incontinence is obviously to relieve the condition once and for all by producing a result which satisfies the patient without producing complications; it should be possible to achieve this in most cases. Relief of the symptoms is not always absolutely complete because it is not always possible to put the vesico-urethral junction back to its original undamaged condition, but it is possible to improve symptoms to such an extent that the patient is relieved of her difficulties. However, even if the diagnosis of stress incontinence has been correct and an apparently well-conceived operation has been performed, not all patients will be sufficiently improved or they may, perhaps, be no better or even worse. All gynaecologists who deal with stress incontinence have experience of patients who have undergone multiple operations without improvement. In this situation, adequate investigation is essential, preferably by reference to a special clinic or department. The surgeon should avoid re-operating in the same way as before without first making sure why the first operation has failed to correct the cause of the symptom.

It may be necessary to use a sling operation if scarring prevents the use of the type of retropubic operation described above. The vaginal wall becomes so inflexible that it will not reach the back of the pubis. A combined suprapubic/vaginal procedure then has a better chance of success. It must be remembered that this may be the last chance of surgical success. It is a technically difficult operation in which the urethra is at great risk.

Operative technique of the retropubic sling operation

The patient is placed in the urological lithotomy position. The incision extends from a point 2 cm above the anterior superior spine on one side in the form of an open V to a similar point on the other side, with the apex of the V at the upper border of the symphysis pubis. The upper and lower wound edges are each undercut about 2 cm to expose the external oblique aponeurosis (Fig. 5.19). Fascial strips are then cut starting from each side where the external oblique muscle becomes fascia. They should each be about 1.0 cm wide, side by side and continuous over the mid-line. This gives an adequate length of fascia on both sides. Next, the upper wound edge is undercut so that it can be lifted upwards, allowing the rectus muscles to be separated. Almost certainly there will be

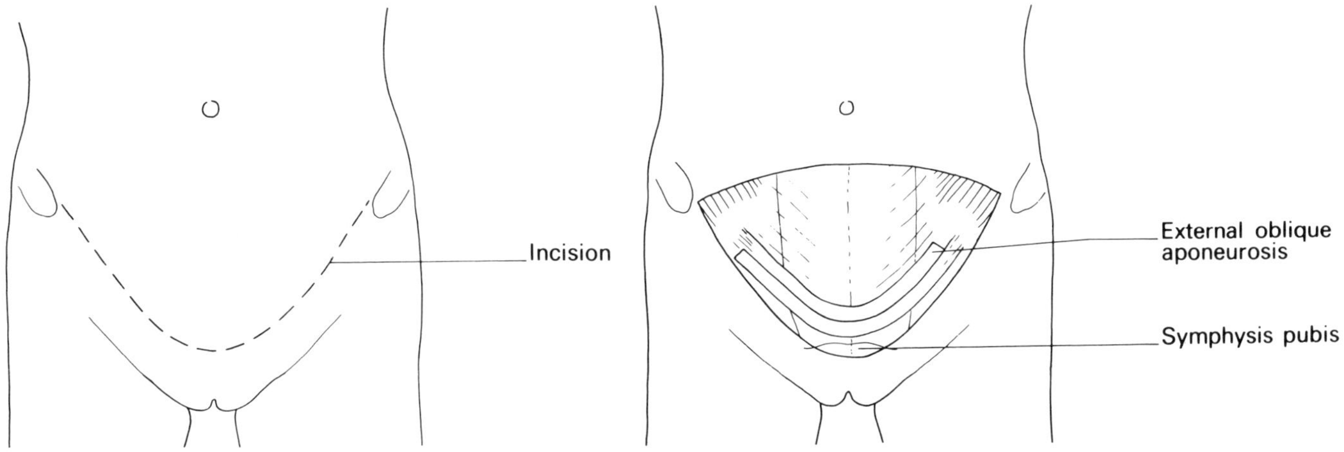

Fig. 5.19. Location of fascial strips.

difficulty from now on as regards exposure of the urethra simply because of previous operations. A 24 F balloon catheter in the urethra is a great help, but it is often an even better help if the surgeon admits early on that he is almost certainly going to open the bladder by accident and therefore opens it intentionally. This may well involve also opening the peritoneum which has become adherent to the scar tissue just above the symphysis. This opening can be closed again as soon as the anterior bladder wall has been freed. Usually there is no transversalis fascia left after previous operations, only scar tissue. If the opening in the bladder wall is enlarged a little, an index finger can be inserted and the anterior bladder wall held between the finger and thumb. With a knife or sharp dissection scissors in the other hand, the scar tissue is divided close to the back of the pubic bones and symphysis so that the bladder and the urethra are exposed down to the pelvic floor (Fig. 5.20).

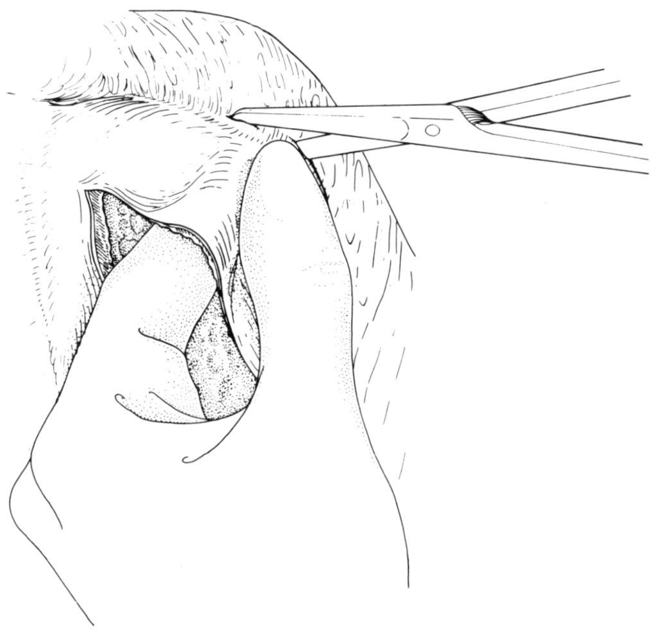

Fig. 5.20. Dissection of the retropubic space with the bladder open.

Now, the perineal operator makes an inverted U-shaped incision in the anterior vaginal wall similar to that used for the vaginal repair operation. He dissects the vaginal wall free from the urethra including about 2 cm of the bladder base, guided by the balloon in the bladder. Both surgeons must concentrate at the same time on freeing the upper urethra and the vesico-urethral junction. This should be done with great care so as not to damage it even more. It is essential here to avoid entering the urethral lumen, so use should be made of the in-dwelling urethral catheter and of the index finger in the bladder which can cause the base to protrude downwards a little so that the perineal surgeon can identify it. Progress may be slow but it is safer that way. The most difficult part is the separation of the urethra from the vaginal wall in the mid-line just below the vesico-urethral junction. To avoid injuring the urethra it may be necessary to take part of the thickness of the vaginal wall because the fascia has become solid scar tissue as a result of previous vaginal operations (Fig. 5.21). This is one of the reasons why a U-shaped incision is used in the vaginal mucosa. It is wise to keep away from the mid-line as incisions in this region always lead to difficulty in identifying the right layers when there is a lot of scar tissue.

The objective is to have enough room to allow two slings to be passed under the upper urethra so that they lie flat against the vesico-urethral junction and side by side. This implies that about 4 cm of bladder base and urethra should be freed by dissection. When this is achieved, the suprapubic operator passes an artery forceps from the retropubic space outwards through the transversalis muscle and fascia at the lateral border of the rectus muscle to grasp the end of the fascial strip from that side and draw it through so that it passes almost directly down to the upper urethra (Fig. 5.22). He does the same on the other side so that both strips can be passed down under the urethra and vesico-urethral junction and up again to the pectineal ligament. The strips must not be twisted and should be arranged by the perineal surgeon so that they lie flat. They can then be fixed in that position side by side by thin sutures which pass through the periurethral tissue super-

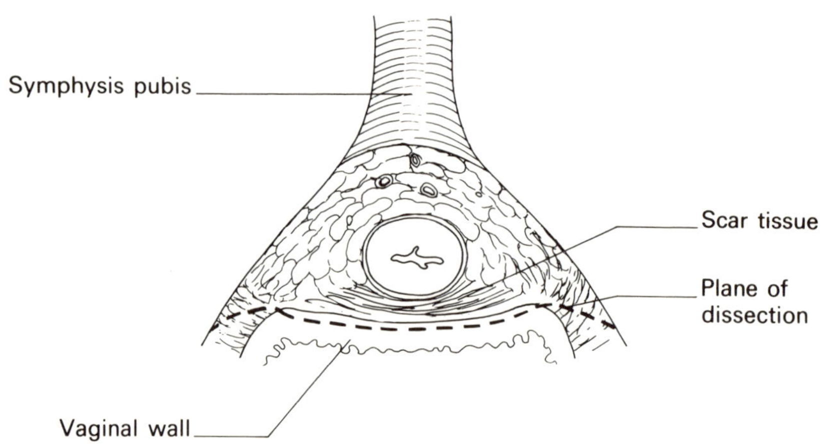

Fig. 5.21. Dissection of vaginal wall from urethra in presence of scar tissue.

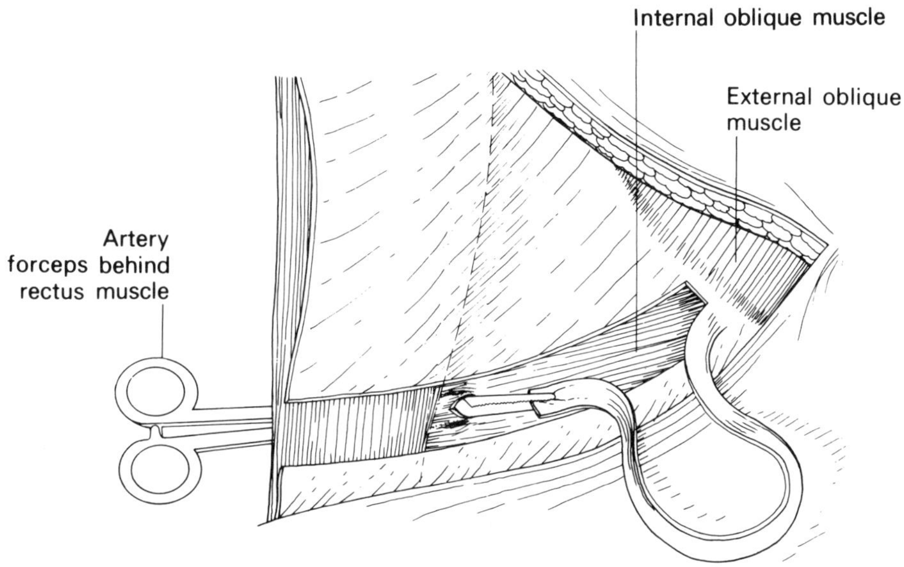

Fig. 5.22. Fascial strip drawn down behind rectus muscle.

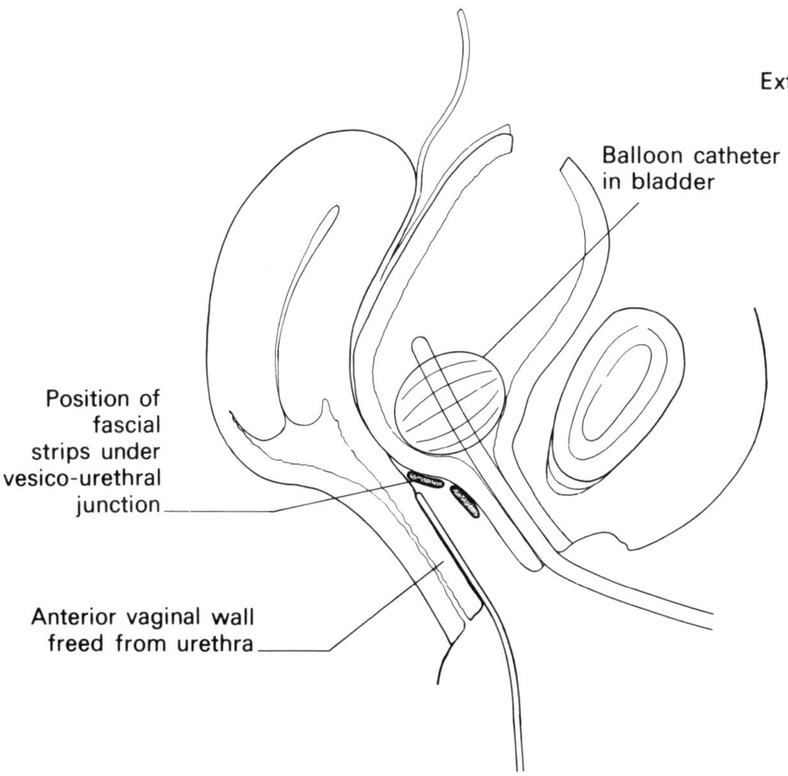

Fig. 5.23. Fascial strips placed side by side beneath urethra.

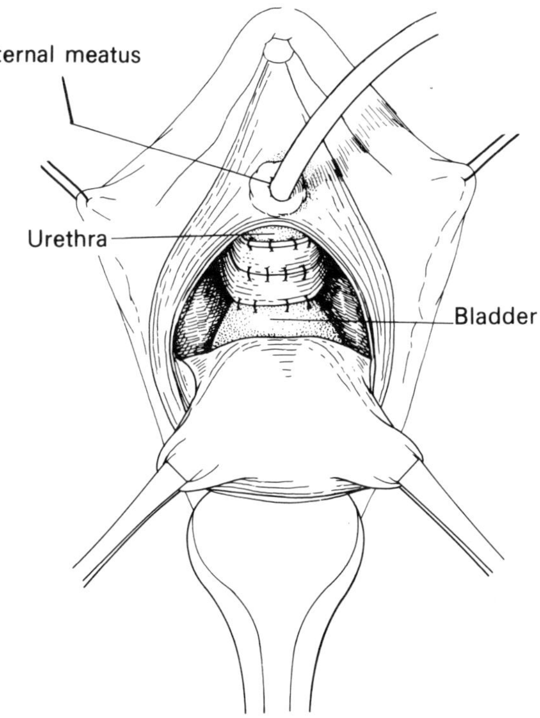

Fig. 5.24. Fascial strips sutured side by side beneath urethra.

ficially (Figs 5.23 and 5.24). The surgeon then pulls on the strips to lift the vesico-urethral junction into position and sutures each end to the pectineal ligament on the opposite side. The exact position is determined by the abdominal surgeon who should be able to put his index finger tip between the upper urethra and the symphysis. This is in order to combine as much lifting as possible with the minimum of direct compression. Surplus fascia is removed.

The anterior vaginal wall is then closed loosely and the urethral catheter removed. A light pack should be placed in the vagina and changed daily for about

5 days to control oozing and to prevent the space between the urethra and the vaginal wall from filling with blood or serum. A suprapubic drainage catheter is fixed in the bladder and the wound is closed with a small drain in the retropubic space for 48 hours.

If some variety of suprapubic sling operation has already been performed so that the external oblique fascia is inadequate, a strip of fascia lata from the thigh can be used as a sling from one pectineal ligament to the other. Fascia is to be preferred to artificial material because the latter can occasionally behave like a foreign body with disastrous results. The round ligament has also been used, but it is not so good a urethral support as a strip of fascia.

Post-operative treatment

This is of extreme importance. The suprapubic catheter is kept in place until acceptable micturition is possible. This should not be attempted for the first two weeks. Since a moderate degree of over-correction can be allowed in recurrent cases so as to be sure of success, a slow stream and residual urine must always be expected to begin with. Residual urine and the concomitant risk of infection may persist in some patients and must be reckoned with because it must be remembered that this is the last chance of achieving something approaching normal micturition. An alternative may otherwise be urinary diversion. Self-catheterization may be helpful here as a temporary solution and occasionally can be continued for a longer period. It may even be preferable to urinary diversion as a definitive form of treatment in some cases. There is less operative risk, there is less risk to the upper urinary tract compared with an ileal bladder and it is socially more acceptable.

STRESS INCONTINENCE ASSOCIATED WITH OTHER CONDITIONS

The diagnosis 'stress incontinence' implies that the patient has no other urinary symptoms. There are patients, however, whose symptoms are not so clear-cut, where one finds indications of overflow incontinence, of neuropathic incontinence or of urge incontinence – or even a mixture of these types. These cases can be very difficult to assess. Here it is essential to use every possible urodynamic aid to work out exactly what is happening in the bladder and urethra. Only then is it possible to know whether or not an operation might improve matters.

DRUG TREATMENT OF STRESS INCONTINENCE

There is little doubt that oestrogen is of some help in the post-menopausal patient with stress incontinence. Its effect is to stimulate the growth of squamous epithelium and increase its blood supply. It also has some effect in increasing tone in pelvic musculature. Urethral pressure studies while at rest, however, show no significant alteration after prolonged oestrogen administration. It is not, in fact, known why it has a beneficial effect, but it is always worth remembering in a mild case and perhaps should always be used post-operatively in post-menopausal patients.

As mentioned in Chapter 2, there is a rich autonomic supply to the urethra; sympathetic nerve endings in particular are numerous. Attempts have therefore been made to treat stress incontinence with drugs the purpose of which is to increase the intraurethral pressure. Sympathetic stimulators have been tried but their theoretical basis seems doubtful in clinical use. The orientation of the smooth muscle fibres in the urethra suggests that their effect can only be on the submucosal vascular plexus. There is, of course, no drug which has a specific action on the urethra itself. These drugs have little therapeutic effect in ordinary doses, the first measureable effect on the intraurethral pressure comes when the dose is so high that the patient has side-effects.

REFERENCES

Asmussen M (1980) Aspects of continence, incontinence and micturition in women based on simultaneous urethro-cystometry. Chapter 10 in *Gynecologic Urology and Urodynamics*, ed. D Ostergard. Williams & Wilkins, Baltimore.

Burch JC (1961) Urethro-vaginal fixation to Cooper's ligament for correction of stress incontinence. *Am. J. Obstet. Gynecol.* **81,** 281.

Enhørning G (1961) Simultaneous recording of intravesical and intraurethral pressures. *Acta Chir. Scand.* Suppl. 276.

Ingelman-Sundberg A (1952) Urinary incontinence in women. *Acta Obstet. Gynecol. Scand.* **31,** 266.

Millin T (1947) *Retropubic Urinary Surgery*. Livingstone, Edinburgh.

Nichols DH (1978) Effects of pelvic relaxation on gynecologic urologic problems. *Clin. Obstet. & Gynecol.* **21,** 759.

Richardson AC, Edmonds PB, Williams NL (1981) Treatment of stress urinary incontinence due to paravaginal fascial defect. *Obstet & Gynecol.* **57,** 357.

Stanton SL, Tanagho EA (1980) *Surgery of Female Incontinence*. Springer Verlag, Berlin.

Chapter 6 Neuropathic Dysfunction

Any malfunction in the various parts of the central nervous system or the peripheral nerves concerned may interfere with micturition. Malfunction may be caused by direct nerve cell damage, inflammatory conditions which damage nerves, neurotoxic drugs and drugs influencing impulse transmission in nerve tissue. It may be anything from slight dysfunction of a small portion of the mechanism which produces minimal symptoms (such as abnormal sensation) to irreversible damage with loss of urinary control.

Most of the patients with severe neuropathic micturition problems never come to the gynaecologist. He sees only a small fraction who have comparatively mild symptoms. Nevertheless, the meaning of neuropathic dysfunction must be based on an understanding of all the links in the chain. The gynaecologist, for example, may have to see a patient in whom urinary symptoms are the first sign of multiple sclerosis or he may have to treat some gynaecological condition in a patient with established neuropathic dysfunction. Most important, he must be able to exclude neuropathic dysfunction before he starts thinking in terms of 'idiopathic' symptoms or stress incontinence.

Malfunction of the process of urinary control may be simplified by thinking of it in two parts:

1 cerebral and upper spinal dysfunction;
2 dysfunction in the lower part of the reflex arc.

CEREBRO-SPINAL DYSFUNCTION

A lesion in the brain or spinal cord above S 2 alters but does not abolish the lower part of the micturition reflex arc. It makes its action more or less independent of conscious and unconscious cerebral control. Depending on the extent of the lesion, the patient loses control of when micturition will occur; the reflex tends to work automatically as a result of filling of the bladder or other forms of stimulation such as cough or movement of the legs. In these cases there is either urgency with incontinence or loss of sensation with periodic involuntary micturition. Examples of this are seen in multiple sclerosis, cerebral haemorrhage and thrombosis, and in various lesions affecting the spinal cord such as fracture-compression, cervical or thoracic disc prolapse, spinal abscess and tumour. If reflex micturition starts, the patient is unable to stop and the bladder empties itself. The whole picture gives an impression of a *hyperactive lower urinary tract.*

DYSFUNCTION OF THE LOWER PART OF THE REFLEX ARC

A lesion which involves the S 2, 3 and 4 segments of the cord or the nerves which originate there interferes with the micturition reflex. Examples of this are seen in some congenital spinal abnormalities, in trauma to the lower spine and in central lumbar disc prolapse. These conditions often also affect the pelvic floor by involving the pudendal nerve (S 3 and 4). The symptoms vary from hypo-activity to complete inactivity according to the extent of the lesion. If it is total then normal micturition does not occur. The bladder fills without normal sensation and is inert so that incontinence results from passive rises in intra-vesical pressure. The patient may only be aware of it through sensation from the abdominal wall and from the perineum.

In gynaecological practice, varying degrees of hypoactivity of the lower urinary tract are seen after radical operations for gynaecological cancer.

If the afferent (sensory) fibres from the lower urinary tract are interrupted or disturbed, the bladder fills until it is grossly distended without any painful sensation. The patient progressively loses the ability to empty the bladder properly with the result that there is residual urine in increasing amounts. Overflow incontinence is the inevitable result. Examples of this are occasionally seen in lumbar disc prolapse and tabes dorsalis, where the posterior columns of the cord are affected, and in the peripheral nerve lesions of long-standing diabetes and pernicious anaemia.

If the efferent (motor) fibres are affected but the afferent (sensory) fibres are intact, the patient will feel the sensation of urge to void but have difficulty in emptying the bladder. This can be improved by straining but there is in most cases still residual urine. If the pudendal nerve is involved as well, there is loss of sensation in the pelvic floor and the perineum with additional symptoms of faecal incontinence and urinary stress incontinence. Examples of this are seen in trauma and lumbar disc prolapse with all degrees of variation of its effect on afferent and efferent impulses.

EXAMINATION OF THE NERVOUS SYSTEM IN A CASE OF POSSIBLE NEUROPATHIC DYSFUNCTION OF THE LOWER URINARY TRACT (Fig. 6.1)

It goes without saying that a detailed history is essential. This alone can lead to a strong presumptive diagnosis in many patients. Details are necessary of how and how often micturition occurs, whether the reflex is normal and under voluntary control, whether there is involuntary leakage and under what circumstances this happens, and whether there is the normal feeling of bladder distension. The next step is to enquire about the anus because the nerve supply of the external (subcutaneous) anal sphincter and the pelvic floor also comes from S 2, 3 and 4. Any bowel dysfunction is important and whether this occurred at the time micturition symptoms began or appeared independently. The autonomic nerve

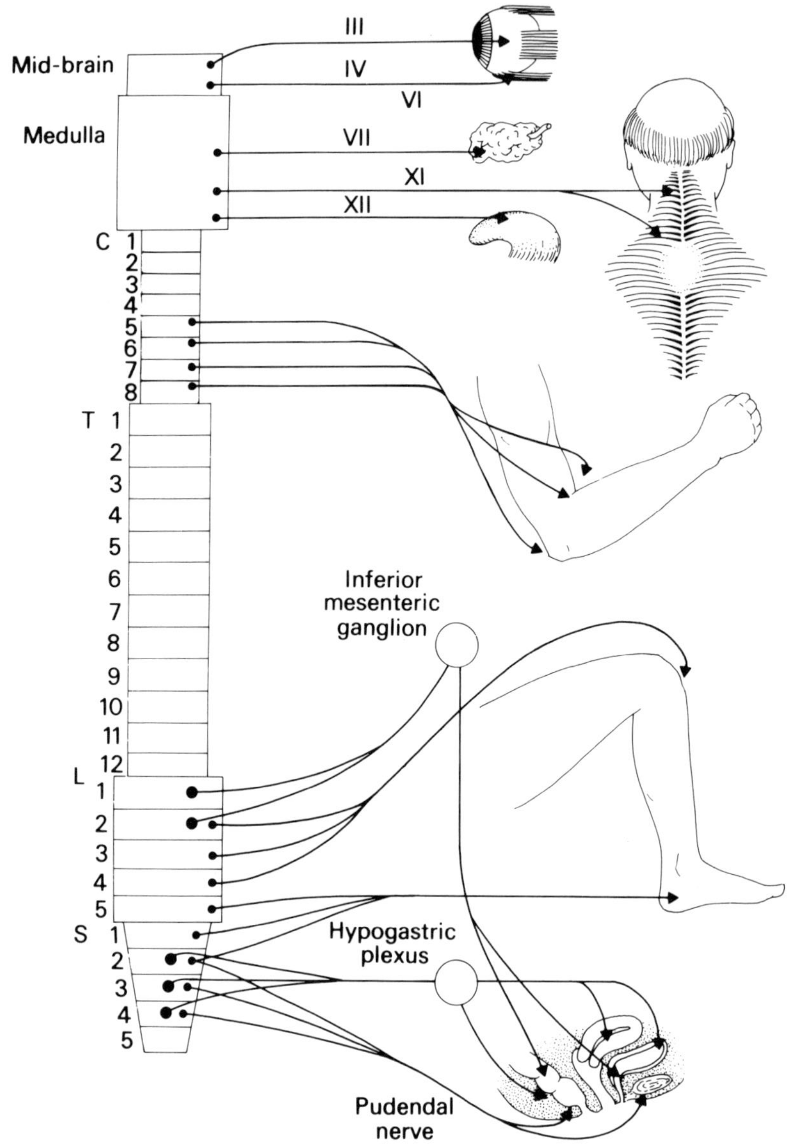

Fig. 6.1. Simplified diagram to illustrate examination of the nervous system.

supply to the rectum comes from the same segments as those which are related to the lower urinary tract. Alteration in sexual function can also be important since erectile tissue and glandular function require the same nerve supply as the bladder, urethra and urogenital diaphragm.

While this part of the history is being taken, the gynaecologist will have gathered information about whether cerebral function is intact and he can pass on to enquiries about the working of the rest of the nervous system. There is no need to go into detail about this; it suffices to inquire if there is any difficulty in eating or in walking. This will reveal both motor and sensory lesions in the arms or legs.

The most important part of the cord that concerns micturition is the S 2, 3 and 4 segments which also supplies motor impulses to the perineal muscles and the superficial anal sphincter. Sensory fibres reach S 2, 3 and 4 from the lower limb around the knee. The peripheral motor nerves which come from S 2, 3 and 4 are responsible for the ankle movements of flexion, extension, inversion and eversion. The anal and bulbo-cavernosus reflexes give special information about the cord at the S 2, 3 and 4 level. Paralysis of the superficial anal sphincter produces a funnel appearance because the outer part of the anal canal is wide open so that it is possible to see the rectal mucosa above the pectineal line if the buttock is drawn to one side. Rectal examination reveals that only the internal sphincter is acting and that the patient cannot voluntarily contract the superficial subcutaneous sphincter – that is squeeze the examining finger. The anal reflex can be activated by scratching the skin adjacent to the anus. The bulbo-cavernosus reflex consists of contraction of the perineal muscles initiated by pressure on the clitoris or by touching the urethral or bladder mucosa, for example by pulling on an indwelling catheter.

These two reflexes have been considered important because they use the same spinal segments as the micturition reflex arc. However it cannot be assumed that the micturition arc is intact if these reflexes are present because the peripheral nerve supply of the bladder and urethra are not involved in the tests. Furthermore, if these two reflexes are abolished, the neurological lesion must be so extensive that it will be obvious.

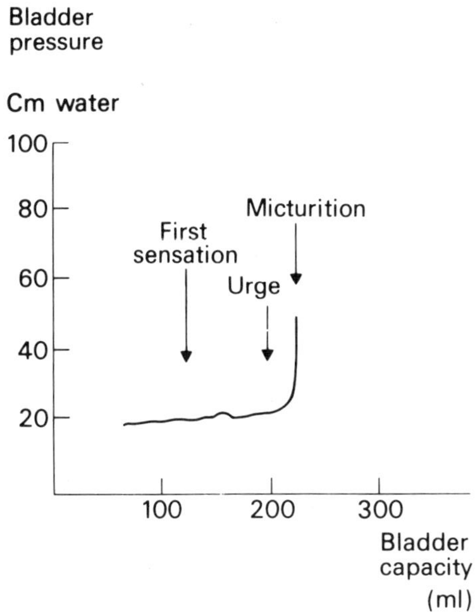

Fig. 6.2. Cystometrogram in patient with cerebral or upper spinal dysfunction.

Cystometry

This is the basic urodynamic examination in all cases of possible neuropathic dysfunction. It demonstrates first sensation, urge and bladder capacity. Furthermore, it can demonstrate a hyperactive micturition reflex. Cystometry cannot give an exact diagnosis by itself, but it can lead the gynaecologist to a definite suspicion of a neurological lesion.

Generally speaking, the bladder capacity is low in patients with cerebral and upper spinal dysfunction (Fig. 6.2). Micturition around the urethral instrument simply starts involuntarily with or without urgency. If the patient has urgency, the difference in volume between first sensation and the point where she feels a strong desire to void is small. She is quite unable to suppress micturition and the bladder is emptied more or less completely.

If the motor and/or the sensory part of the reflex arc is defective, the pattern of overflow incontinence can be seen. The rise in bladder pressure must not be confused with a detrusor contraction. There is no first sensation and some patients only feel discomfort in the abdominal wall and the perineum. The maximum bladder capacity is reached at the point when overflow incontinence occurs. This is usually at a much higher volume than average except, of course, in patients who happen to be examined in the post-operative phase after a radical hysterectomy (see Chapter 10).

In dysfunction of the lower part of the reflex arc, normal voluntary micturition does not occur. No urge is felt but the patient may be able to pass some urine by straining. Otherwise she is incontinent at night and for the most part during the day.

TREATMENT OF NEUROPATHIC DYSFUNCTION

The only condition which is treated by the gynaecologist is dysfunction after radical surgery in the pelvis. This is described in Chapter 10. If there is a definite suspicion or evidence of a lesion of the nervous system, the patient should be referred to a suitable specialist which in practice is usually a urologist and/or a neurologist. In recent years many gynaecologists have developed a special interest in this subject and there is much research in progress to try to find drugs which will diminish hyperactivity in the lower urinary tract.

DETRUSOR-URETHRA DYSSYNERGIA

The word 'dyssynergia' means lack of co-operation between two or more forces, so the term 'detrusor dyssynergia' really has little meaning. The terms 'detrusor/urethra' or 'detrusor/sphincter' dyssynergia are better in that they imply that the normal interplay between the bladder and urethra is disrupted. There has been much discussion about this, mostly based on the findings from simple cystometry and electro-myography, without any final agreement.

It is possible that it is a biological artefact, that is to say something which happens normally but which has been interpreted as a pathological phenomenon. It can be seen as a normal physiological process during controlled provoked micturition when using simultaneous measurements at the stage when the bladder reaches maximum capacity. The patient feels great discomfort and urgency and can just manage to prevent micturition (see Fig. 2.29). The urethral pressure begins to rise and fall ('unstable urethra') while the bladder pressure slowly increases without urine leakage. The condition is limited in duration and the normal woman will soon not be able to inhibit micturition. It can also sometimes be seen when the subject is asked to start micturition before maximum bladder capacity is reached. She begins the initiation of micturition by the normal fall of urethral pressure followed a little later by a slight rise in bladder pressure, but before the closure pressure becomes zero a spasmodic contraction of the urethra occurs. In other words the normal sequence of events has been interrupted, perhaps because of the strangeness of the situation on the examination couch. It can often be seen in another situation under the same experimental conditions when the subject is asked to stop micturition when it is already in progress. A spasmodic contraction of the urethral musculature occurs simultaneously with detrusor contraction, thus interrupting the passage of urine. This can occur under physiological conditions but it is not certain if or when it can become pathological.

In normal women urine never passes out of the urethra as a result of a detrusor contraction by itself. There must be a simultaneous decrease of the urethral pressure before any urine can escape. However, it is possible that some patients with neurological disease produce uncoordinated signals to the bladder and urethra which lead to dyssynergia and which may even perhaps result in leakage of urine.

REFERENCES

Asmussen M (1980) Aspects of continence, incontinence and micturition in women. Chapter 10 in *Gynecologic Urology and Urodynamics,* ed. D Ostergard. Williams & Wilkins, Baltimore.

Krane RJ, Siroky MB (1979) *Clinical Neuro-Urology*. Little Brown, Boston.

Ostergard DR (1979) Review: the effect of drugs on the lower urinary tract. *Obstet. & Gynecol. Surv.* **34,** (No 6), 424.

Chapter 7 Idiopathic Dysfunction

The term 'idiopathic dysfunction' includes all those cases where no definable pathology is found. This includes the so-called 'urethral syndrome'.

The main symptom of idiopathic dysfunction is usually urgency, which does not go so far as urge incontinence. The patient always wants to be in the neighbourhood of a toilet, but this is in fact unnecessary because she can suppress the sensation of urge. She does not wake up at night to pass urine. Cystometry shows that the only difference from normal is that she feels first sensation and urge at a lower bladder volume (Fig. 7.1). She has normal maximum bladder capacity because she can inhibit the onset of micturition before this is reached. She can initiate micturition normally and there is no residual urine. If she cannot suppress the urge to micturate at a low bladder volume and micturition then occurs, this should at once raise suspicion of a neurological lesion.

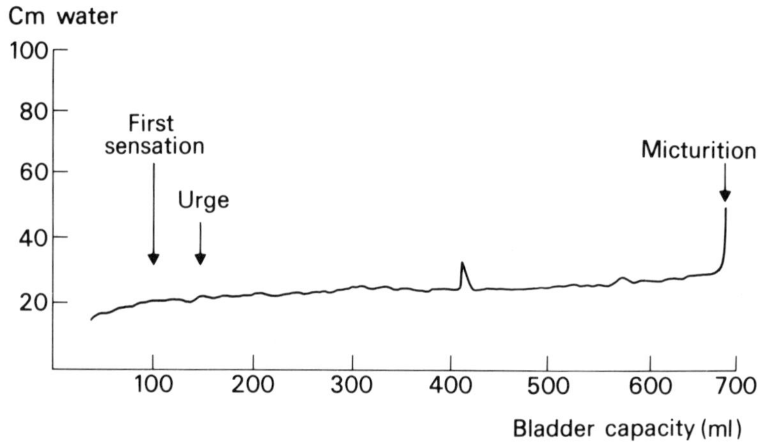

Fig. 7.1. Cystogram of patient with idiopathic dysfunction.

The micturition chart reveals great variations both in time intervals between micturition and in the volume voided. During the day the chart can give the impression that there is a neurological basis, but the patient is never incontinent. At night she does not usually wake up to micturate but if she does, the volume passed is much greater than during the day. She is not a 'slave of her bladder' like a patient with a neuropathic hyperactive bladder.

These patients must be investigated with care because they are often very nervous. Artefacts can easily be produced at cystometry, for example, by using too rapid filling, and even by carrying out cystometry at the first visit before the patient is used to her surroundings.

The symptom complex has been called the 'urethral syndrome' simply because the symptoms are centred on the urethra, but there may be associated perineal or low back pain and muscle cramps. Special attention must therefore be paid to the investigation of the urethra. Non-specific urethritis can explain the condition but it is seldom easy to demonstrate organisms which are pathological. Anaerobic organisms, chlamydia and virus infections are all possibilities.

Certain things seem to be mentioned again and again in the history. Perineal exposure to cold and 'chills' seem to have an aetiological significance in some women, while others connect their symptoms with sexual intercourse. Certain items of diet or a change of diet can have an effect and exaggerated 'personal hygiene' is known to be a cause. Many of these patients have already received courses of sulphonamide from their doctors before being referred to the gynaecologist. Symptoms persist or have recurred and the urine is found to be sterile. Occasionally patients will say that sulphonamide will immediately relieve the symptoms and this leads to self-medication with one or two tablets. Whether there is an occult infection in these women is not known; unfortunately, it only applies to a small minority.

It is of great importance that these patients be put through the whole process of investigation of the genital and lower urinary tracts. The gynaecologist must know for certain that the urinary tract is normal, especially because the symptoms are often so definite that he expects to find something abnormal. The patient must be convinced that everything that can be done is being done because she is often afraid that there may be some serious condition affecting her lower urinary tract. Urethral obstruction in some form has often been supposed to be a cause, chiefly because urethral dilatation can have a beneficial effect, but it is impossible to demonstrate it. The trabeculation of the bladder wall which used to be taken as a sign of obstruction has now been shown to have little to do with it. Furthermore, simultaneous pressure recordings from the bladder and urethra in these patients do not indicate increased urethral closing pressure at rest.

PSYCHOLOGICAL CAUSES

There is very convincing evidence that the mind can have considerable influence on the mechanism of the bladder and urethra. An example of this is the frequency and urgency of micturition which affect candidates before an examination and which immediately disappear as soon as the examination begins. The gynaecologist should be aware of the importance of a psychosomatic background to urinary symptoms and should understand the principles which guide its investigation. He is most likely to be able to help because he has already investigated the physical part of the problem and has the patient's confidence. There is usually no question of psychosis, but rather *hysterical manifestations, depression* or *neurosis*.

A patient should be referred to a psychiatrist only if there is a suspicion of a psychosis, for example a depressed patient who shows suicidal tendencies. The hysterical personality consciously or unconsciously exaggerates normal sensations to the status of symptoms. Urgency comes into this category and also pain. Both of these are absolutely real to the patient, so they should be taken seriously.

The objective is to enable the patient, through discussing her problems with someone she accepts as an expert, for the first time to think of her problems objectively.

Chronic depression in patients with urgency is common because they lose all hope that they can ever come out of a miserable situation. Invalidism is accepted, sometimes to a certain extent because it may have advantages. Urinary symptoms can be an apparently valid excuse for avoiding unpleasant experiences. A somewhat spineless attitude to life is often a characteristic of these patients, who feel that events are too much for them.

There is no doubt that a simple explanation of these mechanisms can be helpful, but, in some cases, the result can be resistance and aggressiveness. If, however, the patient can be made to understand the mechanism by which a dripping tap will induce urgency or how a sudden distraction will abolish an urgent desire to micturate, much can be gained. Even though she may still have a feeling of urgency, she will know that it can disappear and that it is not a sign of serious disease.

The gynaecologist should be aware that the object of this interview is not to solve all the patient's psychological problems, only her urinary ones. Further information may be found in Stone & Judd (1978).

TREATMENT

Most attempts at treatment have been based on the belief that these symptoms have a physical basis which cannot be demonstrated but which nevertheless exists. Urethral dilatation has been used with some success but may have to be repeated. Symptoms can often be relieved by dilatating the urethra up to about 30 F, but the urethral pressure profile does not alter at all. Sulphonamide medication with or without dilatation has been used on the basis that there is some occult infection. Warm Sitz baths have their advocates and the application of silver nitrate or other astringent to the urethral mucosa has been much used. Oestrogen therapy is always to be tried after the menopause or if there is any reason to think that ovarian function is inadequate. Electrical stimulation of pelvic muscles has been tried with equivocal results.

Any drug treatment of idiopathic dysfunction is empirical because the cause of the symptoms is unknown. There is extensive research in progress to find a suitable drug. There is, of course, no drug which acts specifically on the urethra. Diazepam can be useful but may have to be continued for a long time. This is undesirable, so it is better to adopt a more specific anti-depressive drug which can be used continually and so avoid the danger of habituation to diazepam. The dose should be increased until it is effective or until there are side-effects.

Operative treatment of idiopathic urgency

Young women are occasionally seen who have urgency to such a degree that they are barred from all social activity. Drug and psychiatric treatment are of no avail. Attempts have been made to relieve their symptoms by a denervation operation.

It has been suggested that, if there is improvement of symptoms following injection of local anaesthetic into the hypogastric plexus, there might be an indication for hypogastric neurectomy. The test is performed in the same way as a paracervical block; 5–10 ml of 0.5% lignocaine is injected through the lateral fornix about 2 cm from the top and about 2 cm deep (Fig. 7.2). This is done on one side first and its effect on the cystometric curve recorded. If no effect is obtained, local anaesthetic is injected on the other side and the cystometrogram repeated. Two approaches have been used, transabdominal and transvaginal. The latter is to be preferred because the difficulties of dissecting out the hypogastric plexus deep in the pelvis under the uterine artery and ureter are considerable and an adequate result can be obtained by the simpler vaginal approach (Fig. 7.3). One

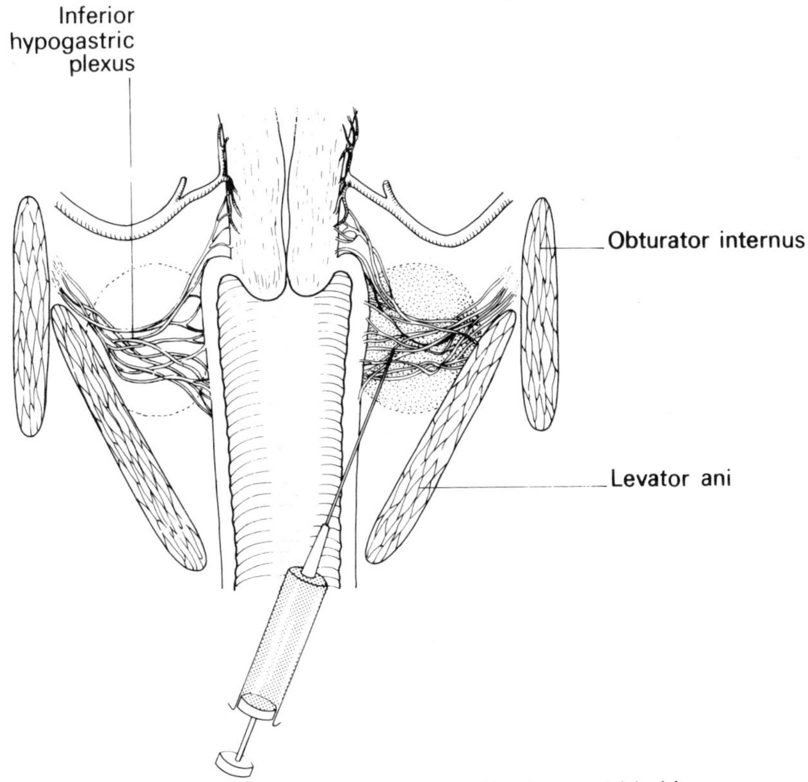

Fig. 7.2. Injection of local anaesthetic into hypogastric plexus.

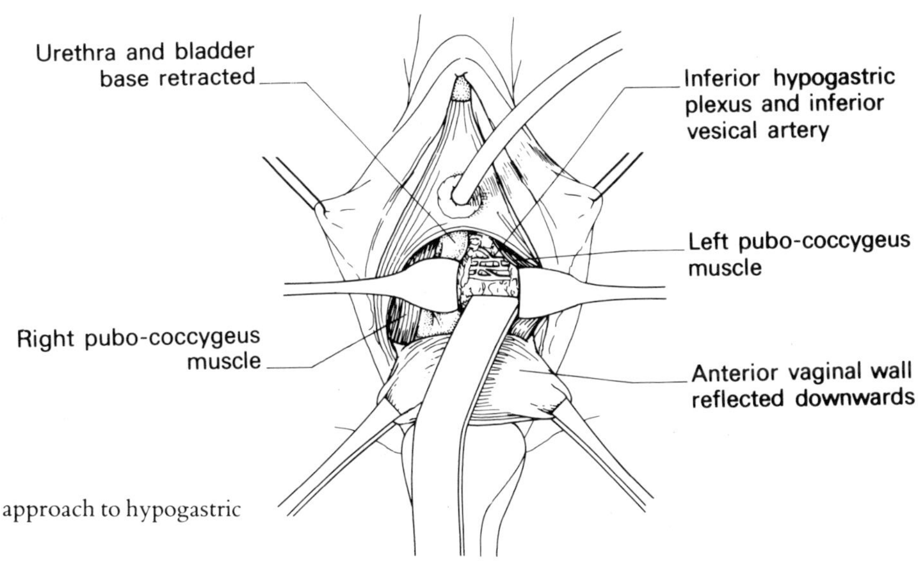

Fig. 7.3. Vaginal approach to hypogastric plexus.

side may be enough. Denervation on both sides can result in bladder paralysis with residual urine and overflow incontinence. In addition, it can interfere with urethral function by direct injury to its blood supply.

The authors have encountered several cases of extreme urgency where, after a series of operations and complications, some form of urinary diversion was the only alternative. These cases included examples of colo-cystoplasty which had been done to increase bladder capacity. This has no place in the treatment of idiopathic symptoms because it does nothing to relieve the urgency.

ACUTE URINARY RETENTION

The most dramatic manifestation of idiopathic dysfunction is acute retention of urine. The patients are almost always young women between 15 and 30 years of age. They often have a previous history of retention and symptoms of urgency and frequency of micturition. Clinical examination shows no gynaecological or neurological abnormality and the urinary tract and urine, when it appears, are normal. It has been considered to be a hysterical manifestation and indeed indications of hysteria can be found in the majority of these patients. Traditional teaching recommends avoidance of catheterization because there is a tendency for acute retention to recur. To the patient, catheterization is an objective, probably not because it is pleasurable in itself but because the resulting relief of discomfort and muscular spasm is satisfying. It is better to use a sedative combined with a cholinergic drug, after which micturition will occur spontaneously.

When the acute episode is over, the urinary tract should be investigated and cystometry or simultaneous bladder and urethral pressure recordings made. Having excluded mechanical and neurological causes, attention should be turned to the psychological side. It will usually be found that these patients are psychologically ill and in need of help.

Other causes of acute retention are acute urethritis, urethral or pelvic tumour and incarceration of an enlarging retroverted uterus. Extreme constipation can compress the urethra enough to make micturition impossible.

REFERENCES

Bull TL (1963) *Gynecologic Surgery and Urology*. CV Mosby, St Louis.

Doyle PT, Briscoe CE (1976) The effects of drugs and anaesthetic agents on the urinary bladder and sphincters. *Brit. J. Urol.* **48,** 329.

Ingleman-Sundberg A (1959) Partial denervation of the bladder. *Acta Obstet. Gynecol. Scand.* **38,** 487.

Krane RJ, Siroky MB (1979) Hysterical urinary retention in the female. In *Clinical Neurourology*. Little Brown, Boston.

Ostergard DR (1979) Review: the effect of drugs on the lower urinary tract. *Obstet. & Gynecol.* Survey 34 (No 6), 424.

Smith PJB (1977) The menopause and the lower urinary tract. *Practitioner,* **218,** 2.

Smith PJB (1977) Age changes in the female urethra. *Brit. J. Urol.* **44,** 667.

Stone CB, Judd GE (1978) Psychogenic aspects of urinary incontinence in women. *Clin. Obstet. Gynecol.* **21,** 807.

Tanagho EA, Lyon RP (1971) Urethral dilatation versus internal urethrotomy. *J. Urol.* **105,** 242.

Chapter 8

Injury to the Lower Urinary Tract during Gynaecological Operations

Palpation of the urinary tract at laparotomy is a normal and important part of the exploration of the whole peritoneal cavity, which is the classical preliminary step in any abdominal operation which is not an emergency. This teaching is still valid in principle, but it is perhaps more important for the general surgeon to explore the pelvis and exclude gynaecological pathology than vice versa. It seems, at first sight, reasonable for gynaecologists to assume, in the absence of symptoms, that they will find no pathology in the upper abdomen and therefore leave it alone and confine themselves to the pelvis.

However, there is no getting away from the fact that the surgeon who carries out a gynaecological operation has opened the peritoneum and is therefore in a position to discover previously unsuspected pathological conditions in the abdominal cavity such as large benign and malignant tumours, gall stones and enlarged lymph nodes.

SYSTEMATIC EXPLORATION OF THE ABDOMINAL CAVITY AND THE UPPER URINARY TRACT

Before any gynaecological operation in which a subumbilical approach to the pelvis is used, a hand should be passed into the upper abdomen to carry out a systematic exploration designed to exclude obvious pathology. The operator must learn to do this gently, because the hand must be introduced to the full extent of the forearm to places where rough handling may do harm.

It is a good plan to begin on the right by pulling the great omentum to the patient's left side to allow exploration of the caecum and appendix. The principles are shown in Fig. 8.1.

The ascending colon is then followed upwards with the hand on its lateral side until the liver is felt. The lower aspect of the liver is then felt with the back of the fingers and the gall bladder palpated with the finger and thumb (2). The fingers then feel for the liver's anterior edge and pass between it and the costal margin so that the diaphragmatic surface can be felt with the fingers and the palm of the hand (3). As the hand passes medially, the fingers must be withdrawn a little to negotiate the ligamentum teres and then passed onto the upper surface of the left liver lobe (4). It is easy to come down again under the liver edge to feel its lower aspect, the pre-pyloric and pyloric regions of the stomach and the beginning of the duodenum (5). It is not necessary to palpate the spleen. The transverse and

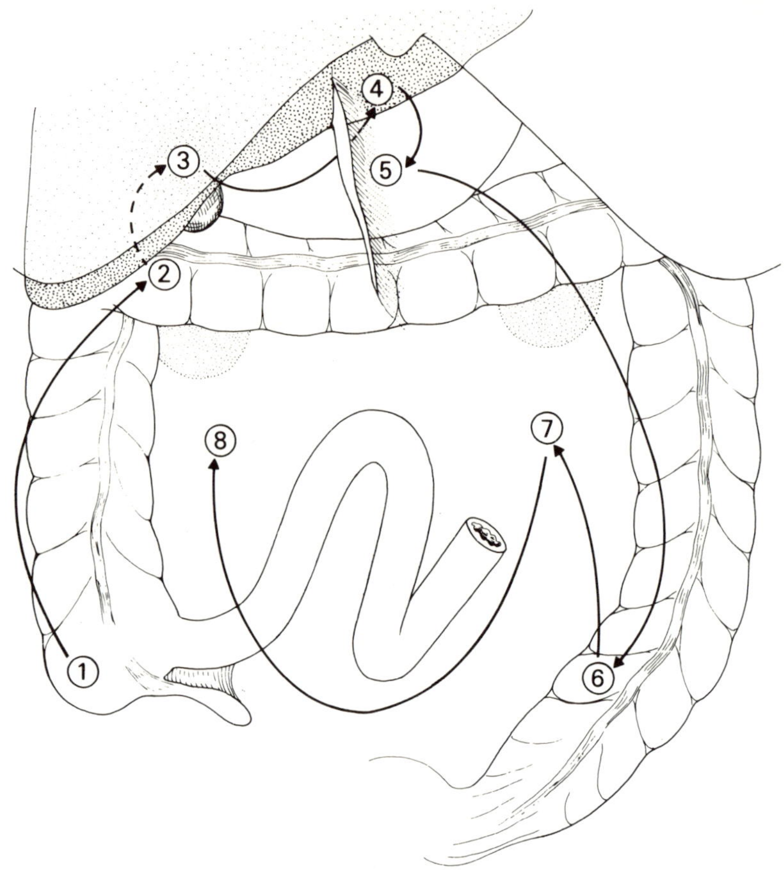

Fig. 8.1. Systematic exploration of abdominal cavity.

descending colon is then palpated until one reaches the sigmoid colon (6). The next step is to withdraw the hand and pass it behind the great omentum, first on the left (7) and then on the right of the root of the mesentery (8). The hand slides above the sigmoid colon and behind the great omentum and small intestine and is made to follow the inner side of the descending colon in an upward and backward direction (see Fig. 8.2). The lower pole of the kidney lies a little higher on the left

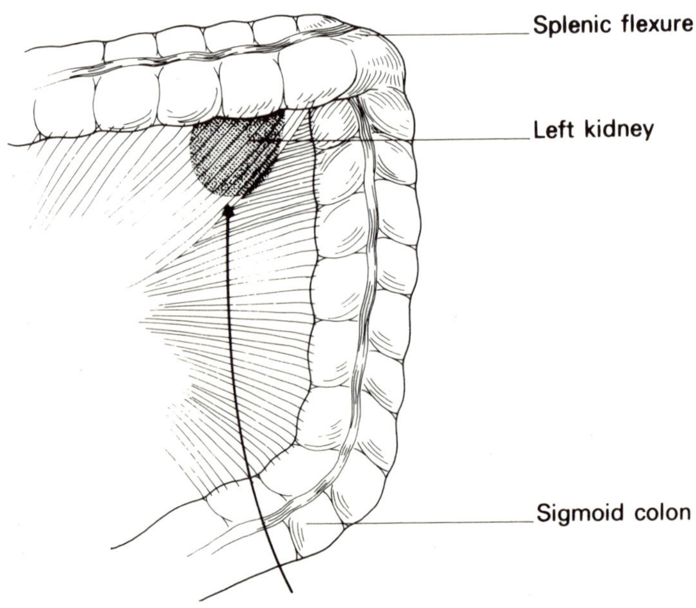

Fig. 8.2. Palpation of left kidney.

side compared with the right but can be felt more easily. The region of the renal pelvis and upper ureter can be felt, but the upper pole is difficult to reach, because the peritoneum comes forward to cover the tail of the pancreas and form the base of the great omentum.

On the right side, the hand is passed upwards behind the great omentum and adjacent to the ascending colon (see Fig. 8.3). One must be careful to begin with the hand on the right side of the root of the mesentery, which can be difficult if, for example, there are adhesions in the appendix region. The posterior abdominal wall goes surprisingly far backwards as one gets higher, in contrast to the lumbar spine, which lies very near the anterior abdominal wall in most women. The hand follows the ascending colon upwards and again reaches the under aspect of the liver. The lower pole of the kidney is then palpable through the posterior peritoneum if one moves the hand directly backwards. The upper half of the kidney is difficult to feel adequately, because it is obscured by the duodenum and the fold of peritoneum formed by the right side of the great omentum. Two fingers can be passed upwards along the medial border of the lower kidney pole to the region of the renal pelvis, but it is not possible to feel very much in normal patients. A stone in the renal pelvis is easily felt here, and a stone in the upper ureter is palpable through the posterior peritoneum against the quadratus lumborum and psoas muscles.

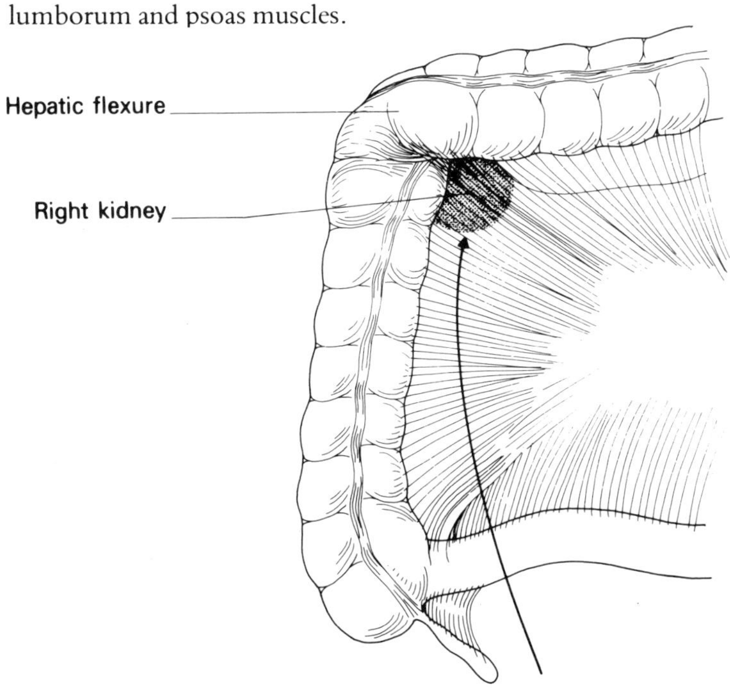

Fig. 8.3. Palpation of right kidney.

DIRECT INSPECTION AND PALPATION OF THE LOWER URINARY TRACT

The ureter

One recognizes the ureter not only by the obvious fact that it is a muscular tube running in the right direction, but also by the well-known property known as 'vermiculation'. This means that it makes a worm-like peristaltic movement when it is stimulated by a pinch from a pair of dissecting forceps. Ureters can do this even if they are moderately dilated. The grossly dilated hydro-ureter is atonic and will not react to stimulation.

The normal ureter can be picked up and 'rolled' between the finger and thumb and gives a characteristic 'snap' when it escapes from the fingers. This point is especially important when it is being identified before oophorectomy and hysterectomy. These signs are not so easy to elicit after infections such as pelvic peritonitis, appendicitis and diverticulitis, or in the presence of spreading tumour.

The right ureter. The right ureter can usually be seen at the pelvic brim through the posterior peritoneum. After incision of the peritoneum it is easy to follow it upwards to the lumbar portion or downwards into the pelvis. If it is not visible, it can be found by incising the peritoneum along a line overlying the right common iliac vein as shown in Fig. 8.4.

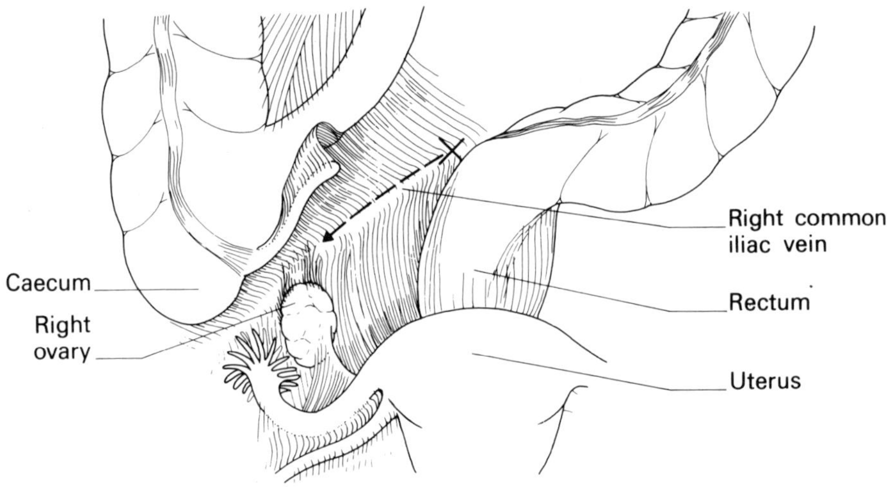

Fig. 8.4. The right ureter at the pelvic trim.

Lumbar ureter on the left side. The left lumbar ureter differs from the right in that it is often impossible to see it through the peritoneum. It is difficult to find it by incising the posterior peritoneum above the root of the sigmoid mesentery because it lies behind many blood vessels passing to and from the descending and sigmoid colon and is obscured behind fat and lymph vessels. In addition, the site of the root of the sigmoid mesentery is very variable and of little use as a landmark. It is far easier to find the ureter if one lifts up the colon where the descending part becomes looser because of the beginning of the sigmoid mesentery and incises the peritoneum here on the lateral side so that the colon can be reflected medially. There is one important point to remember, however, which may make all the difference when one is looking for the ureter; it is loosely attached to the peritoneum so that it is always reflected forwards with it and does not remain lying on the posterior abdominal wall (Figs. 8.5 and 8.6).

This fact is made use of by the urologist when he is exposing the lumbar ureter from the loin. He opens the space between the peritoneum and the posterior abdominal wall and feels for a stone in the ureter on the back of the peritoneum.

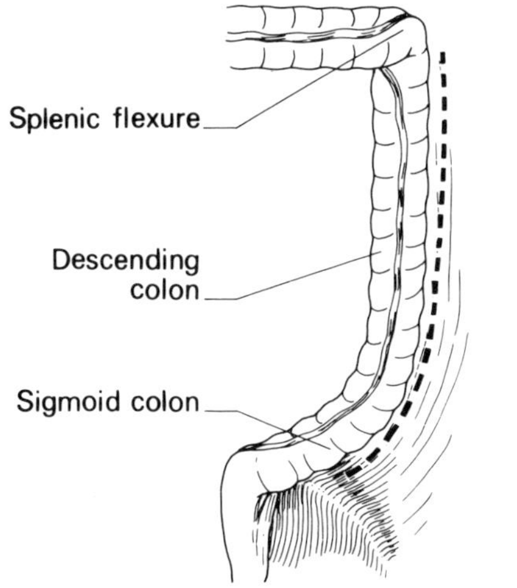

Fig. 8.5. Exposure of left ureter by reflecting the descending colon medially.

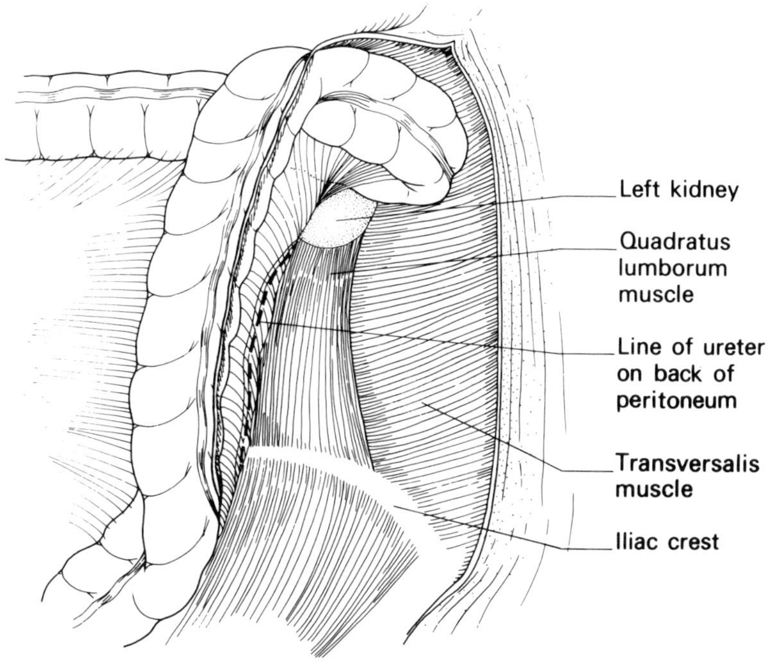

Fig. 8.6. Exposure of the left lumbar ureter.

Below the pelvic brim, both ureters can be felt through the peritoneum against the pelvic wall for a short distance parallel to the infundibulo-pelvic ligament until they disappear just before they reach the side of the cervix. Here they run in the lateral (cardinal ligament) and anterior retinacula (vesico-uterine ligaments) and are therefore difficult to palpate from within the peritoneum.

BLADDER INJURY

Abdominal operations

Hysterectomy, Caesarian section and other abdominal operations.

Opening the peritoneum

There is sometimes an injury during opening of the peritoneum in the early stages of a pelvic operation. If the bladder is distended, its dome comes up into the lower end of the wound by obliteration of the prevesical pouch of peritoneum and can be damaged by the scissors as the surgeon cuts the peritoneum downwards in the mid-line towards the symphysis pubis. The bladder should always be emptied before any pelvic operation, not only because of the chance of this accident but also so that it takes up as little room as possible. If an in-dwelling catheter has been placed in the bladder preoperatively, it must be allowed to drain freely because even 100 ml in the bladder during the operation is enough to make injury more likely. If the bladder has not been emptied, the accident can always be avoided by the manoeuvre by which the surgeon and his assistant both put an index finger behind the peritoneum on either side of the line of incision. If the bladder is distended or displaced into the suprapubic region by tumour it will be felt. In other words, the peritoneum is not divided until it is felt to be free (Figure 8.7). It is not always safe to hold up the peritoneum with artery forceps on each side of the initial opening and cut downwards without first making sure that neither bladder nor intestine is hiding under the lower end.

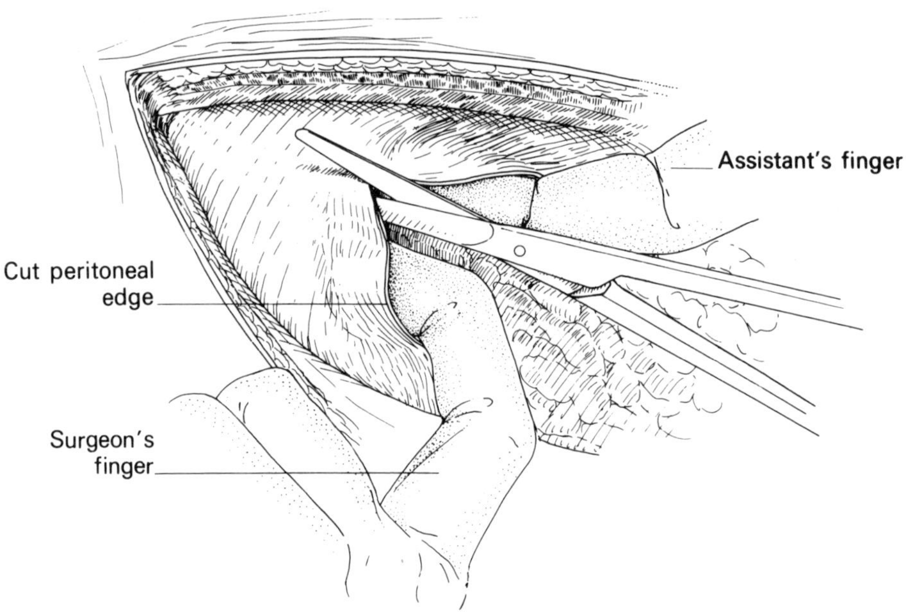

Fig. 8.7. Index fingers holding peritoneum and feeling for bladder or adherent intestine.

Previous suprapubic or retropubic operations such as operations for stress incontinence, perhaps with suprapubic postoperative drainage, produce a situation where injury to the bladder can be difficult to avoid if the retropubic space must be opened again. As stressed in Chapter 5 in the description of the 'last resort' operation for stress incontinence, if the surgeon cannot easily avoid opening the bladder in the preliminary dissection then it is best to admit this and open it intentionally. This takes a considerable weight off the mind and also can shorten the preliminary dissection. After all, the bladder will probably be opened in any case at the end of the operation to put in suprapubic drainage. The same is true, in fact, of the peritoneum which is always attached to the scar remaining after suprapubic drainage and is usually opened in the preliminary dissection.

With the bladder open, a finger can be inserted to feel whether bladder wall and bladder base are adherent to the back of the pubis and this greatly simplifies the dissection.

Separating the bladder base

The commonest site of injury is at the bladder base when it is being separated from the cervix and upper vagina. The upper part of the separation is usually done by blunt dissection using a pledget swab on a holder. Some surgeons use even blunter dissection by pushing the posterior wall of the bladder away from the uterus with a thumb covered with gauze. It is not difficult by this method to go through the thin perivesical fascia so that the thumb begins to tear the muscle of the bladder wall without the surgeon realizing it, because the gauze obscures vision and dulls the feeling of increasing resistance lower down the anterior wall of the uterus. In the region of the anterior fornix of the vagina the areolar tissue becomes much tougher and is sometimes tougher than the bladder wall. For this reason sharp dissection of the bladder from the uterus under vision is safer (Fig. 8.8). The dome can be held by non-toothed tissue forceps while the areolar tissue is divided by scissors, keeping close to the uterus and vagina all the time.

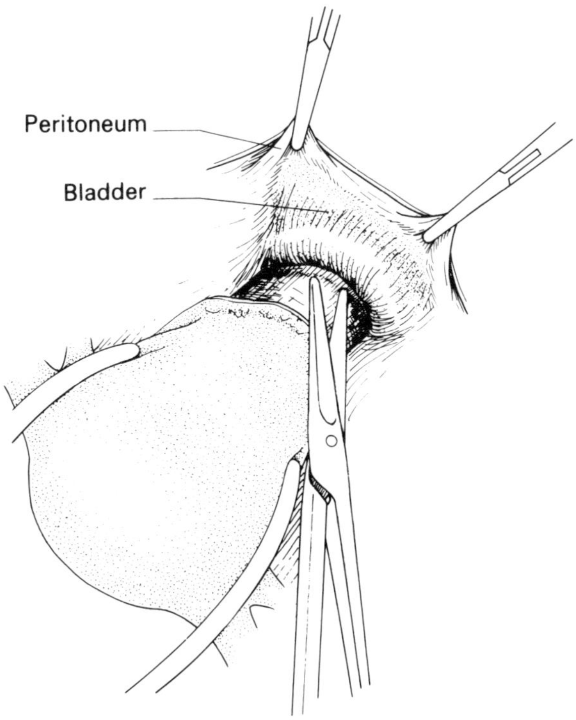

Fig. 8.8. Separation of bladder from urterus and anterior vaginal wall by sharp dissection.

If the patient has been operated on before—for example, a Caesarian section, large cone biopsy, prolapse operation or a sub-total hysterectomy—and it is necessary to remove the cervical stump, the separation of the bladder can then be very difficult. The solution to this problem is to put an instrument into the bladder via the urethra so that the wall can be accurately identified. A curved male urethral sound size 22 F is ideal for this purpose. It is large enough not to perforate the bladder wall and can be manipulated from the vulva to demonstrate the limits of the bladder (Fig. 8.9).

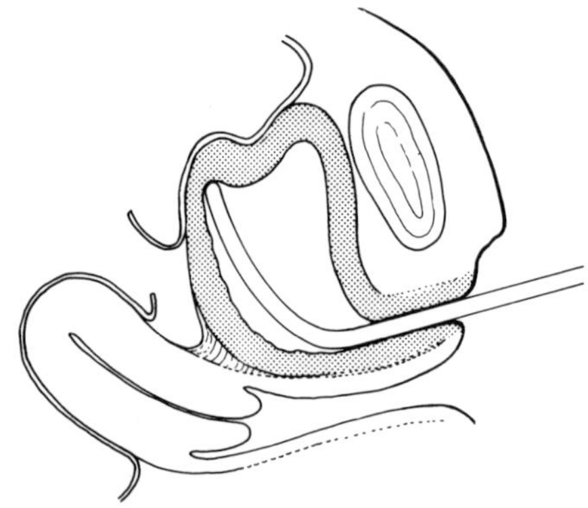

Fig. 8.9. Large male urethral sound used to demonstrate limits of bladder wall during preliminary dissection.

Vaginal operations: prolapse and cystocoele repair

Every surgeon who has operated on cases of recurrent prolapse or cystocoele is fully aware of the difficulties which sometimes occur during this dissection.

The site of injury is in the same region of the bladder wall as was the case in abdominal operations. It lies just above the interureteric bar which marks the upper limit of the trigone. Injury occurs when the vaginal mucosa and submucosal layer of connective tissue is divided from the thin perivesical fascia. The vaginal mucosa and fascia are both thick, especially before the menopause or if the patient has a marked cystocoele. They should both be incised in the mid-line and the incision gradually deepened until, using the handle of the knife, it is possible to open up a space on each side between the perivesical fascia and the vaginal wall in the relatively loose connective tissue. The right layer is avascular apart from small veins at the lateral border of the anterior vaginal wall. It is easy to open so blunt dissection does no harm here. If the surgeon cuts too deeply in the midline, he will go through the perivesical fascia into the bladder muscle where there is always considerable bleeding and a danger of going through the bladder mucosa. If the perivesical fascia has been opened, blunt dissection is highly dangerous as it produces more haemorrhage and more damage to the bladder muscle, with a risk of fistula formation immediately or later and of haematoma formation. What was meant to be a delicate plastic operation with minimal bleeding and disturbance of blood and nerve supply can easily become a mess. Recognition of anatomical layers is made difficult and correction of the prolapse or cystocoele becomes difficult with possible consequences in the form of micturition dysfunction.

If the gynaecologist inadvertently finds himself in this situation he should stop the dissection immediately and try another place in the midline a little above or below the point at which he is operating. This will enable him to find the right layer which can then be opened up as desired.

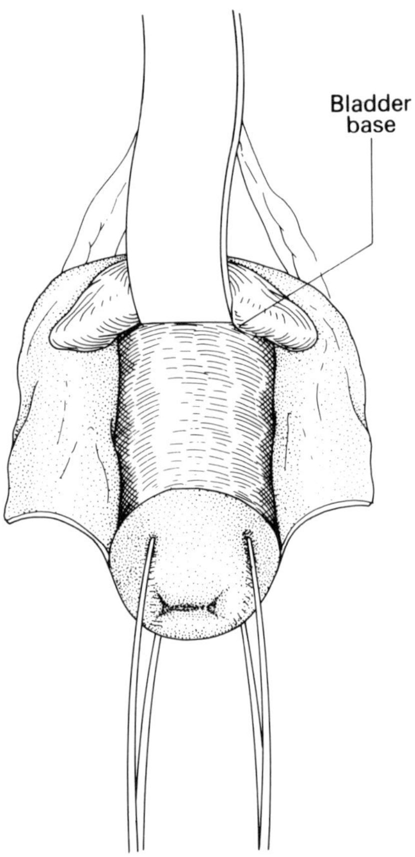

Fig. 8.10. Retractor holding bladder up when vaginal wall is to be closed.

The use of sutures in the bladder wall during a prolapse operation with the object of invaginating it is not to be recommended. Invagination contributes nothing to bladder support, it merely traumatizes the bladder wall. The wall will itself contract and take up any slack. The bladder should be held up out of the way by the assistant while the trimmed vaginal mucosa and fascia is closed (Fig. 8.10). In this way one avoids the risk of placing sutures in the bladder wall so tightly and so far laterally that there is a serious danger of constricting the ureter. This is no idle threat: complete anuria brought about by constriction of both ureters has been described.

Vaginal hysterectomy

If this operation is combined with anterior colporraphy, the principles

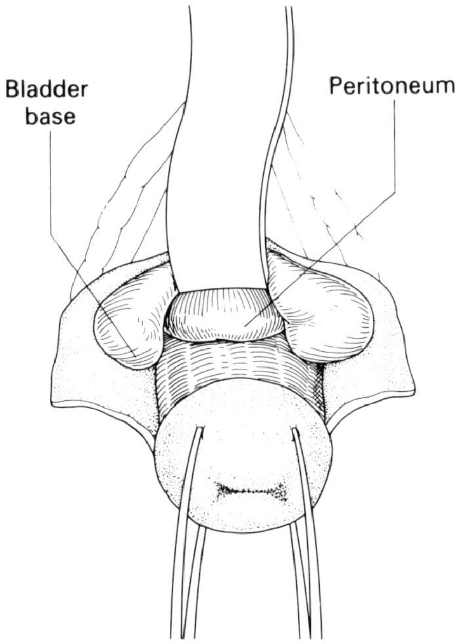

Fig. 8.11. Exposure of peritoneum during vaginal hysterectomy. The bladder base is lifted up by a retractor.

concerning treatment of the bladder described above should be followed. If not, the operation starts over the cervix with a curved incision which passes through the sub-mucosal fascia. The bladder is then freed from the anterior aspect of the uterus by sharp dissection with scissors in the midline, in the reverse direction to that described under abdominal hysterectomy. The dissection is kept close to the uterus until the peritoneum is seen. The peritoneum is tightly adherent to the uterine wall so it is easy to see where it should be opened so that damage to the perivesical fascia can be avoided (Fig. 8.11). The opening is enlarged enough to allow introduction of the deep curved retractor which holds up the bladder. This also has the effect of lifting up the ureters. As long as the operator then keeps close to the sides of the cervix, he is well away from the urinary tract.

If the ovaries have to be removed at the same time there is a risk of ureteric damage because the uterus and adnexa must be pulled downwards and this in turn displaces the ureters downwards so that they may be dragged into the narrow opening. This risk can be lessened by doing an episiotomy which gives much better access and vision.

PRINCIPLES GOVERNING REPAIR OF SURGICAL INJURIES TO THE BLADDER

These consist of holes in the wall or injuries to the muscle with intact mucosa. The principles of treatment are the same.

Always repair the injury as soon as it is discovered

If it is not repaired at once it will be twice as big when one comes back to it later as a result of retraction and movement. Also, it may be forgotten.

Close the opening with one layer of interrupted thin atraumatic absorbable sutures, size 0, put in fairly loosely 0.5 to 1.0 cm apart (Fig. 8.12)

The bladder is not an inert cistern which must be made watertight. The edges of the opening should be approximated with minimal interference with blood supply. The ordinary process of healing will do the rest. Therefore avoid continuous and use interrupted sutures and use only one layer. Do not pull them tight.

Sutures take in the whole thickness of the bladder wall including mucosa

It wastes time avoiding the mucosa and the sutures get a better grip if they go through all layers.

If the injury is in the retropubic space, put in a suction drain from suture line to surface by the shortest extraperitoneal route

The drain is put down in case of urinary leakage. Urine must be allowed to come to the surface. If it collects in the perivesical tissues, infection and fistula will be the inevitable result.

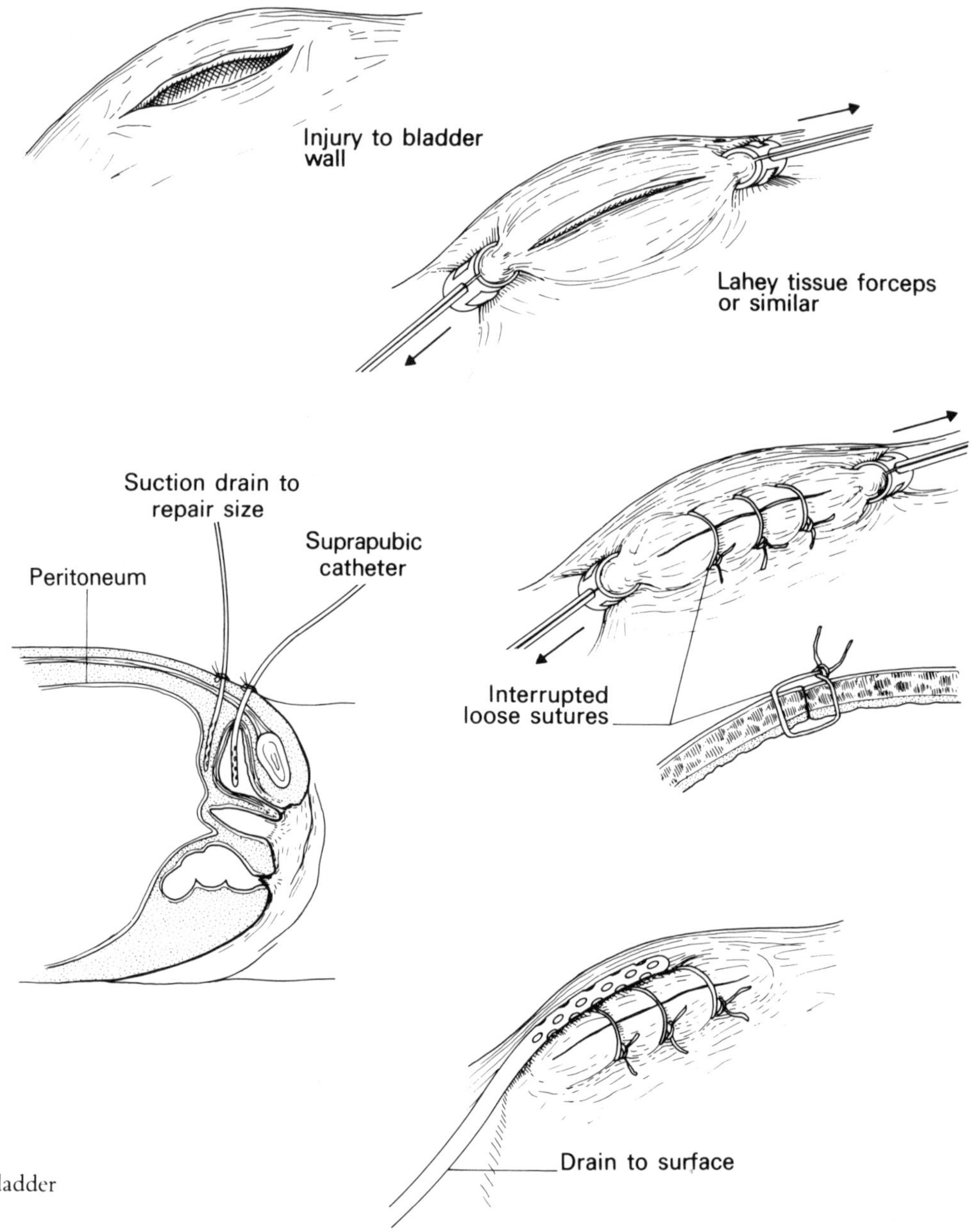

Fig. 8.12. Steps in the repair of a bladder injury.

If the injury occurs during a vaginal operation a drain is unnecessary because possible leakage has direct access to the vagina.

Keep the bladder empty for at least 6 days by catheter drainage

Bladder drainage is necessary to avoid tension on the sutured wound while healing is going on.

THE URETER

The ureters in the pelvis in abdominal operations

For many gynaecologists the ureter is a mysterious tube which everybody talks about but few have actually seen dissected free in the pelvis. If one has not seen and identified a structure, it can easily be damaged; if one learns to see it and/or feel it, it is easy to avoid it.

Most injuries to the ureter occur during simple hysterectomy because it is the commonest gynaecological operation where the ureters are in danger. Obviously, benign and malignant pelvic tumours, pelvic infection, post-radiation fibrosis and endometriosis can make this dissection and identification extremely difficult.

There are two points of danger:

Just below the pelvic brim. When the ovary is lifted up, the peritoneum of the infundibulo-pelvic ligament will be stretched and the ureter may be drawn up with it because of its loose connection to the peritoneum (Fig. 8.13). The ureter may be clamped with the ovarian vessels or the clamp may be put so close that the suture-ligature produces direct or indirect damage. To avoid this, the ureter should always be identified either by sight (vermiculation) or feel (the snap) before the ligature is placed. In cases of ovarian tumour this method is sometimes impossible and it is then necessary to identify the ureter above the pelvic brim and follow it down to the danger point. Identification of the ureter can sometimes be so difficult that it is advisable to stop the operation and put up a ureteric catheter as described in Chapter 9. If there is strong indication of uteric involvement or

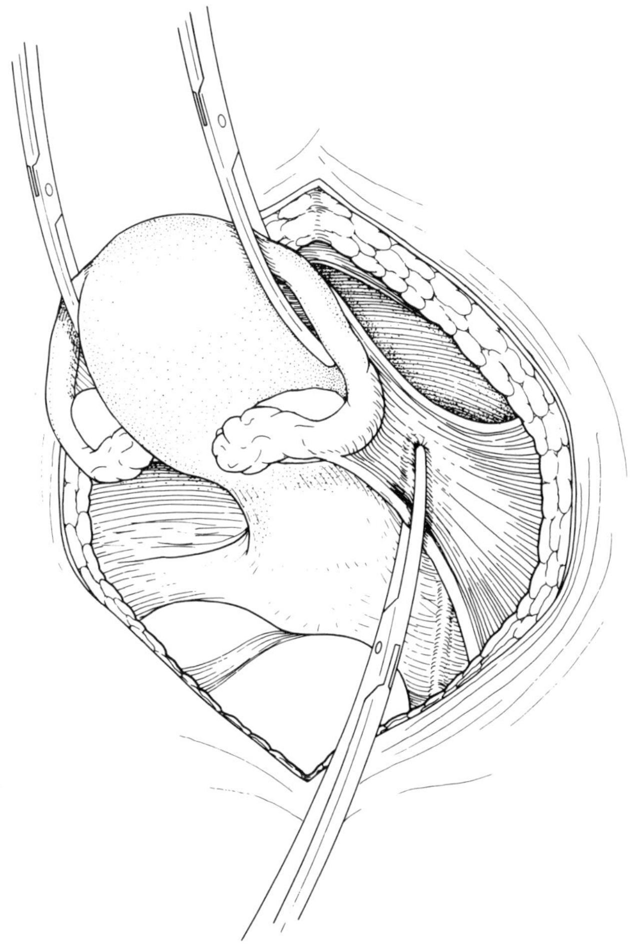

Fig. 8.13. Lifting the ovary may draw up the ureter.

displacement on the pre-operative intravenous urogram, the surgeon should not hesitate to put up the catheter before operation. This is one of the reasons why the gynaecologist must be familiar with the cytoscope and ureteric catheterization. If there is any question of damage to the uteric wall by dissection or by tumour involvement, or if there is great risk of post-operative haematoma or infection, the catheter can be left in for several days with the lower end coiled up in the bladder. This allows urine to pass unhindered to the bladder in the critical post-operative phase and lessens the possibilities of fistula and stricture formation.

The point where the uterine artery crosses the ureter. This is the most likely point for injury to occur because the ureter lies close to the side of the cervix. This relationship is maintained no matter how the uterus is manipulated during operation or in the displacement involved in uterine prolapse, because the uterine artery pulls the ureter down by lying directly over it (Fig. 4.2). Myomas in the cervix can cause bizarre displacements so that, for example, the ureter may lie between the uterus and the bulk of the myoma.

Damage may be direct by cutting, crushing in a clamp, inclusion in a ligature or kinking by ligature.

In order to be safe the surgeon should always know where the ureter is before he clamps the uterine artery during a hysterectomy. It is not necessary in every hysterectomy to dissect out the ureter so that it can be followed until it has passed the danger spot where the uterine artery crosses it. If the surgeon is in any doubt about the safety of clamping the uterine vessels he can always palpate the ureter between the index finger and thumb, using his right hand to feel the left side and vice versa. It can be identified by the characteristic 'snap' and its direction: there is no other similar structure in the neighbourhood. It has been a general rule that if the surgeon keeps close enough to the uterus there is no need to worry about the

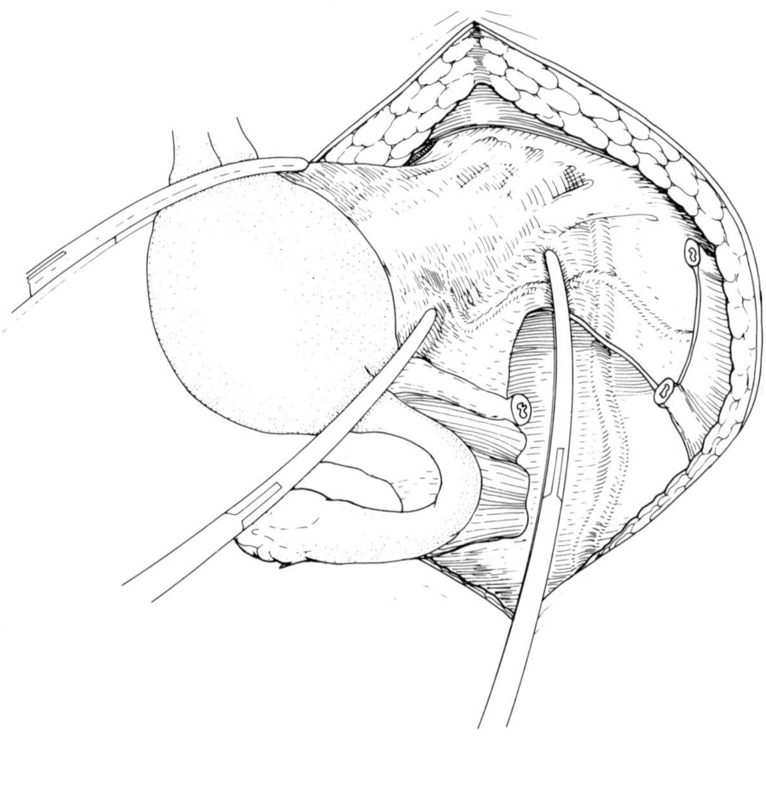

Fig. 8.14. Correct placing of clamp when attempting to control uterine artery bleeding.

ureter. This is basically true and it is a fact that the distal ureter, where it passes into the anterior retinaculum (vesico-uterine ligament), is generally speaking only in danger in radical hysterectomy. This rule, however, does not always hold because one can get troublesome arterial or venous bleeding in this region, either because the clamp on the uterine artery loosens or is pulled off, or because the ligature is too loose and slips off. Danger to the ureter immediately becomes a reality if clamps are placed blindly in the depths of the wound in a panic attempt to control this bleeding (Fig. 8.14). This must never be done without first identifying the ureter either by the fingers or under vision. The first method is often the easiest because it is difficult to clear the wound of blood and because the field of vision is not nearly so large and clear as in a radical hysterectomy. If it is venous bleeding that is the problem, it normally stops as a result of compression and because both the uterine arteries are clamped. If however, one artery is still open the vein can be compressed by a swab on a holder while the artery is ligated. If the bleeding is arterial and clamping or ligation is a risk to the ureter, there is then only one safe thing to do. *All gynaecologists should be able to do this.* It is not difficult and should without doubt be done more often when trouble is encountered. The manoeuvre is one of the first steps in radical hysterectomy.

Lift up the round ligament, pass the two index fingers back to back down the sidewall of the pelvis, moving them apart from one another and so opening up the loose tissue on the lateral pelvic wall between the peritoneum and the division of the common iliac into the external and internal iliac arteries. This is avascular loose connective tissue. Follow the internal iliac (hypogastric) artery under vision to its division into the obliterated unbilical, superior vesical and uterine arteries. This manoeuvre only takes a few seconds. The uterine artery is about as thick as a match and there is never any difficulty in identifying it at this point. It is then ligated in continuity here (Fig. 10.7).

This manoeuvre should also be done as a preliminary step in extended hysterectomy because of the common variations in vascular anatomy in the pelvis. It destroys no significant blood supply to other organs and achieves so much in the way of safety. There is no need to worry about the blood supply of either the ureter or the bladder.

Another advantage of this manoeuvre is that the ureter is beautifully demonstrated attached to the pelvic peritoneum after this has been reflected medially. It can be seen to pass under the uterine artery and into the anterior retinaculum (Fig. 10.5).

The ability to carry out this little manoeuvre gives the surgeon a most satisfactory feeling of confidence, both as regards control of haemorrhage and where preservation of the pelvic ureter is concerned.

PRINCIPLES GOVERNING REPAIR OF SURGICAL DAMAGE TO A URETER

Although repair of an injury to the lower urinary tract can certainly be said to be a urological operation, a urologist is not always available at short notice. It is therefore sometimes necessary for the gynaecologist to be able to do his own repairs. In fact, any gynaecologist who is capable of performing delicate plastic operations on the fallopian tubes can carry out these repairs easily as long as he keeps to the basic principles. Two things are fundamental in deciding what to do; the extent of the damage and the site.

Injury by cutting with scissors, ligation, clamping or constriction

The main point is to decide whether the injured part of the ureter is viable or not.

If the damaged area is too big to allow repair without stricture formation or if there is any doubt at all about its viability, *all damaged tissue should be removed,* if necessary dividing the ureter completely. It must be remembered that the complication rate after leaving a doubtfully viable portion which then becomes necrotic is much greater than the complication rate after removal and repair of the gap. The situation is then reviewed when the area is thoroughly cleaned up. One should never be afraid of removing badly damaged tissue to the extent that an incomplete division is converted into a complete division. The injury is then treated as if the ureter had originally been completely divided.

A cut in the ureteric wall which does not open the lumen should be sewn together with very fine sutures passing through the muscle and periureteric fascia. No catheter is necessary in the ureter but it is wise to place an extraperitoneal drain from the site of injury to the surface to take care of any urine leakage if it should occur.

Incomplete division

Incomplete division by a cut which opens the lumen is repaired by fine sutures in the same way. If this injury is in the immediate vicinity of the bladder, the thick periuteric fascia tends to produce much fibrosis which makes stricture formation more likely here than higher up. The surgeon should therefore take no chances when the lumen has been opened and it is wise to put in a splint in the form of a 6 F soft plastic catheter or a ureteric catheter of the same size without its stilette before the stitches are inserted. This is best done by making a small opening in the bladder wall extraperitoneally between holding sutures so as to expose the ureteric orifice so that the catheter can be passed up to the renal pelvis. Attempts to pass the catheter both ways through the site of injury involve the risk of increasing the damage. The lower end is coiled up in the bladder and fished out at a later date with a pair of forceps through the urethra. Alternatively, the lower end can be brought out of the suprapubic wound and sewn to the skin and fixed with tape (Fig. 9.7).

The ureteric splint catheter is removed on the 6th day and the extraperitoneal drain on the following day if there is no leakage.

Complete division

Re-implantation into the bladder is safer if the division is within about 10 cm of the ureteric orifice. This is because of the danger of stricture formation described above and also because it is difficult to mobilize the lower end of the ureter enough to allow adequate access for a good anastomosis.

Complete division higher up can usually be managed by re-anastomosis.

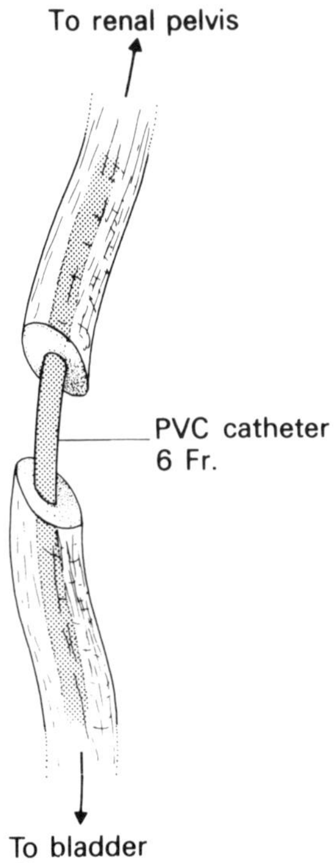

Fig. 8.15. Re-anastomosis of ureter.

RE-ANASTOMOSIS OF A URETER

Cut ends obliquely with sharp scissors

An oblique cut makes the ends a bit larger to sew.

Put in a catheter from the renal pelvis to the bladder

An in-dwelling catheter acts as a splint, makes suturing much easier and takes care of drainage for the first few days. It should be about size 6 F, either soft PVC or a ureteric catheter without stilette, and can either be coiled up in the bladder or brought out suprapubically (Fig. 8.15).

Put in 4-0 holding sutures about 2 cm from each end

These are used to pull the ends together while they are being sutured and afterwards are used to fix the ureter to avoid tension during the first few days. They should pass through the periureteric fascia and the muscular coat but should not enter the lumen (Fig. 8.16).

Sew the ends together with four sutures, north, south, east and west

These should be the same fine absorbable material and pass through the periureteric fascia and muscle without entering the lumen (Fig. 8.17).

Anchor holding sutures to fascia covering psoas, periarterial fascia or whatever is available in the neighbourhood

This avoids tension due to periatalsis (Fig. 8.18).

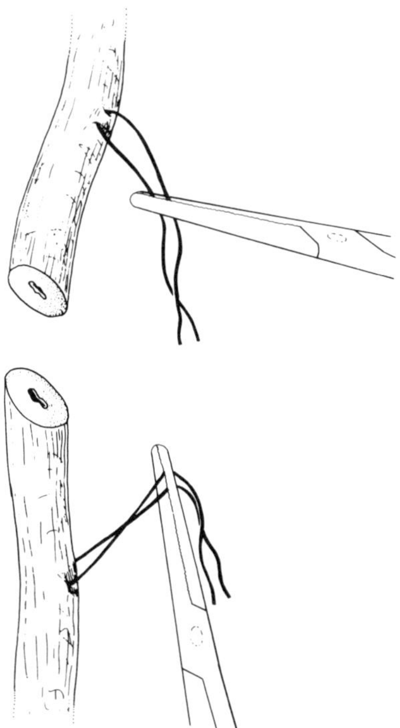

Fig. 8.16. 4-0 holding sutures used to anchor anastomosis.

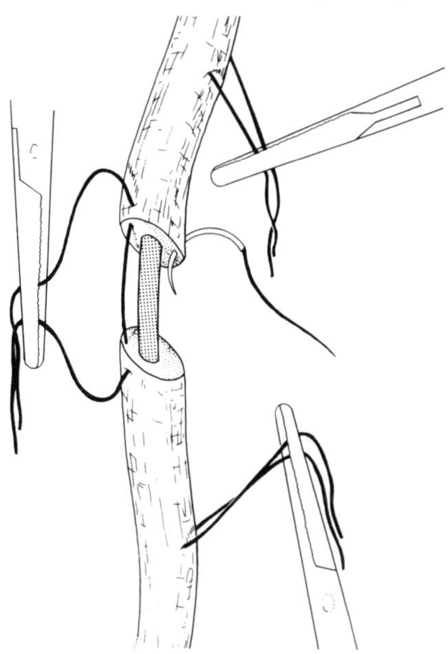

Fig. 8.17. Suturing ends of severed ureter.

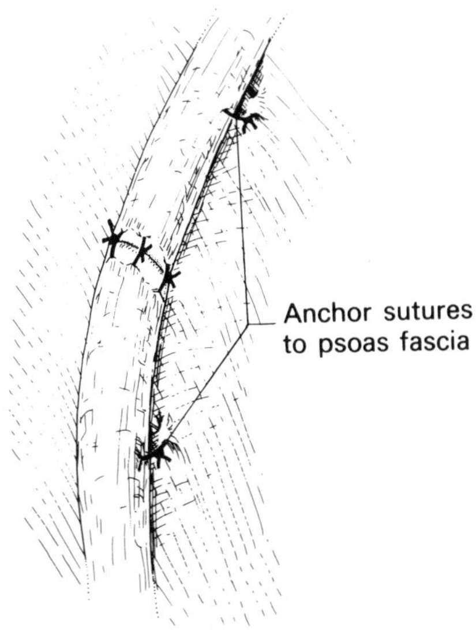

Fig. 8.18. Anchoring holding sutures to avoid tension on anastomosis.

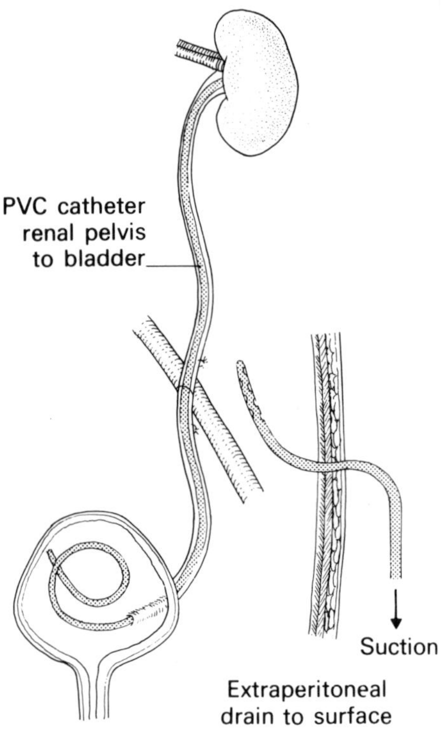

Fig. 8.19. Drainage after re-anastomosis of severed ureter.

Place extra-peritoneal suction drain from anastomosis to skin and drain bladder by urethral balloon catheter

This renders urine leakage from the anastomotic site harmless (Fig. 8.19).

Remove the ureteric catheter by the 6th day and the extra-peritoneal drain a day or two later if there is no leakage

After-treatment

If there is persistent leakage, the extra-peritoneal drain should be retained because the leakage usually stops by the end of the third post-operative week. If it still continues after this, a urologist should be called in. The anastromosis may have broken down and the kidney be in danger. Treatment must be as for a urinary fistula (Chapter 12).

All cases should be followed up by intravenous urography or isotope renography in order to reveal stenosis if it should occur.

RE-IMPLANTATION OF URETER INTO THE BLADDER

Mobilize the lateral wall of the bladder

The paravesical space is opened up on the same side by blunt dissection. Ligate the ureteric stump.

Open bladder transversely on the same side of the dome

This gives good access to the inside of the lateral wall (Fig. 8.20).

Incise mucosa 3 cm below where the ureter will conveniently pass through the bladder wall

It is quite unnecessary to choose the most dependent part; make the ureter go through where it is most convenient.

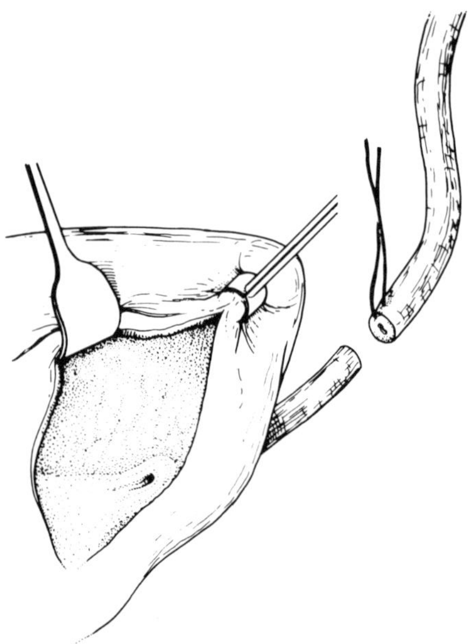

Fig. 8.20. Opening in bladder wall to give access to region behind and above ureteric orifice.

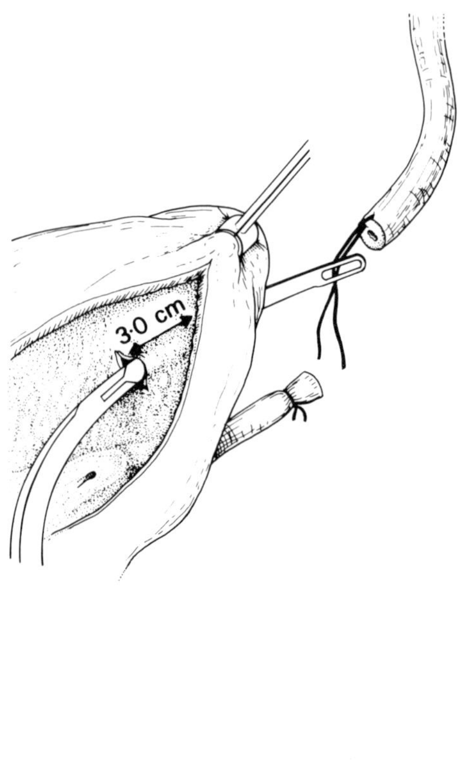

Fig. 8.21. Submucosal tunnel is made before forceps draw end of ureter through bladder wall.

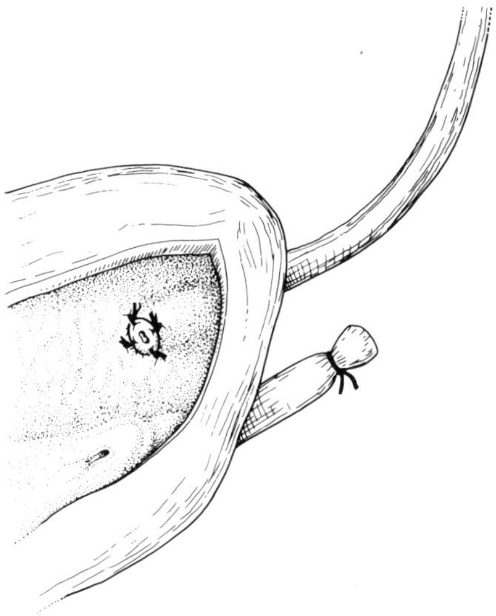

Fig. 8.22. The ureter is sutured to the bladder mucosa.

Make a sub-mucosal tunnel for 3 cm and then burrow through the bladder wall, pick up end of ureter and draw it inside the bladder
Use long, thin, curved forceps for this (Fig. 8.21).

Suture end of ureter to bladder mucosa
Sutures pass through the whole thickness of the ureteric wall. It is easier if the ureter is opened a few millimetres (Fig. 8.22).

Place one suture to anchor ureter to outside of bladder wall
This is an added safety precaution to avoid tension due to peristalsis.

Close bladder with suprapubic catheter and extraperitoneal suction drain to anastomotic site

Put in an in-dwelling ureteric catheter (as above) if there is any doubt about a good anastomosis
This is a safety precaution which is not always necessary.

After treatment

If a ureteric catheter has been inserted, it can be removed on the 6th day and the extraperitoneal drain on the following day if there is no leakage. The suprapubic bladder catheter should be retained until acceptable micturition has been achieved. This is best not attempted until 14 days after operation because manipulation of the bladder wall produces considerable oedema and healing of the anastomosis may be delayed as a result.

If there is persistent leakage after the ureteric catheter has been removed, it is best to wait another 10 days in the hope of closure. Intravenous urography and cystoscopy should be used to see if the implantation site is intact with the ureter in place. If this shows that the anastomosis has come apart then re-operation is probably the best solution.

All cases of re-implantation should be followed up by intravenous urography or renography. The results are, however, very good as a general rule, with no problems such as ureteric reflux or stenosis. Furthermore, necrosis is not seen in spite of the fact that the arterial supply to the lower end of the implanted ureter must have been partly destroyed.

Another method

If the ureter will not reach the bladder without tension, the bladder must be drawn up to reach the ureter. The gynaecologist is well advised to avoid 'flap' operations because they are difficult to perform and the complication rate is high if they are not accurately performed. After radical pelvic operations, flap operations become dangerous because necrosis of the flap may result from inadequate blood supply. In addition there is often considerable oedema of the bladder wall in the post-operative phase. It is better to mobilize the bladder wall on the same side, as described above, and then do the same thing on the other side. This certainly gives some welcome extra mobility

Next, the bladder is opened in the dome so that two fingers can be inserted to lift up the whole side wall. It can be stretched slowly so that it will reach the pelvic brim and can be sutured to the fascia over either the psoas muscle or the vessels with strong sutures which take in the whole thickness of the bladder wall (Fig. 8.23). This as adequate to allow anastomosis of a ureter divided at or just below the pelvic brim. Tunnelling and fixation of the ureter is carried out by the method described above. Tension in the ureter caused by peristalsis must be relieved by fixing it to the surroundings 2 or 3 cm above the anastomotic site. An in-dwelling ureteric catheter with the lower end curled up in the bladder is also a safety precaution and can well be retained longer than in the simple re-implantation. It can be left in place for as long as 10 days. Closure of the bladder and insertion of the suction drain is done as described above.

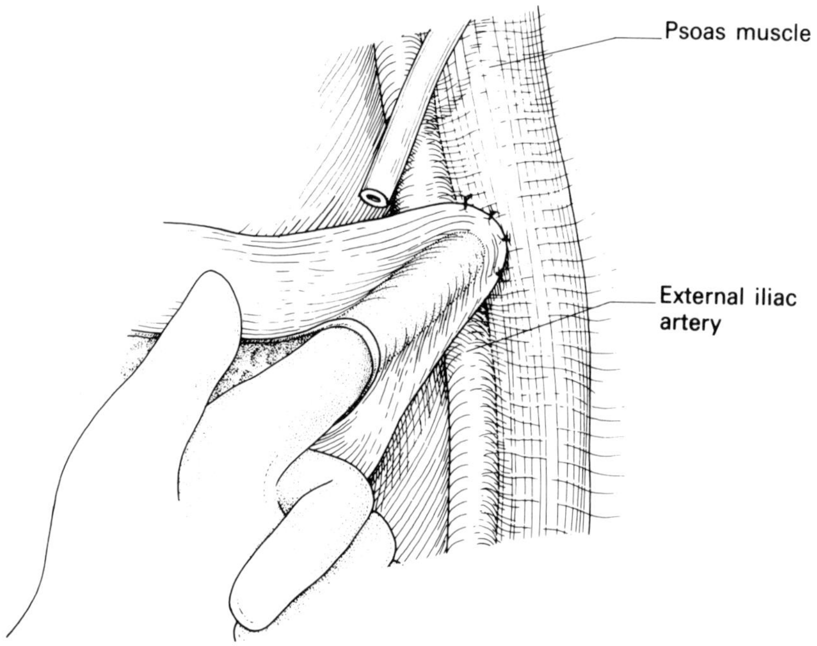

Fig. 8.23. The bladder wall can be stretched so that it can be sutured to the fascia of the psoas muscle or any convenient fascia at the brim of the pelvis.

One should always bear in mind that peristalsis will begin in the ureter soon after the operation when urine production gets going and 'vermiculation' will drag the end away from any anastomosis which is under tension. The stitches are pulled out of the ureteric wall. Even the holding, tension-relieving sutures will have often worked out of the ureteric muscle by the fourth day irrespective of how they are put in or what sort of material is used. By this time, of course, the ends should have been joined by young fibrous tissue so that they will hold.

After treatment

As mentioned in the section on radical hysterectomy, it can be an advantage to use a stiffer male type of plastic balloon catheter so that the bladder can be drained and kept completely empty for at least 10 days. The ureteric catheter and the suction drain can both be removed on the 6th day; they should be retained longer if there is any leakage. It is seldom that there is any persistent leakage through the suction drain; if it continues after the 6th day it may indicate that the ureter has come out of the bladder.

The gynaecologist should be conservative as regards the length of time urinary drains and catheters are retained. This is a safety precaution; urologists may advocate early removal on the grounds of infection risk but it is still better to retain a drain too long than to remove it too soon.

Damage during vaginal operations

The ureter is damaged most often during vaginal hysterectomy. If damage has occurred, it is impossible to do an adequate repair from below. The abdomen must be opened so that a repair based on the above principles can be carried out. Damage to the ureter which is not discovered at operation is described under urinary fistula (Chapter 12).

Ureteric obstruction

Causes

Obstruction can develop after a pelvic operation if forceps are applied or stitches are put in too close to the ureteric wall. The stitch angulates the ureter enough to obstruct it.

Short and long term effects

The immediate effect of both partial and complete obstruction of a ureter is dilatation of the segment immediately proximal to the site of obstruction. Dilatation spreads upwards to the renal pelvis and calyces at a rate dependent upon the degree of obstruction and the rate of secretion. A hydroureter and hydronephrosis are produced. The collecting tubules which empty into the calyces become distended, permitting pyelovenous and pyelo-lymphatic backflow. The secretion of urine gradually ceases. After 2 to 4 weeks of obstruction complete recovery of function becomes impossible.

Urinary infection together with obstruction greatly increases both the speed and degree of renal damage and leads to infection of the renal parenchyma, acute pyelonephritis. Pyelo-venous reflux introduces the possibility of spread of bacteria to the bloodstream in the form of bacteriaemia and septicaemia. Persistent obstruction combined with ascending infection can be rapidly fatal in spite of intensive antibiotic administration. It is the most serious urological complication associated with gynaecological surgery. Treatment is discussed under radical hysterectomy (Chapter 10).

Operation after radiotherapy

These operations which have just been described for re-anastomosis and re-implantation of the ureter are based on the existence of a normal blood supply to the lower urinary tract. *They cannot be performed with the same chance of success after irradiation of the pelvis.* Vascularity and tissue viability are then so poor that necrosis of the bladder becomes a real danger and the possibility that the ureter will not unite with the bladder and may come to lie loose in the pelvis a week later must be borne in mind. This is discussed in Chapter 11.

Urethra

When any preliminary dissection involving separation of the vaginal wall from the urethra is being done, the gynaecologist should not damage the urethra at all. If he is in the right layer the urethra can be separated intact. Anything which interferes with the nerve or blood supply will endanger normal function.

Damage to the urethra occurs most frequently during vaginal operations but can happen during an abdominal dissection, especially after previous retropubic surgery. Also, sutures may be placed too close to the urethra or inadvertently in the urethral wall itself.

If the urethral musculature is damaged, the surgeon should repair the injury at once using fine absorbable sutures. It is a good idea to do this with a fair-sized catheter (24 F) in the urethra, for this avoids constriction of the lumen.

REFERENCES

Mattingly RF, Borkowf HI (1978) Acute operative injury to the lower urinary tract. Chapter 7 in *Clinics in obstertrics and Gynecology*, **5,** 123, ed. S Stanton.

Smith P, Roberts M, Slade N (1970) Urinary symptoms following hysterectomy. *Brit. J. Urol.* **42,** 3.

Symmonds RE (1976) Ureteral injuries associated with gynecologic surgery: prevention and management. *Clin. Obstet. Gynecol.* **19,** 623.

Yossef AF (1960) *Gynecologic Urology*. Thomas, Springfield.

Zincke H, Malek RS (1974) Experience with cutaneous and transuretero-ureterostomy. *J. Urol.* **111,** 760.

Chapter 9 Urological Operations which the Gynaecologist may need

Any gynaecologist may find himself confronted with a urological emergency as a result of complications after a pelvic operation. Urological help may not be available, so he must not only be able to understand what is happening but also know enough to be able to deal with the emergency. The emergency often occurs as a result of the development of obstruction in one or both ureters or because of a so-called 'ascending' infection combined with obstruction.

It behoves the gynaecologist to know the principles underlying the various forms of urinary diversion even though he may never wish to do any of these operations himself.

The fundamental necessity is usually drainage of urine directly to the surface from either bladder, ureter or renal pelvis.

BLADDER DRAINAGE

In-dwelling urethral catheter

Bladder drainage is necessary after most pelvic operations, because the patient is temporarily unable to micturate. This is partly due to local disturbance in the neighbourhood of the bladder and urethra, partly to the fact that the patient is lying in bed and partly to the effect of postoperative sedation. Until she can sit out of bed on a toilet chair it is unrealistic to expect her to micturate, let alone empty the bladder. This means that drainage may be necessary for about 24 hours in smaller operations and for as much as a week or 10 days after major pelvic surgery.

It is almost impossible to keep the urine sterile in a female patient with an in-dwelling catheter. The organisms normally present in the introitus and outer urethra, quickly colonize the mucus film around the catheter, and small amounts of urine in the base of the bladder become infected. Something can be done to postpone this by preventing in-and-out movement of the catheter, by local antiseptic applications, by forced diuresis and by closed drainage, but to little avail; the urethra is short and the introitus and perineum cannot be sterilized. Any in-dwelling catheter acts as a foreign body, whatever its size or type. In addition, hospital patients rapidly acquire additional infection by proteus, pyocyaneus and other hospital organisms which are already resistant to most antibiotics.

After a few days, urinary leakage around the catheter may become a problem and in the past it has been usual to change the catheter for a larger one. This seldom produces improvement because the leakage is due to involuntary micturition stimulated by the presence of a foreign body in the bladder, combined with the irritation of a lower urinary tract infection. It is better to use a smaller catheter instead of a larger one, if it is essential to continue with the in-dwelling catheter. If a patient can micturate around an in-dwelling catheter, she can certainly do it better without the catheter. There is no getting away from the fact that the in-dwelling urethral catheter in women is always unsatisfactory and can produce many complications such as infection, leakage, mucosal ulceration, stricture formation and even urethral fistula. Intermittent catheterization is a better alternative but very demanding on the nursing staff and must be regarded as a luxury in most departments. This has led to the increased use of suprapubic bladder drainage in post-operative cases and there is no doubt that the infection rate has become less and the complicaiton rate almost negligible. Most important of all, perhaps, is the preservation of the delicate mechanism of the urethra from disturbance by an acute inflammatory reaction.

SUPRAPUBIC CYSTOSTOMY

The technique resembles the taking of a urine specimen from the bladder by suprapubic puncture described in Appendix A. Sterile suprapubic drainage sets are commercially available. After ascertaining that the bladder is at least moderately distended, local anaesthetic should be injected along the track which is placed 1 cm to the side of the mid-line just above the symphysis pubis and should pass backwards and downwards. If a finger is introduced per vaginam to the anterior fornix, the surgeon will readily appreciate the direction in which the track must go. A small incision is made in the skin with a knife and the catheter mounted on its introducer is passed through the rectus muscle, the prevesical space and the bladder wall in succession. Urine will appear when the introducer is removed. The catheter is connected immediately to a closed drainage apparatus and is attached to the skin securely with tape and/or suture.

Self-catheterization if long-term drainage is necessary

As an alternative to the permanent in-dwelling catheter this has much to recommend it. The infection risk can be lower and the patient avoids wearing a urine-collecting bag. A patient can be taught to catheterize herself while sitting on the toilet. She should use a standard disposable plastic female catheter, size 10–12 F. This can be used repeatedly as long as it is cleansed with soap and running water before and after each occasion. She should be encouraged to drink more than usual in order to maintain a diuresis, which lessens the chance of infected residual urine in the bladder. The female bladder and urethra seem to tolerate this treatment very well without the necessity of any form of continuous prophylactic medication. Patients have been able to catheterize themselves successfully for many months. As mentioned in Chapter 6, over-correction of urethral stress incontinence may result in temporary or persistent residual urine. This is an example of a recurrent problem which can be solved by self-catheterization.

DRAINAGE OF A KIDNEY

It may be necessary for the gynaecologist to drain a kidney more or less as an emergency operation. The indication is usually either ureteric stricture with hydronephrosis, ureteric fistula or infection leading to acute pyelo-nephritis or pyonephrosis. The acute situation can be adequately treated by drainage, that is to say ureteric catheterization or nephrostomy as a temporary measure; nephrectomy can then be done later if necessary.

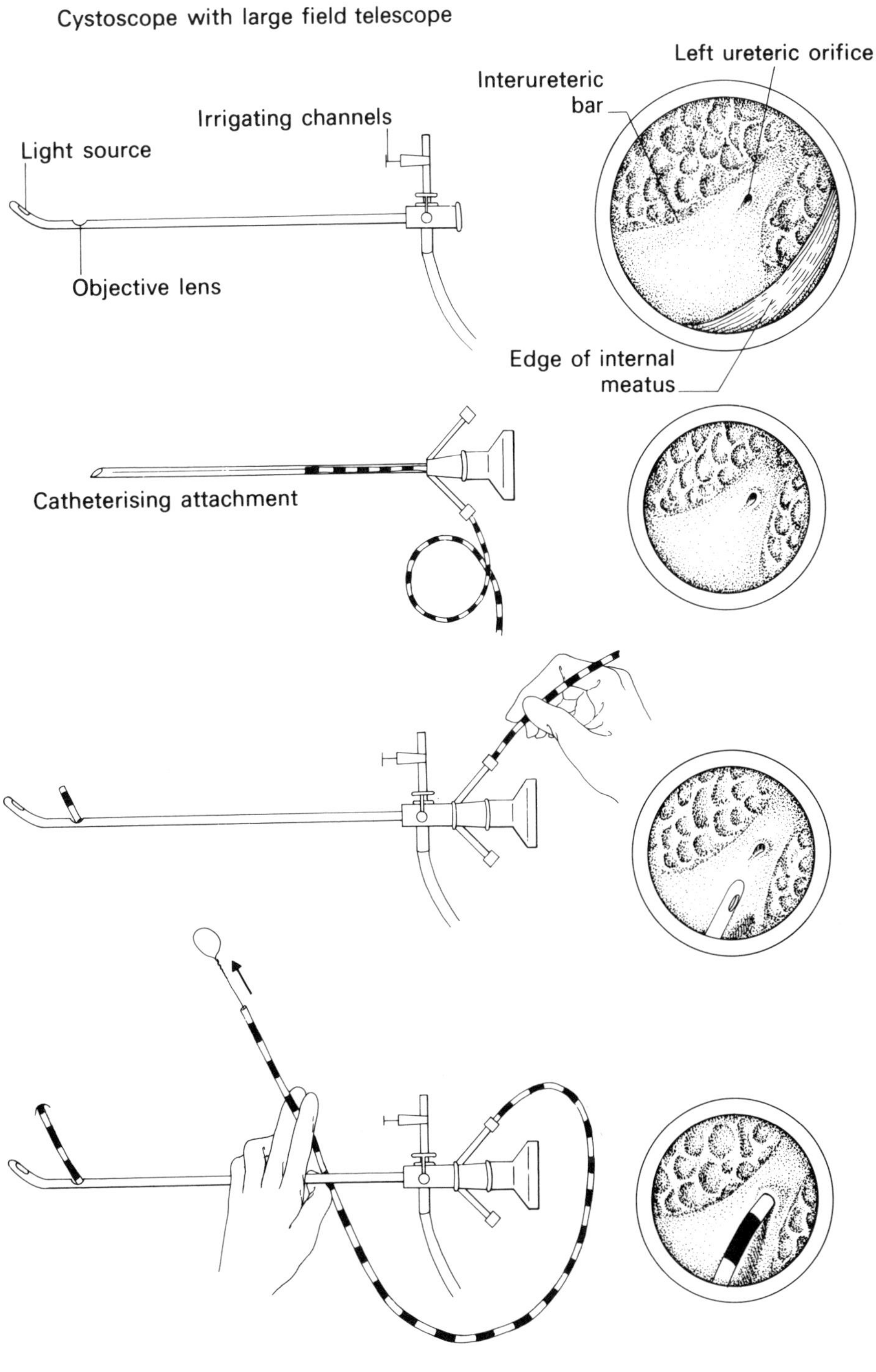

Fig. 9.1. Catheterization of the ureter.

Catheterization of the ureter

The following description covers basic principles (Fig. 9.1). There are several types of cystoscope with different telescopes. The catheterizing cystoscope has a single channel or two channels side by side for catheterization of the two ureters. A rubber nipple is placed on the end of each channel so that irrigating fluid does not run out alongside the ureteric catheter. A large-field telescope should always be used when looking for the orifices; it is not always so easy to find them if a smaller catheterizing attachment is used to start with. Having found an orifice it is a simple matter to hold the sheath in position and change over the telescopes. The catheterizing telescope should be placed in the cystoscope with a ureteric catheter already threaded 10 cm through the nipple. The rest of the long catheter must be maintained sterile. The telescope is locked in position and the fluid irrigation turned on for a few seconds to replace what has been lost while the telescopes have been changed. There is no need to distend the bladder; it is in fact easier with only a little fluid because distention flattens out the normal contours which are used in orientation. The orifice should lie in the telescopic field if the instrument has not been moved and the catheter is then passed in until its tip can be seen through the telescope. The position of the cystoscope is adjusted until the tip points at the orifice. The whole instrument is advanced towards the orifice so that the catheter engages; the instrument is then held still and the catheter is gently passed about 10 cm into the ureter.

Stilette

Ureteric catheters contain a thin wire stilette which makes them more rigid and prevents kinking. It must be removed from the portion of the catheter which lies in the ureter because a ureteric catheter containing a stilette can be pushed through a normal ureteric wall and cause a perforation if it meets an obstruction or bend; a catheter without its stilette will either bend itself double or kink before it penetrates the wall. If the stilette is retained after the catheter has passed 10 cm into the ureter, sooner or later a perforation will occur which will introduce a completely unnecessary element of risk into the little operation. This applies whether the object is to obtain a specimen of urine from the renal pelvis or merely to put something stiff into the ureter so that it can be more easily recognized at subsequent operation.

Taking a specimen

As the catheter is passed into the orifice, the operator should watch through the telescope and count the centimetre markings as they disappear into the ureter. He must always have the position of the tip of the catheter in mind. On average, the renal pelvis will be reached when 25 cm has passed into the ureter and urine will usually then begin to appear from the catheter in a steady drip. If it does not appear, it is worth moving the catheter in and out 1 or 2 cm. If there is still no urine and it is necessary to obtain a specimen, a 2 ml syringe can be attached via a

16 gauge needle so as to produce a little negative pressure by aspiration. An air-lock is sometimes the cause of the lack of urine and this is easily overcome. More negative pressure than can be produced by a 2 ml syringe is unnecessary and harmful, for the eye or eyes of the catheter will simply be sucked against the epithelial lining of the renal pelvis or calyx and cause bleeding. The reason for maintaining the outer end of the catheter sterile is now obvious. Some urologists keep the sterile plastic cover in place over the part of the catheter outside the cystoscope and even use it to collect the specimen of urine which comes from the renal pelvis. This, however, is a counsel of perfection and only works well when the operator has an assistant. If he is alone, it is best to use the right hand to push the catheter through the nipple while the left hand holds the cystoscope in position and at the same time holds the outer end of the catheter up out of harm's way and well away from the operator's head. The stilette can also be easily manipulated in this position. Gadgets attached to the table which are designed to hold the cystoscope are unnecessary.

In-dwelling ureteric catheter

If the catheter is to be left in for more than a few minutes, the cystoscope must be removed (Fig. 9.2). The catheter is first pushed through the instrument so that it curls up in the bladder; the catheterizing telescope is then unlocked and pulled out

Fig. 9.2. Taking out the cystoscope while leaving the ureteric catheter in position.

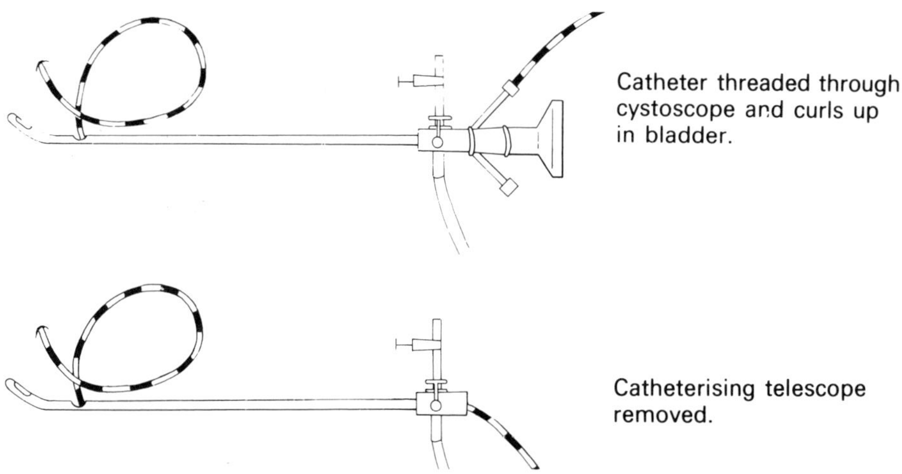

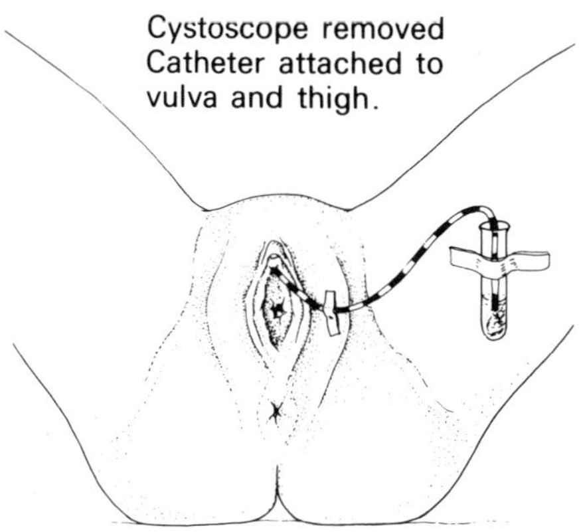

Fig. 9.3. Taking a ureteric catheter specimen.

about 10 cm. The catheter is picked up where it lies in the guide channel and the end drawn through the nipple in the direction of the bladder and held in the left hand which is supporting the cystoscope sheath. The telescope can now be removed completely. The rest of the fluid is allowed to run out of the bladder and the sheath is then completely removed by threading it over the catheter so that the latter remains undisturbed in the bladder. The catheter should be secured by tape to the inside of the patient's thigh near the vulva and its end covered with a sterile towel which is also secured to the same thigh. If a urine specimen from the renal pelvis is required, a sterile test-tube is attached (Fig. 9.3). The legs are taken out of the lithotomy stirrups and placed horizontally while the specimen is being collected.

One must remember that the presence of fresh blood in a ureteric catheter specimen means only that the catheter has scratched the lining epithelium. It must not be taken to mean that there is a source of haematuria such as a tumour in the kidney or renal pelvis. Occasionally, all attempts to obtain a specimen are in vain; it is then a waste of time to wait more than a few minutes if small movements of the catheter do not succeed in starting the flow. The end of the catheter is perhaps caught up in a narrow calyx or, more probably, there is for the time being little urine secretion from the kidney due to a combination of sedation and dehydration. Patients can come to operation in the morning having not drunk any fluid since the middle of the previous day. When it is known beforehand that a ureteric catheter specimen is required, it is advisable to arrange for a certain diuresis either by giving the patient more to drink the day before or by means of intravenous fluid just before the catheterization.

Ureteric catheterization can have several objectives:

To drain the kidney. This emergency operation is occasionally required as temporary treatment of an acute pyonephrosis, for example, during pregnancy.

To obtain a urine specimen. This can be necessary when it is essential to demonstrate infection in the kidney, or the converse, where in the presence of bladder infection it is useful to know that there is no infection in the kidney. In the latter case the surgeon should think twice before doing it; the possibility of carrying infection from an infected bladder up to the kidney is a real one if there is any ureteric obstruction.

To enable the radiologist to do retrograde pyelography. In the early days of radiology this was often necessary but advances in radiological technique have now rendered it almost obsolete. Contrast should be injected up the catheter under continuous observation on the radiological screen. If, for any reason, it has to be done 'blind', then after the preliminary film has been taken, a small amount of contrast is injected – never more than 3 ml – and a picture taken. The reason for this is twofold. First, nobody can ever be quite certain that the catheter tip is really in the kidney or renal pelvis – it can lie in the periureteric tissues, and second nobody can be quite sure that the patient does not have an allergic sensitivity to contrast medium. Ideally, the patient should be awake or at any rate awake enough to react to pain. For if she feels pain when contrast is injected, there is something wrong and the injection should be stopped at once. Another reason for beginning with 3 ml or less is that this amount is usually enough to demonstrate what is required. The capacity of the normal renal pelvis together with the calyces is not more than 3 to 5 ml and the contrast fluid will be mixed with the urine that is already there. It is often assumed that the renal pelvis is empty before the contrast is injected, but this is never the case.

To facilitate identification of the ureter at operation. Many urologists get the impression that gynaecologists are taught to operate without the help of indwelling ureteric catheters and that they are expected to identify and avoid the ureter in all cases either by anatomical dissection or by some manoeuvre which pushes the ureter and periureteric tissue out of the region where clamps are used. To put in a ureteric catheter is to some a confession of failure. This attitude is, of course, based on false precepts, for urologists have no hesitation in making use of this aid when they anticipate difficulty in identifying the ureter in the pelvis or at the pelvic brim – for example, if they operate on patients with periureteric fibrosis or infiltrating pelvic tumours. It is always better to be sure than sorry and nobody need ever worry about the extra time spent before operation in passing the catheter, it is saved (sometimes many times over) later during the operation by the ease and certainty with which the ureter is exposed.

Catheterization of the ureter in fistula and stricture. This should be done with the very greatest care and never with the stilette in the catheter. Soon after a pelvic operation, when a tell-tale leakage of urine appears from a drain, the wound or the vagina, cystoscopy and catheterization of the ureters is an essential part of the localization of the site of leakage. Usually the catheter is obstructed at the site of a ureteric fistula and this serves to localize it. Occasionally it passes the ureteric fistula site and can be passed up to the renal pelvis. It is then best left in-dwelling for a short time, for it can result in closure of a small leak. Special precautions should be taken after radical hysterectomy because the ureter may be temporarily unsupported near the bladder. See Chapter 10.

Percutaneous nephrostomy

This elegant method of renal drainage is the result of a combination of the Seldinger technique with modern radiological methods for visualization of the renal pelvis on a TV screen. Ultrasound and computer-tomography can also be used but are not essential. The method which will be described has been developed so that it is as simple as possible, both as regards catheterizing equipment and radiological apparatus. It should be possible in all hospitals which have equipment for radiological TV screening in one or two planes. Commercially produced percutaneous nephrostomy sets are now available. Percutaneous nephrostomy is indicated in all cases where temporary drainage of a kidney is required. It can even be made a permanent form of renal drainage. The operation

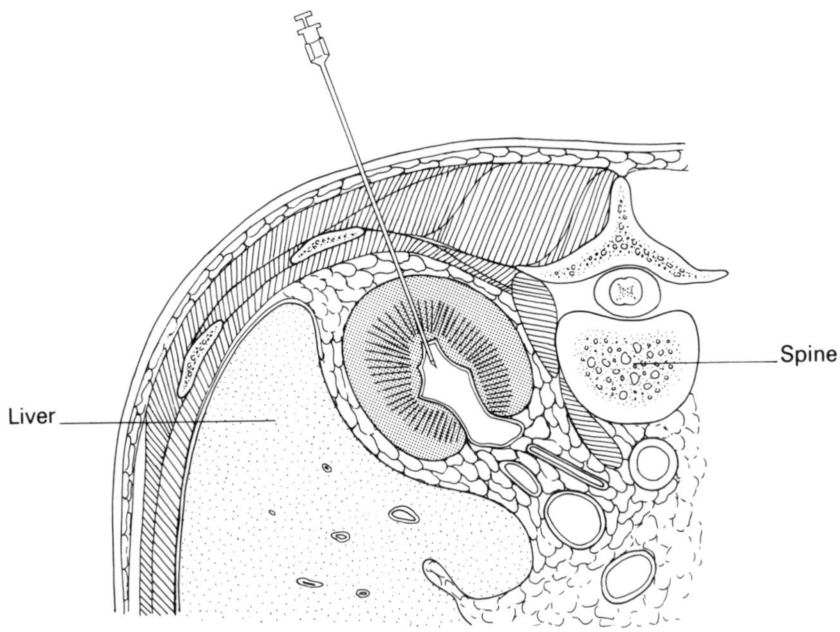

Fig. 9.4. Percutaneous nephrostomy. Insertion of needle into the renal pelvis.

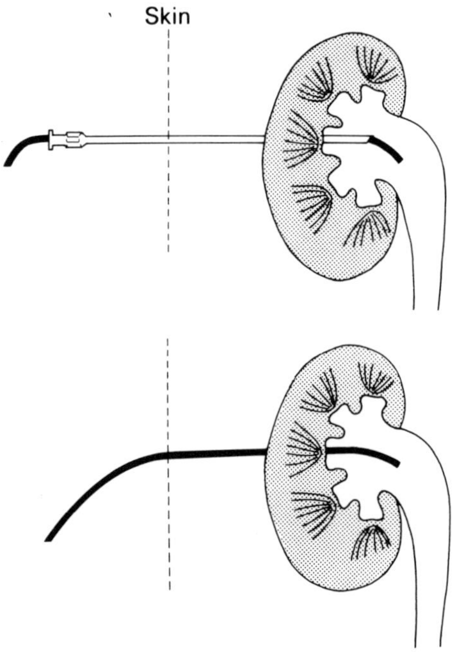

Fig. 9.5. The guide wire is passed through the needle to the renal pelvis. The needle is then removed.

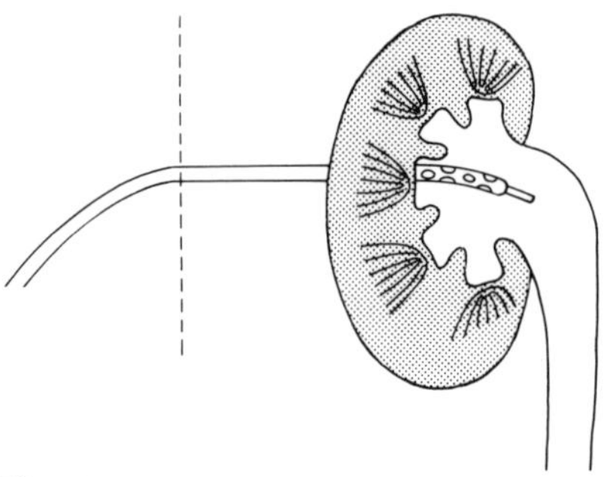

Fig. 9.6. Radio-opaque catheter (8 F) draining the renal pelvis.

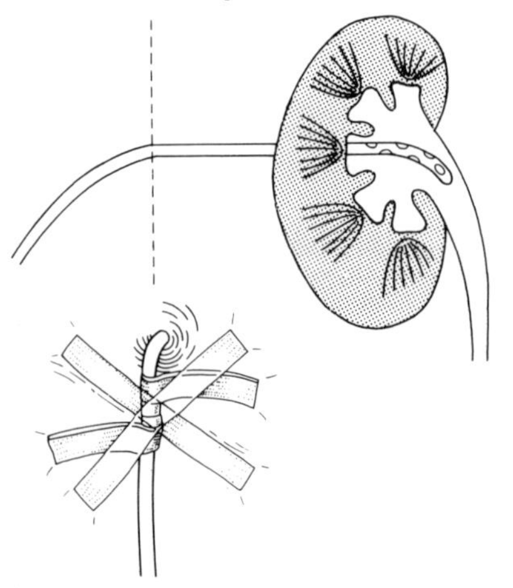

Fig. 9.7. Catheter taped securely to the skin. It should be connected to a closed drainage system.

should be performed in cooperation with a radiologist with experience of the Seldinger technique in arteriography.

The nature of the operation is explained to the patient and she is given adequate premedication. Local anaesthetic is introduced in skin and muscle layers along the track of the needle as described below. The patient lies supine on the X-ray table with the side to be operated on raised about 45° to the horizontal. If renal function is adequate, contrast is injected through an intravenous canula as for intravenous urography and the kidney and renal pelvis visualized on the screen. A point is chosen just below the 12th rib and half way between the lateral border of the erector spinae muscle and the mid-axillary line (Fig. 9.4). This ensures that the needle passes behind the peritoneum and the ascending or descending colon, but at the same time lies laterally enough so that when the catheter is in place it does not get kinked or disturbed by the patient lying on it. A special needle size 4 F and 15 cm long with stilette in place, is then passed through the muscle layers beneath the 12th rib in an upward and medial direction with the help of the X-ray screen until it reaches and passes through the kidney substance into the renal pelvis. Urine will appear when the stilette is withdrawn and the position can be verified on the screen by injecting a little contrast through the needle.

The guide-wire (3 F) is then passed through the needle to the renal pelvis and the needle removed, leaving the guide-wire in position (Fig. 9.5). A 6 F dilator is then passed along the wire through the renal parenchyma and is followed by an 8 F dilator. A little glycerine helps as a lubricant. After the 8 F dilator has been removed, a radio-opaque catheter size 8 F is threaded along the wire and its position in the renal pelvis verified (Fig. 9.6). The guide-wire is then removed and the catheter connected to a closed drainage system. The catheter is taped to the skin and the connecting tube is also taped in a loop to the flank. We have found that modern tape is preferable to a skin suture which is tied around the tube. The suture often pulls out after about a week and encourages infection (Fig. 9.7).

There can be bleeding into the renal pelvis which sometimes is fairly brisk. The best means of dealing with this is to irrigate the pelvis repeatedly with saline through the catheter, sucking it out with a syringe so as to avoid clot formation. As a general rule bleeding, even when it appears at first to be a little frightening, will gradually stop within a few minutes.

After 2 or 3 days on continuous drainage, the 8 F catheter is removed and a 10 F one introduced. This is done by the Seldinger technique in the same position as has been described. The new catheter is taped to the skin and connected to the closed drainage apparatus as before.

Two or three days later the same procedure is used to increase the size of the catheter to 12 F.

Insertion of balloon catheter

After a further 2–3 days, the same procedure is repeated. A stiffer guide-wire with a flexible tip is passed through the catheter to the renal pelvis and the catheter removed. The operator must make sure that the flexible tip is introduced first. A

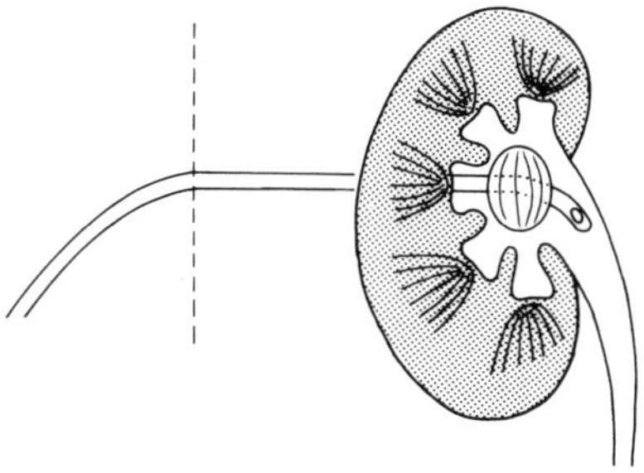

Fig. 9.8. Small balloon catheter (12 F) draining the renal pelvis. It should be securely taped to the skin and connected to a closed drainage system.

14 F dilator is then passed through to the renal pelvis and removed. A balloon catheter size 12 F can then be passed fairly easily along the guide-wire into the renal pelvis (Fig. 9.8). The balloon is inflated with 2 ml of contrast and the tube leading to the valve tied as a precaution against leakage. The position of the catheter is verified on the screen and the guide-wire is then removed. The catheter is then connected to a closed drainage apparatus and taped to the skin. This size 12 balloon catheter can be left in position for about 4 weeks, when it should be changed for a similar sized catheter. X-ray control is unnecessary for this.

It is important that all the steps of this procedure be carried out until the balloon catheter is satisfactorily in position. It is a mistake to be content with the first catheter. It will certainly stop draining and come out sooner or later. With the balloon catheter in the kidney, the patient is mobile and drainage is effective. It can continue in use with periodic changes as long as necessary, weeks or months. When drainage is no longer necessary, the catheter is simply removed and the channel will close spontaneously within 48 hours.

If the catheter should fall out because the balloon collapses, it should be replaced immediately, even if it is in the middle of the night. It helps to have the patient in the same position as that in which the nephrostomy was originally done. If a canula falls out during the first week, replacement is usually impossible and the procedure must be carried out again. After 8–10 days, replacement usually presents no problems as long as it is done soon after the catheter has fallen out.

Kidneys tolerate nephrostomy drainage very well. It can even be used as a permanent method of drainage. In many cases the drainage is so good that no urine passes down the ureter and a uretero-vaginal fistula can become dry. The procedure can be bilateral, for example after irradiation damage where both ureters are involved in a large vesico-vaginal fistula. It is also easy to observe the results of reparative surgery on the lower ureter by doing an antigrade ureterography through the nephrostomy tube.

DRAINAGE OF URETER

Ureterostomy in situ

Not all gynaecologists have access to a well-equipped X-ray department or to a radiologist who has experience of percutaneous nephrostomy. Under these conditions it may be difficult to know what to do with the patient who is admitted to hospital as an emergency with uraemia due to bilateral compression of the ureters by infiltration from an *untreated* carcinoma of the cervix. This is an uncommon but not a rare situation which can be dealt with by first treating the uraemia and then using radiotherapy to reduce ureteric compression. It should be noted that in these cases the ureters are not at first infiltrated but are compressed. It must also be stressed that good results can only be obtained when the carcinoma of the cervix is untreated. The uraemia that results from recurrent carcinoma after full radiotherapy should in most cases not be treated at all.

If – as is often the case – the patient is unfit for open nephrostomy, which carries a much greater risk of bleeding during uraemia, ureteric catheterization from the bladder can be considered. This is usually impossible due to the obstruction and in any case cannot be maintained long enough to allow drainage until the ureteric obstruction disappears.

Ureterostomy in situ offers a simple alternative and need only be done on one side; the other kidney will survive until natural drainage begins again. This may occur shortly after radiotherapy starts.

STEPS OF OPERATION

Under general anaesthesia the patient lies supine on the operation table and an oblique muscle-cutting incision is made parallel to the inguinal ligament, the anterior superior spine lying about the middle of the incision. The peritoneum is not incised but is pushed medially so that a deep retractor can be introduced behind it.

The brim of the pelvis is identified and followed upwards and inwards until the distended ureter comes into view. It will be loosely attached to the back of the peritoneum which is lifted forward. This loose attachment is separated over a short distance so that a ring forceps can be placed around the dilated ureter. A small hole is cut just above the forceps with a pair of scissors and a long polythene tube is passed upwards through the hole to the renal pelvis. A bronchial suction catheter size 14 F is ideal. A balloon catheter may not be long enough. The retractor and ring forceps are removed and the wound closed with interrupted sutures through all muscle layers. The tube is attached to the skin by tape and the end attached to a closed drainage unit.

This provides a satisfactory temporary drainage which can be terminated when the ureter begins to function by simply removing the tube. It is, however, a known fact that once the disease has produced bilateral ureteric obstruction, the prognosis is extremely poor. Any irradiation is, in fact, palliative.

Occasionally the ureteric obstruction is found to be due to previously unsuspected massive lymph node metastases in the lumbar region. This makes the operation impossible and, in any case, the disease is then so advanced that uraemia must be seen as a welcome solution.

Uretero-ureterostomy

A situation can arise where, usually after injury to the lower part of one ureter, a ureteric stricture develops combined with uretero-vaginal or uretero-cutaneous fistula formation. If re-implantation of the ureter into the bladder for some reason cannot be done or has failed – for example because of irradiation damage, and the kidney and ureter on the other side are normal, then the gynaecologist may be tempted to do a simple ligation of the ureter above the brim of the pelvis. This may be justifiable in the presence of metastatic cancer, but can hardly be justified if life expectancy appears to be reasonably good. It may be better to consider an anastomosis of the affected ureter to the other ureter across the midline behind the peritoneum. This requires at least the whole length of the ureter which lies above the pelvic brim because it is always further than one thinks to the other ureter. The track must go forwards in front of the aorta and inferior vena cava and then backwards again to the other ureter. The track is made with a long curved forceps from the normal side and the ureter is drawn through. An end-to-side anastomosis is made with fine sutures. A drain is put in retroperitoneally from the anastomotic site to the flank by the shortest route. One must be aware that this operation does not always produce a fortunate result. The normal ureter can be adversely affected by stricture formation at the anastomosis and leakage from the anastomosis is not unknown.

Cutaneous ureterostomy

This can relieve obstruction of a ureter but is an operation which has a well-earned reputation for producing complications. The ureter is very liable to obstruction, either by kinking at the abdominal wall level or by stricture formation at the uretero-cutaneous junction. As a form of longterm drainage it can still perhaps be recommended for the patient in whom no other solution seems possible. Percutaneous nephrostomy is preferable to it, in that the tube drains better and it is easier to maintain.

Autotransplantation of the kidney

This method can be indicated when the ureter from a solitary kidney is inadequate and the bladder is still functional. It may well be preferable to an ileal conduit. It is carried out in the same way as a renal transplant. The complication rate is lower because there is no possibility of rejection.

Uretero-colic anastomosis

This method of urinary diversion has been superseded by the ileal conduit in most urological patients, but it can still be used with advantage in certain cases of advanced recurrent pelvic cancer with urinary fistula formation. The sigmoid colon and rectum must, of course, be intact. The expectation of life after it is not more than 3 years at the most in an elderly patient because of progressive renal failure. This is of little consequence if expectation of life is only about 1 year or less because of metastatic cancer. The operation can provide urinary continence for the remainder of life without the necessity of using any form of stoma which needs an external appliance. The principles of the operation are described below:

Find the ureters at the pelvic brim. Open the overlying peritoneum and dissect out about 10 cm of ureter below the brim. Divide the ureters and ligate the lower ends (Fig. 9.9).

Place the suture in the end of the ureter through all coats and load each end with a round-bodied curved needle.

Select the piece of sigmoid colon just above the rectum and place tissue forceps on a taenia adjacent to where ureter comes through the posterior peritoneum.

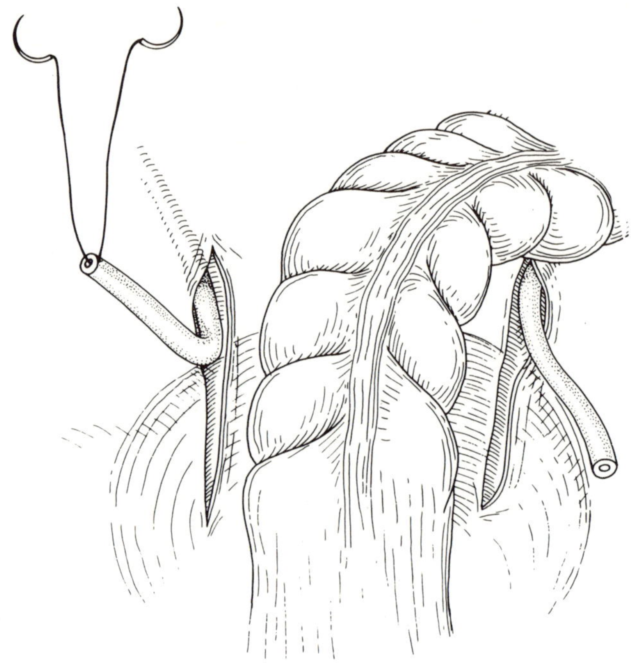

Fig. 9.9. Preparation of ureters before uretero-colic anastomosis.

Incise all coats longitudinally for about 3 cm. Make a small hole in the mucosa at the lower end of the incision.

Pass needles through the hole and out through the bowel wall about 2 cm below the opening. Tie these sutures loosely.

Close the channel with 2 or 3 sutures to bury the ureter for a distance in the wall (Fig. 9.10).

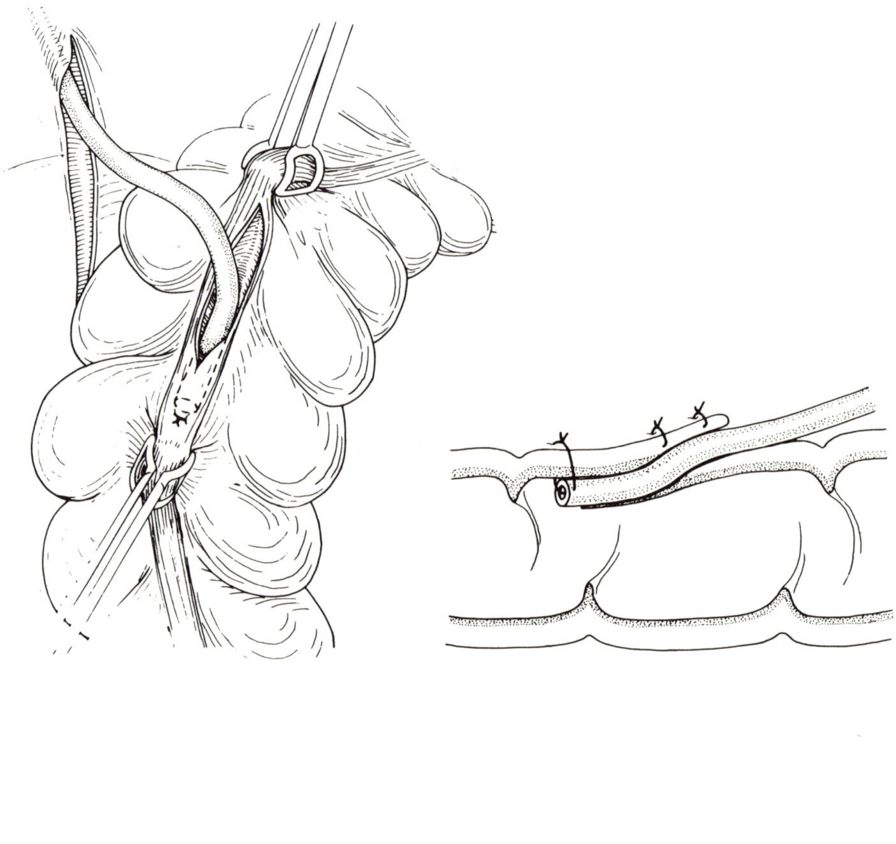

Fig. 9.10. The ureter is made to pass obliquely through a taenia and fixed with the suture which carries two needles. Indwelling ureteric catheters can be used as an added precaution against leakage.

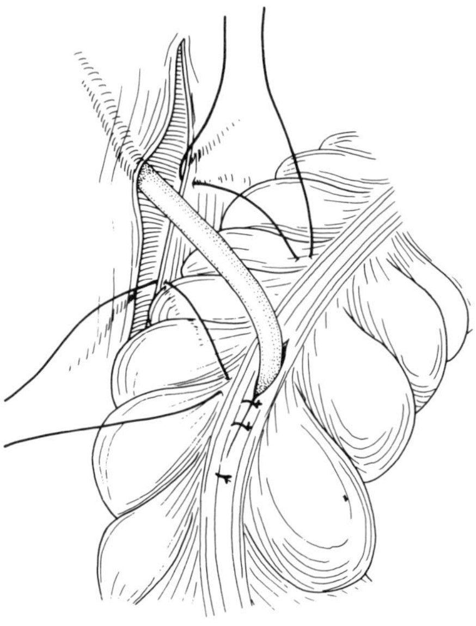

Fig. 9.11. The colon is then fixed to the posterior peritoneum to avoid tension.

Fix the edge of the posterior peritoneum to the adjacent colon. Fix the other edge of the peritoneum to the colon so as to extraperitonealize the anastomotic site (Fig. 9.11 and 9.12).

As in all other kinds of ureteric anastomosis the secret of success is avoidance of tension. In-dwelling ureteric catheters can be used as described under ileal conduit; they are not always necessary but are advisable if there is any doubt about renal function or if the pelvis has been irradiated. They are brought out through the anus and are retained for 6 to 8 days.

These patients tend to develop a hyperchloraemic acidosis because of the re-absorption of chloride and nitrogenous breakdown products.

Ileal conduit

This operation can be of great use in certain problem cases. It may be the only rational treatment of some large fistulae, especially after irradiation, and it is an essential part of an anterior exenteration operation. Gynaecologists will not usually be required to perform this urological operation, but they should understand the principles. Urologists have developed many sophisticated variations with minor differences in ureter implantation, how the sutures are put in, etc. The method which is illustrated is comparatively simple but has been found to be safe.

The day before operation mark where the ileostomy is to be made on the patient's abdomen while she is standing. Avoid the anterior superior spine and the belt area.

Choose a piece of lower ileum about 15 cm long (longer in fat patients) and isolate it as shown in Figs 9.13 and 9.14. The last 20 cm of ileum must be avoided because it is vital for reabsorption of bile products. Make sure that adequate blood supply is retained by identifying the vessels by transmitted light. Divide the mesentery from the lowest 5 cm of the bowel so that the ileostomy can be constructed.

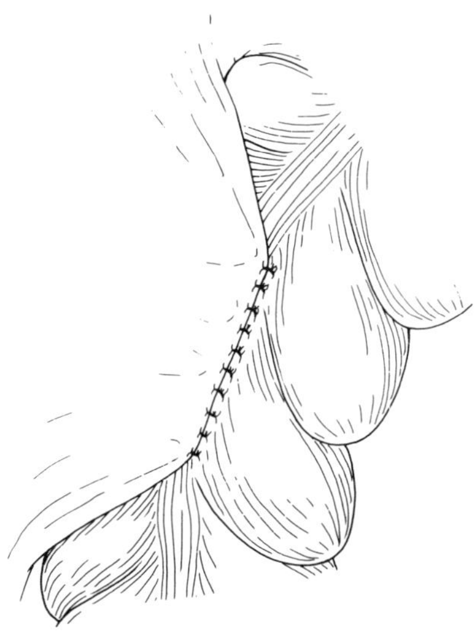

Fig. 9.12. The site of anastomosis is then covered with the other lip of posterior peritoneum.

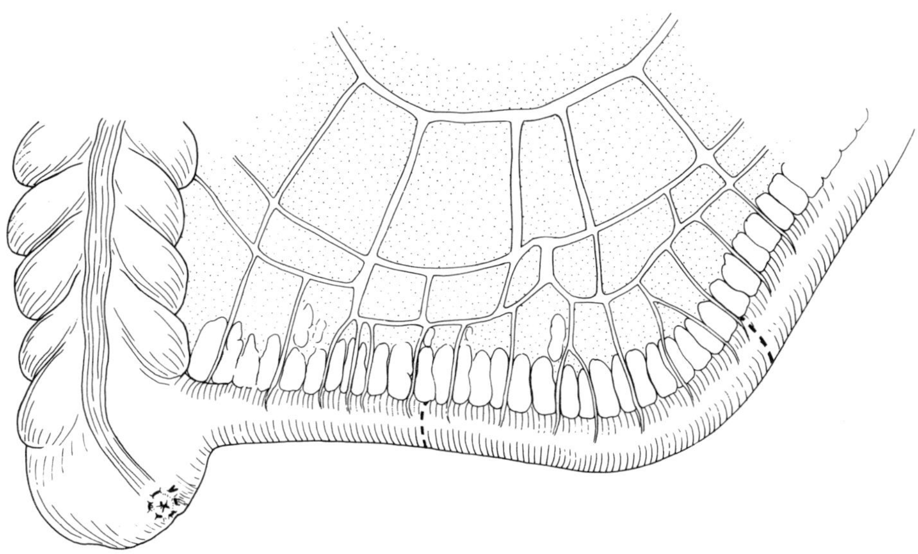

Fig. 9.13. The appendix is removed and a piece of ileum about 15 cm long is chosen.

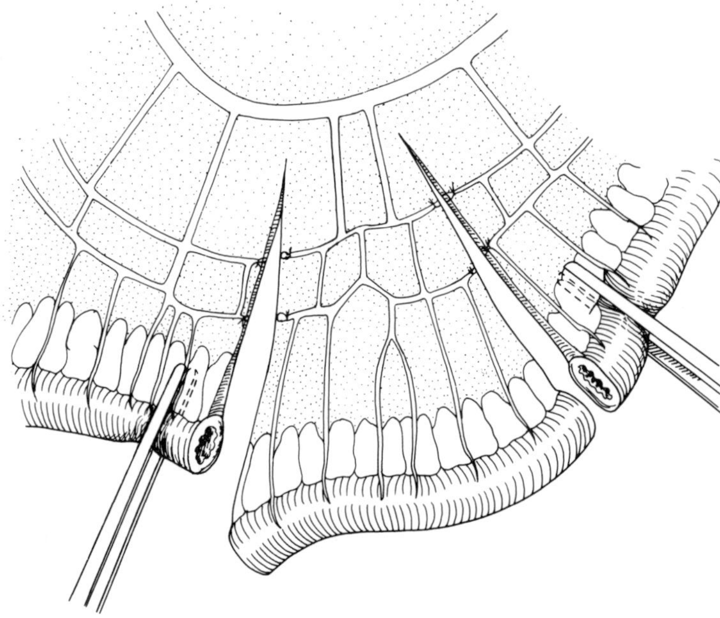

Fig. 9.14. The intestine is lightly clamped and then transected together with its mesentery, preserving 2 vessels at least.

Close the remaining intestine by end-to-end anastomosis and close mesentery (Fig. 9.15).

Close the proximal end of the isolated loop. Bring the ureters out through the posterior peritoneum to the right of the root of sigmoid mesentery so that they will easily reach the end of the isolated loop (Fig. 9.16).

Catheterize both ureters and put sutures in the ends. A needle is loaded on each end of each suture (Fig. 9.17).

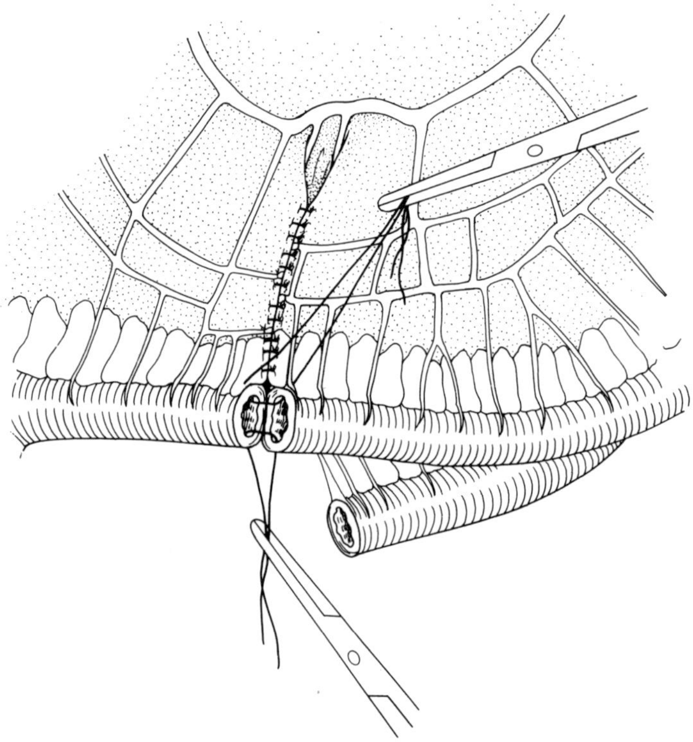

Fig. 9.15. The mesentery is sutured together and an end-to-end anastomosis of the ileum performed.

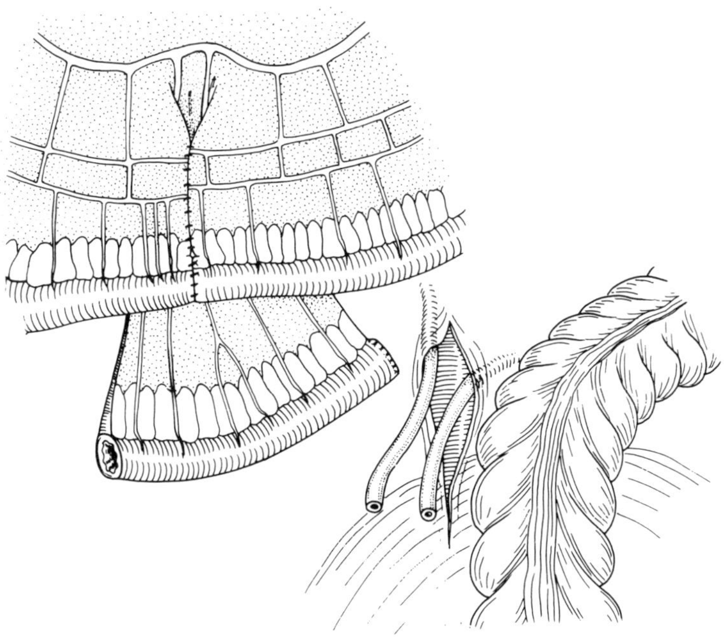

Fig. 9.16. The proximal end of the isolated loop is closed and the ureters are brought out through the posterior peritoneum so as to lie side by side.

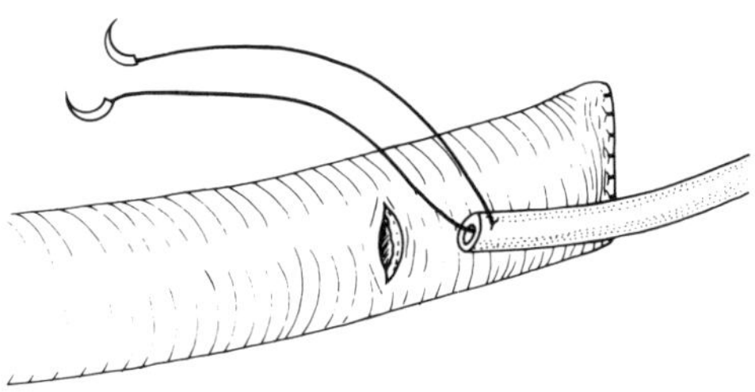

Fig. 9.17. A suture with a needle at both ends is placed in the end of the ureter and a small hole is made in the ileum.

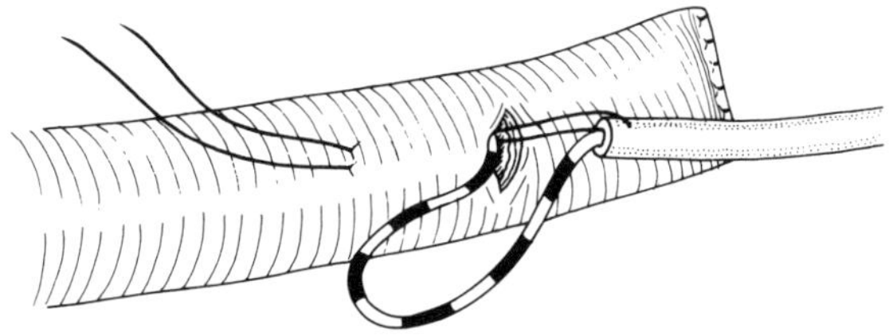

Fig. 9.18. The ureters are catheterized and the catheters threaded through the hole in the ileum. The sutures are put through the ileal wall from within.

Make two small holes transverse to the length of bowel and pass catheters and then sutures into the lumen of the bowel (Fig. 9.18). The needles are passed through the wall from within outwards about 2 cm below the openings and the sutures tied, thus fixing the ends of the ureters. There must be no tension. Close the holes in the intestinal wall with small sutures which do not pass through the ureter (Fig. 9.19).

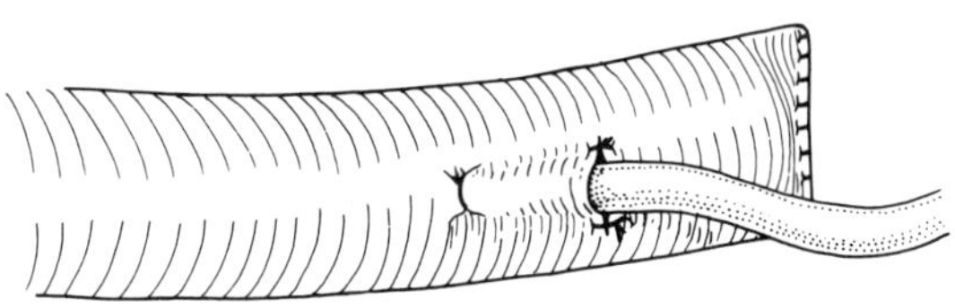

Fig. 9.19. The openings in the wall are closed with small sutures.

Fix the proximal end of the loop to the edge of the hole in the posterior peritoneum and suture the other edge of the peritoneum to the bowel wall so as to cover the ureters (Figs 9.20 and 9.21).

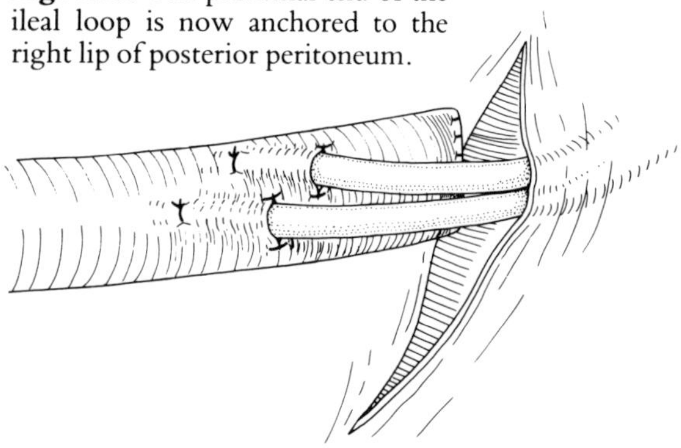

Fig. 9.20. The proximal end of the ileal loop is now anchored to the right lip of posterior peritoneum.

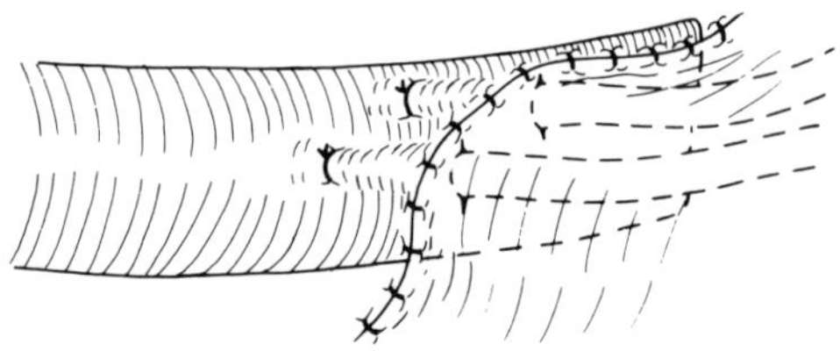

Fig. 9.21. The site of anastomosis is covered by the left lip of posterior peritoneum.

Make an opening in the parietal peritoneum of the abdominal wall to correspond with the mark on the skin (Fig. 9.22).

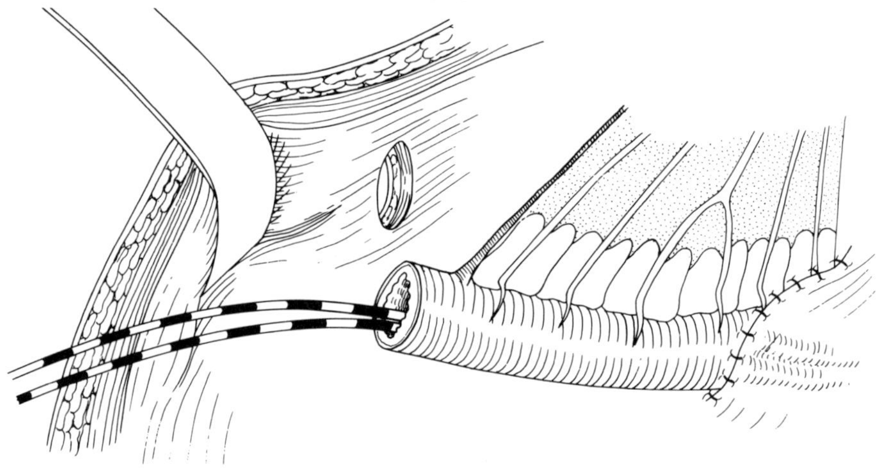

Fig. 9.22. An opening is made in the abdominal wall by removing a circle of tissue.

Pick up the skin where it is marked and cut out a circle 3 cm in diameter including fascia (Fig. 9.23).

Bring bowel and catheters out through the opening as shown.

Suture as shown and then turn down a cuff of wall and suture to skin around opening (Figs 9.24 and 9.25).

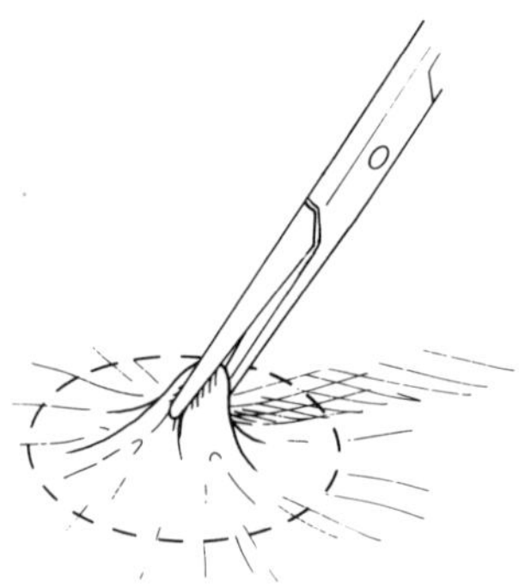

Fig. 9.23. A circular piece of skin is excised.

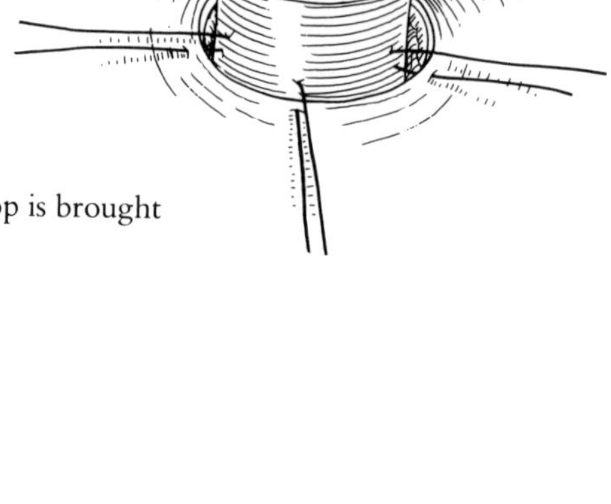

Fig. 9.24. The end of the loop is brought through the skin.

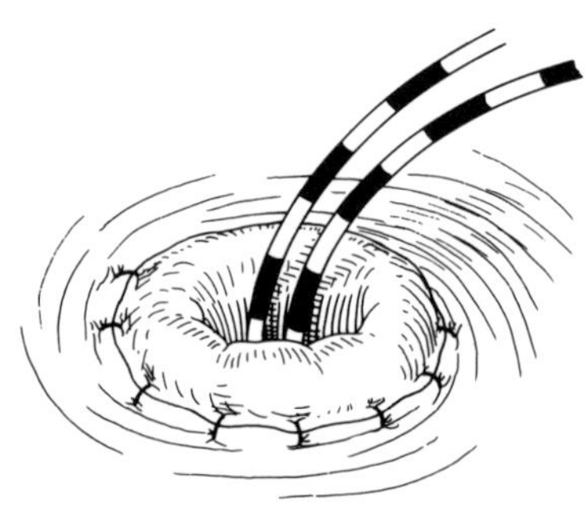

Fig. 9.25. The intestinal mucosa is sutured to the skin edge to form the ileostomy.

Open nephrostomy

The patient is placed on the table in the lateral position with the kidney to be operated on uppermost (Fig. 9.26). The patient's pelvis is fixed to the table by strapping so that the lower lumbar region of the back is vertical and the waist is over the place where the table can be broken or where the kidney rest is situated. The upper arm is lifted onto a support so that the back of the chest is also vertical. The table is now 'broken' so that the upper flank is put somewhat on the stretch. This must not be overdone; excessive lateral flexion is a great strain on the back, can compress the inferior vena cava and make inflation of the lower lung difficult.

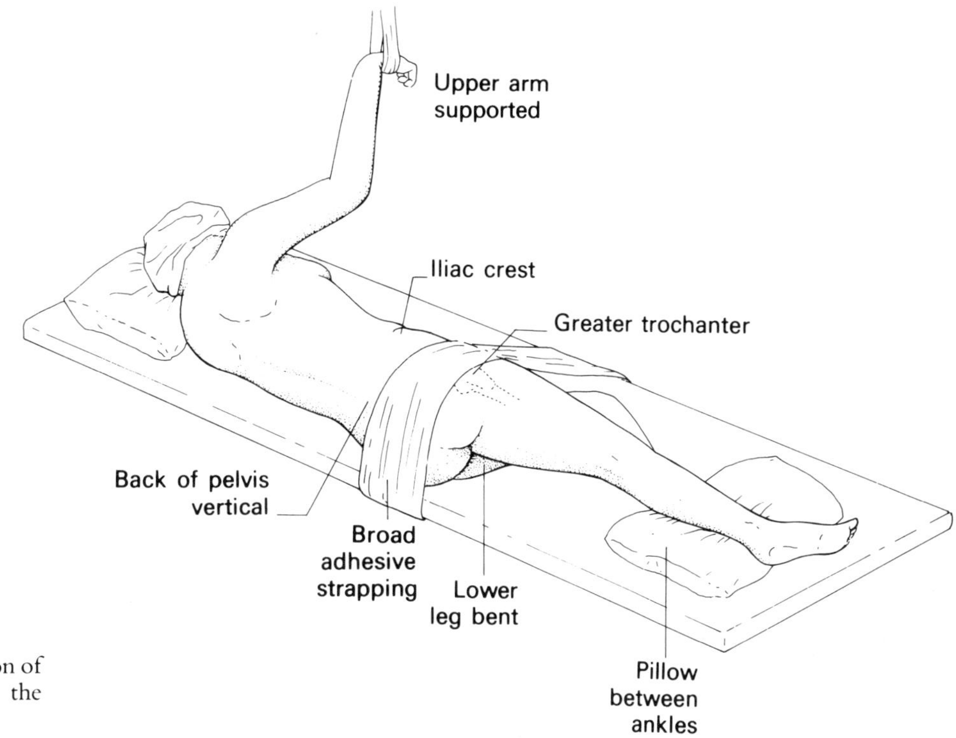

Fig. 9.26. Open nephrostomy: position of patient on operating table before the kidney bridge is raised.

An incision is made 1 cm below and parallel to the 12th rib from the lateral edge of the erector spinae muscle to the middle of the flank in the mid-axillary line. The muscles are divided in the line of the incision (Fig. 9.27). It helps to incise the lumbo-dorsal fascia just lateral to the erector spinae margin, and insert 2 fingers which separate the perirenal fascia and peritoneum from the inner aspect of the transversalis muscle before dividing the muscle in the line of the incision (Fig. 9.28). The 12th rib is then retracted upwards. The perirenal fascia is now divided just in front of the quadratus lumborum muscle and parallel to it (Fig. 9.29). This will be well behind the posterior limit of the peritoneum. The posterior leaf of the perirenal fascia is lifted up and the posterior aspect of the kidney freed from it by finger dissection. The renal pelvis lies posteriorly behind the main vessels and medial to the lower half of the kidney. The kidney should be turned forwards with the aid of a deep retractor so that two holding sutures can be placed in the renal pelvis (Fig. 9.30). The pelvis is opened with a knife blade

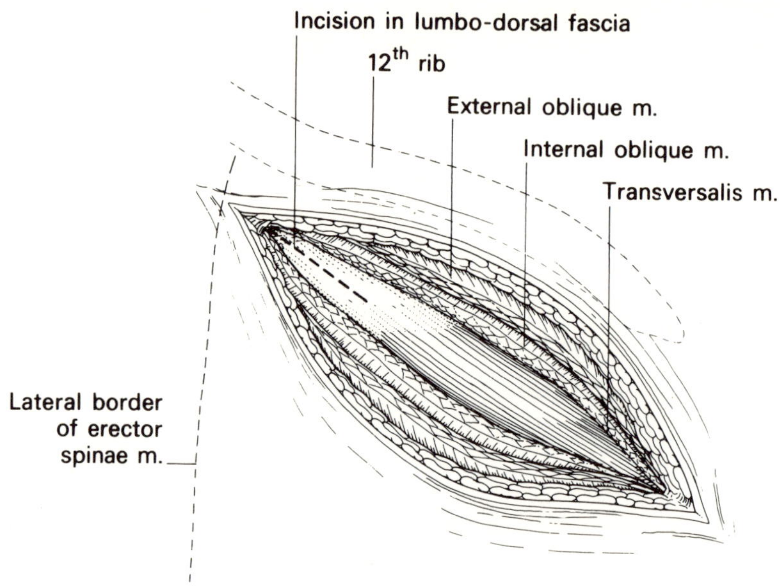

Fig. 9.27. Incision for open nephrostomy.

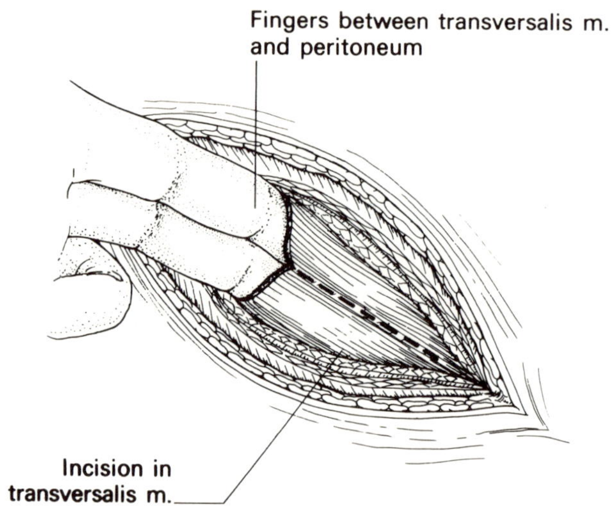

Fig. 9.28. Two fingers beneath the transversalis muscle help to guide the division of its fibres and to keep peritoneum out of harm's way.

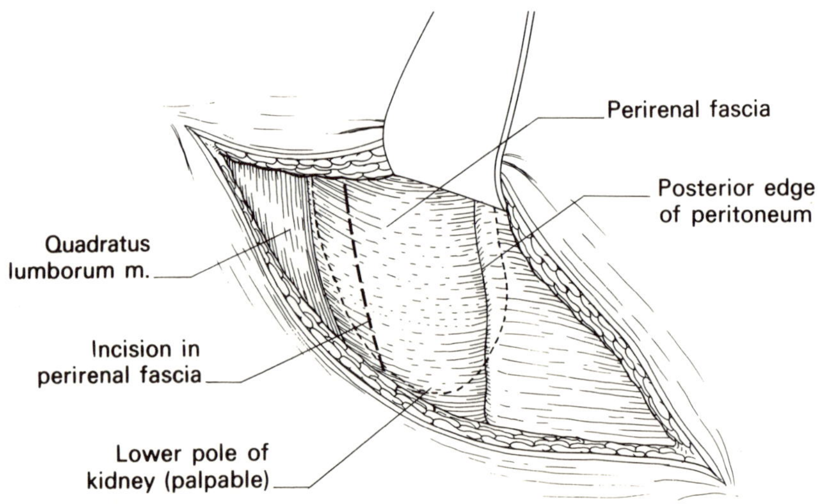

Fig. 9.29. Incision of perirenal fascia in order to expose the kidney.

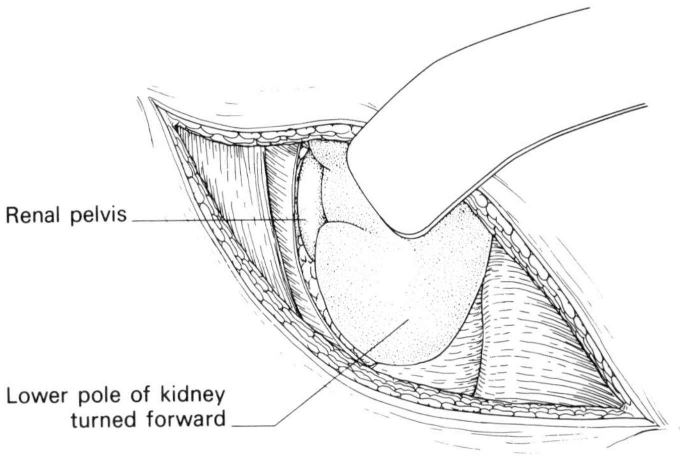

Fig. 9.30. The lower pole of the kidney is turned forward without lifting it out of the wound.

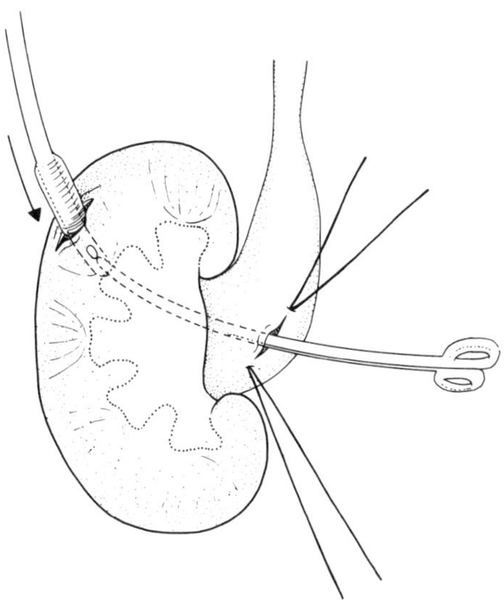

Fig. 9.31. Method of introducing the balloon catheter by drawing it into the pelvis by means of forceps passed from the pelvis outwards through a calyx.

between the sutures and the contents aspirated. A specimen of urine is taken for bacteriological examination. A curved ureteric stone forceps or similar thin well-curved forceps is passed through the opening in the renal pelvis, into a convenient calyx and out again through the renal substance and capsule. The end of a balloon catheter about size 16 F is then grasped in the blades of the forceps and pulled through the calyx into the renal pelvis. The balloon is inflated and the incision in the pelvis is closed by tying the holding sutures together (Fig. 9.31).

The bridge of the table is now lowered and the wound is closed by sewing the muscle layers with interrupted sutures. A drain is unnecessary because of the presence of the catheter.

The above description applies to operation on a kidney with a renal pelvis which is of normal size or nearly normal. In this case it is too dangerous to pass an instrument directly through the kidney substance into the pelvis because it is impossible to locate a calyx and the chance of damaging a large blood vessel is great. It is therefore necessary to expose the pelvis and open it so that an instrument can be passed from within outwards, this is the only safe way.

Nephrostomy by trocar and cannula

In many cases which the gynaecologist must deal with as emergencies, the kidney and renal pelvis are distended either by infected urine or by pus. This makes the operation much easier. If the surface of the distended kidney is palpated with a finger, thinner areas of the already thinned out parenchyma will be felt. These areas are really calyces. One of these which lies conveniently placed towards the lower pole and near the lateral border should be chosen and a trocar and canula size 20 F passed through it into the interior. If the surgeon is in doubt about the direction in which to introduce the instrument, he can allay his doubts by passing the fingers of the other hand behind the lower half of the kidney until he feels the distended pelvis. This gives him something to aim at. The trocar is removed and the purulent urine sucked out (a specimen should be taken for bacteriological examination). The canula is next removed and a balloon catheter, size about 16 F, introduced.

Surgeons often wonder why it is necessary to introduce the catheter through the kidney substance instead of directly into the renal pelvis. Experience has shown that a direct pyelostomy is difficult to maintain even with a balloon type catheter. If the catheter should come out it is quite impossible to put it back because the opening in the renal pelvis quickly closes or alters position. The track through the kidney substances does not do this so quickly, so that it is possible to change the catheter when necessary.

Consultation with a urologist

The urological operations described above are naturally best performed by a urologist. Their description is included here so that no gynaecologist finds himself in a helpless position if he cannot get urological help. The clinical course of urinary tract complications after pelvic operations can be extremely rapid if there is a combination of obstruction and infection.

REFERENCES

Blandy J (1978) *Operative Urology*. Blackwell Scientific Publications, Oxford.

Fernstrøm I, Andersson L (1977) Percutaneous puncture nephrostomy. *Encyclopaedia of Urology*, Suppl. 5. Springer Verlag, Berlin.

Swinney J, Hammersley DP (1963) *Handbook of Operative Urological Surgery*. Livingstone, Edinburgh.

Yeates WK (1965) Genito-urinary system. In *Clinical Surgery*, ed. Rob C & Smith R. Buttherworths, London.

Chapter 10 Gynaecological Cancer Surgery and the Lower Urinary Tract

'By all means cure them of their cancer, but don't do it by making them into urological cripples'.

This well-known saying draws a vivid picture of the quandary in which the gynaecological cancer surgeon finds himself. He must be radical without compromise if there is to be a real chance of curing the patient. At the same time he must avoid complications, especially urinary tract complications, which can very easily make the patient's life a misery or become so serious that they threaten her life.

Speaking generally, the frequency of complications in cancer surgery varies with the extent of the operation. If extensive surgery is combined with radiotherapy, the complication rates of both forms of treatment must be added to one another. There is then almost no way of avoiding some sort of trouble – the objective becomes the reduction of trouble to an acceptable level by all known means.

It is out of place here to discuss the pros and cons of radical cancer treatment. Suffice it to say that radical surgery has been proved to be capable of achieving results which can compete successfully with any other method. There are many clinics in the world where it is standard practice. A method of radical operation is described here which has been developed as a clinical research project. It is used to illustrate the pre-operative, operative and post-operative precautions which are necessary to protect the lower urinary tract from injury.

A more detailed definition of gynaecological cancer surgery consists of:

Primary radical hysterectomy with lymph node dissection.
Extended hysterectomy.
Total vaginectomy.
Anterior exenteration i.e. radical hysterectomy with lymph node dissection with cystectomy and urinary diversion.
Posterior or total pelvic exenteration.
Removal of central recurrence with or without lymph node dissection.
Removal of big malignant pelvic masses (for example, ovarian tumours).
Vulvectomy.

PRIMARY RADICAL HYSTERECTOMY WITH LYMPH NODE DISSECTION

THE WERTHEIM, OKABAYASHI OR MEIGS OPERATION

This operation is performed in many countries under the name of Wertheim's operation. It is named after the Viennese surgeon, Ernst Wertheim, who, at the beginning of this century, was the first to systematize the method. It was by no means so extensive as the modern operations described by Okabayashi and by Meigs. All surgeons develop their own more or less individual variations as a result of education, experience, technical skill and research.

The operation will be described in detail because it is the key to many of the other operations in gynaecological cancer surgery in so far as they involve danger to the lower urinary tract. The special urological problems are best overcome if the various steps in the operation are carried out systematically. If a surgeon has understood and mastered the steps of this operation, he will be equipped to deal with any of the difficulties involving the lower urinary tract which may crop up in simpler gynaecological operations. The manoeuvres which involve opening up the 'dry spaces', the exposure of the vessels near the pelvic wall and the removal of fat which obscures the operative field can all sometimes be of great use in the commoner operations. He is also equipped with a much more detailed knowledge of pelvic anatomy which gives him confidence and makes possible improvization, if this is necessary.

Long-lasting absorbable sutures and ligatures are used throughout the operation. The only exception to this is where vascular sutures are occasionally necessary and here we use the usual atraumatic sutures.

The operation consists of extirpation of the uterus (with or without adnexectomy) including the uterine ligaments or retinacula and a part of the vagina, together with the pelvic lymph nodes up to the aortic bifurcation and including the external iliac and obturator nodes. The surgeon has to dissect the bladder free from the anterior wall of the uterus and vagina and to dissect free the last 10 cm of the ureter before it enters the bladder.

This is a difficult operation which requires detailed knowledge of pelvic anatomy and its variations. The surgeon must especially understand how the so-called 'dry' spaces are disposed in the pelvis and it is an advantage to work to a standardized series of operative steps which follow one another in a logical manner, the next step always based upon the successful execution of the previous one.

Previous gynaecological infections such as salpingitis, tubo-ovarian abscesses, infection in the tumour with lymphatic reaction, or lymph node metastasis with direct infiltration into the surrounding organs, can make this operation extraordinarily difficult and occasionally impossible. The risk of complications is certainly increased and the surgeon must realize this and be prepared to stop before he has gone too far.

A 'lateral approach' from the pelvic wall is used so that the dissection starts as far away from the tumour as possible by displaying the dry spaces and removing lymph nodes. The lateral approach is the key move in the operation because it allows the logical display of detailed pelvic anatomy which makes the later steps of the operation so much easier. Removal of the lymphatic drainage field early in the operation also ensures that there is no spread of tumour cells above the pelvis as a result of surgical manipulation. The risk of bleeding is minimized because the major vessels are secured near the pelvic wall at an early stage. It also enables the surgeon to isolate the autonomic nerve supply and the blood supply to the bladder and to preserve them as much as possible. Above all, it facilitates the dissection of the ureters so that damage is easier to avoid.

Preoperative preparations

Pre-operative intravenous urography should always be performed unless the patient is allergic to iodine. In this event, isotope renography is used. The object is to discover pre-existing ureteric abnormalities such as hydroureter or double ureter and to have a standard of comparison for post-operative pictures.

Local infection and tumour necrosis increase the risk of post-operative pelvic infection considerably. Antibiotics (including metronidasol) should be given for as many days as necessary. The tumour should be treated locally both by antibiotics and a suitable antiseptic solution for 2 days before the operation.

Packing the vagina in order to facilitate dissection of the bladder and ureters is not advocated because the packing occupies valuable space in the lower pelvis and is unnecessary if the surgeon utilizes the lateral approach. After the vaginal toilet is completed, the urethra is disinfected by squeezing in some antiseptic gel and a small balloon catheter is passed into the bladder, which is emptied. In addition, 50 ml of 0.01% aqueous chlorhexidine is put into the bladder for 10 min to counteract post-operative infection. Some surgeons will wish to put a little methylene blue into the empty bladder to make possible damage more obvious. The catheter is attached to a sterile closed drainage apparatus and must be allowed to drain continuously during the operation.

The patient is then laid supine on the operating table.

Step 1. Incision and exploration

A midline incision extending from the symphysis pubis to above the umbilicus is generally used (Fig. 10.1). A low transverse incision with or without division of the recti (the so-called Pfannenstiel incision) may give inadequate exposure in the region of the common iliac arteries especially if something goes wrong. After opening the peritoneum, the pelvis and abdomen are explored. The stage and operability of the tumour is confirmed by gentle intrapelvic palpation.

A search is made for pelvic or lumbar lymph node metastases. If there is doubt about an enlarged gland, a frozen section is advisable. The cause can be earlier pelvic inflammatory disease, reaction after a lymphogram or reaction to infection in the tumour in addition to the presence of metastasis. If the para-aortic or common iliac nodes are found to contain tumour metastasis, experience shows that radical lymph node dissection has no purpose.

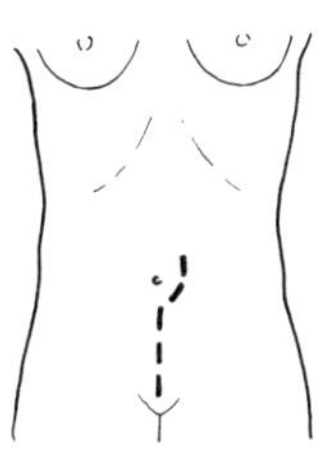

Fig. 10.1. Mid-line incision extended upwards alongside the umbilicus as a paramedian incision.

However, under these circumstances, and with the abdomen open, it is well worth while removing the primary tumour by doing an extended hysterectomy if this is possible without cutting through tumour tissue. This operation has a low urinary complication rate and post-operative radiotherapy is not significantly delayed. Also, one avoids local radium insertion in the cervix and can concentrate radiotherapy on an unshielded chimney field straight away.

Step 2. Opening pelvic peritoneum

The table is tilted head-down about 10° and the small intestine packed off. Care should be taken not to pack too tightly because this compresses the inferior vena cava and increases venous pressure in the pelvis. This in turn produces oozing during the whole operation from the exposed wound surfaces. Forceps are placed on each side of the uterus and the bladder is held up out of the way by a stitch to the skin at the lower end of the abdominal wound (Fig. 10.2). The round ligament and infundibulo-pelvic ligament are ligated and divided as in a standard hysterectomy, this means not too far laterally so as to preserve enough peritoneum to cover the bare area afterwards. Here care is needed to avoid the ureter at the pelvic brim (Fig. 10.3). The incision in the peritoneum is continued upwards alongside the infundibulo-pelvic ligament around the brim of the pelvis. The medial leaf of the peritoneum is reflected medially and the ureter is identified loosely attached to its deep aspect.

Step 3. Identification of paravesical and pararectal dry spaces

The peritoneum between the bladder and the uterus is divided and the round ligament is lifted up so that the index and middle fingers of each hand can be inserted back to back to open up first the paravesical and then the pararectal 'dry' spaces right down to the pelvic floor. These are called 'dry' because they consist of loose connective tissue and fat into which the bladder and rectum can expand.

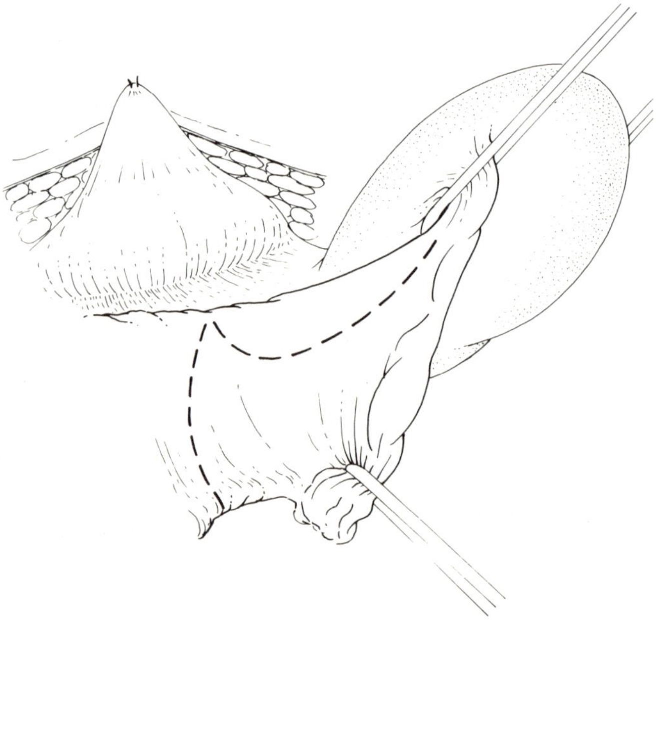

Fig. 10.2. Forceps are placed on either side of the uterus which is pulled upwards and to the right. The bladder is held out of the way by a holding suture attached to the lower end of the abdominal wound. The dotted line shows the line of incision in the broad ligament. Only the upper part is used if the ovaries are to be preserved. This is an important argument in favour of the operation in young women.

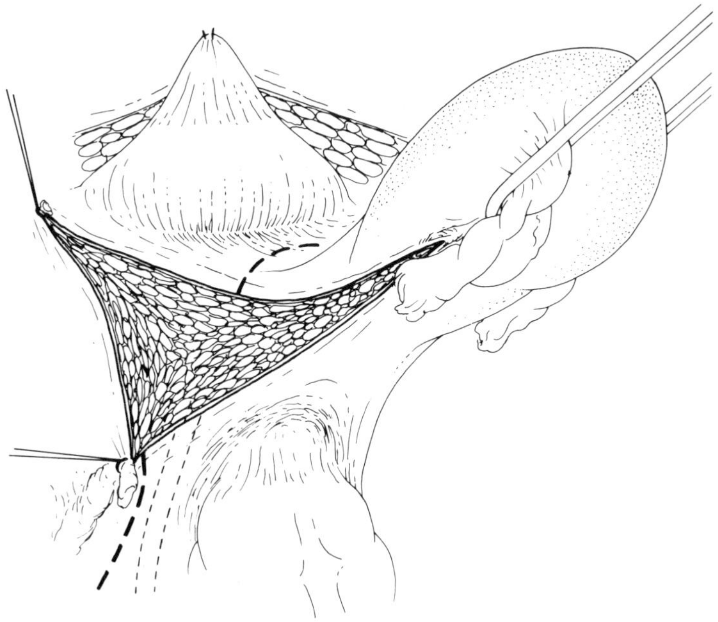

Fig. 10.3. Incision in peritoneum prior to opening paravesical and pararectal dry spaces. The ureter is identified at the pelvic brim. The peritoneum between the uterus and the bladder is also divided as far as the mid-line. In this case the ovaries are not preserved.

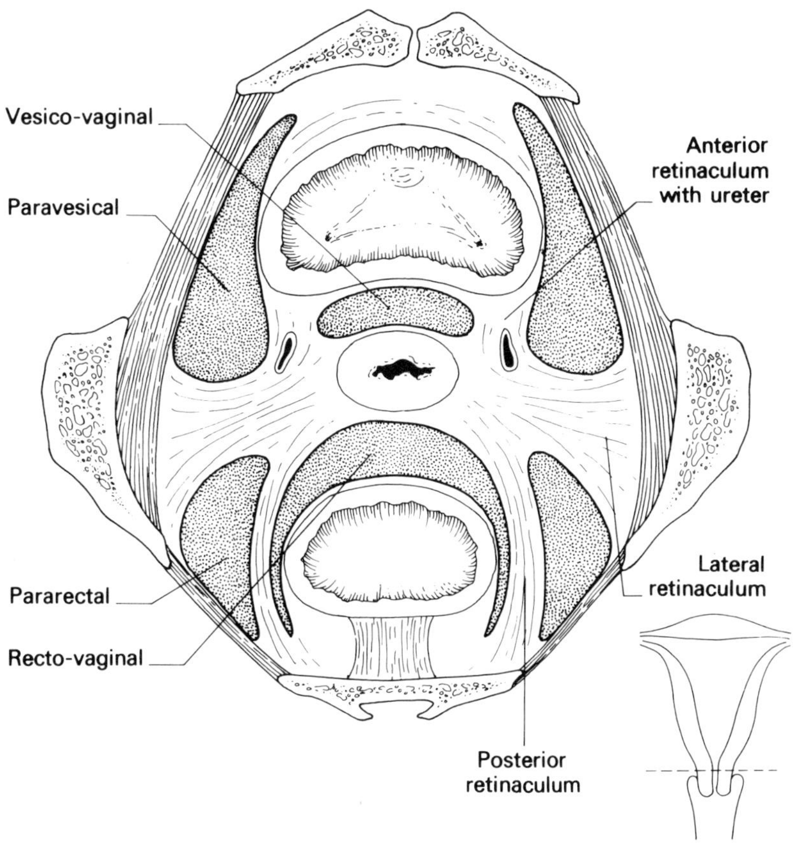

Fig. 10.4. Diagrammatic cross-section of the pelvis at the level of the cervix which shows the so-called 'dry spaces' with the anterior, lateral and posterior retinacula between them.

There are no major vessels to bleed. These two spaces are separated by the lateral part of the three retinacula which hold the uterus in position in the pelvis. This structure has acquired many names such as Mackenrodt's ligament, the cardinal ligament, the web, etc. We prefer the term lateral retinaculum because it is not a ligament but consists of a complex collection of blood and lymph vessels and the autonomic nerve supply to the genital and urinary tracts surrounded by fat.

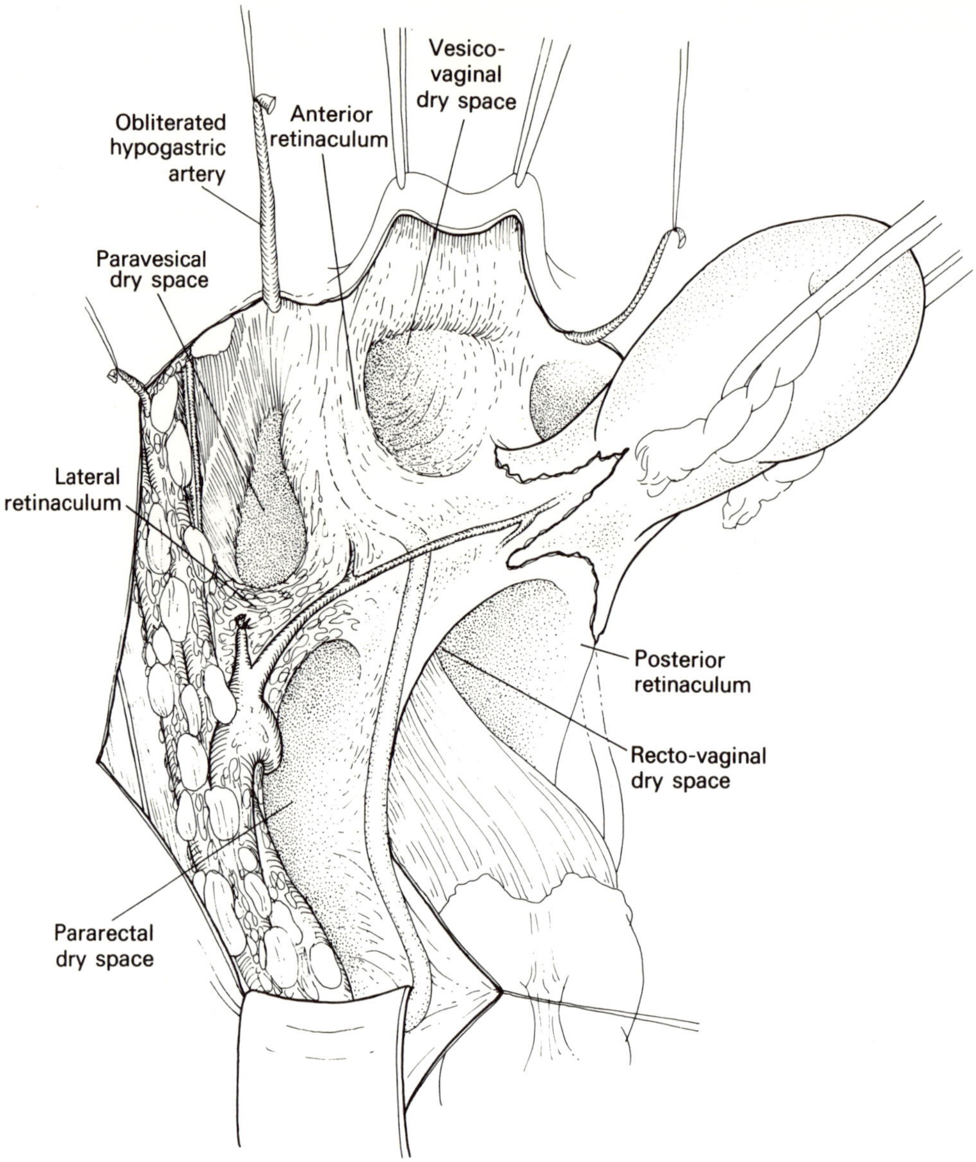

Fig. 10.5. The dry spaces on the left side as seen at operation with the uterus lifted upwards and to the right. The spaces have been cleared of fat and the obliterated hypogastric artery ligated and divided. Note how the ureter is pulled up by the uterus as it passes along the posterior retinaculum, under the uterine artery and into the anterior retinaculum.

The gross anatomy of these spaces and of the retinacula is shown in Figs 10.4 and 10.5. Figure 10.6 shows the attachment of the lateral reinaculum to the pelvic wall.

Step 4. Identification of the major blood vessels

The first move is to find the obliterated hypogastric artery and loosen it with forceps from the lateral vesical wall to which it is attached. It can then be followed back to the point where the uterine artery takes origin. If fat is gently removed by ring forceps from around this point, the arterial division is easily visualized and quite often shows a little branch going to the bladder. It is wise not to ligate the vessels at this stage because the ligatures will be endangered during the lymphadenectomy (Fig. 10.7).

The common and external iliac arteries and their accompanying veins are dissected free from the psoas muscle and pelvic wall by cutting through the pelvic fascia on their lateral aspect and continuing downwards by blunt finger dissection along the lateral pelvic wall until the obturator nerve is seen (Fig. 10.8). There is

Fig. 10.6. Site of attachment of lateral retinaculum to the pelvic wall. The dotted line shows the level of cross-section in Fig. 10.4.

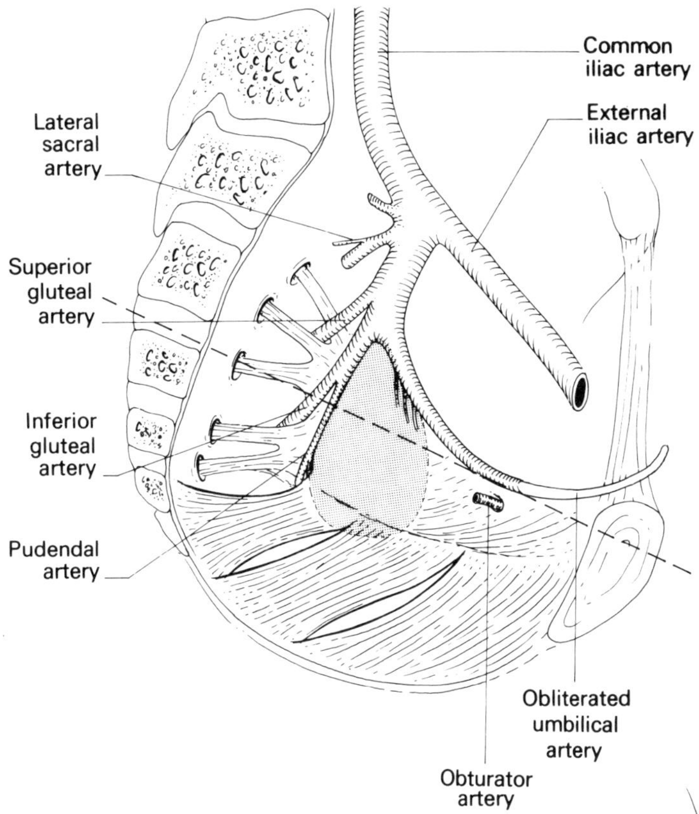

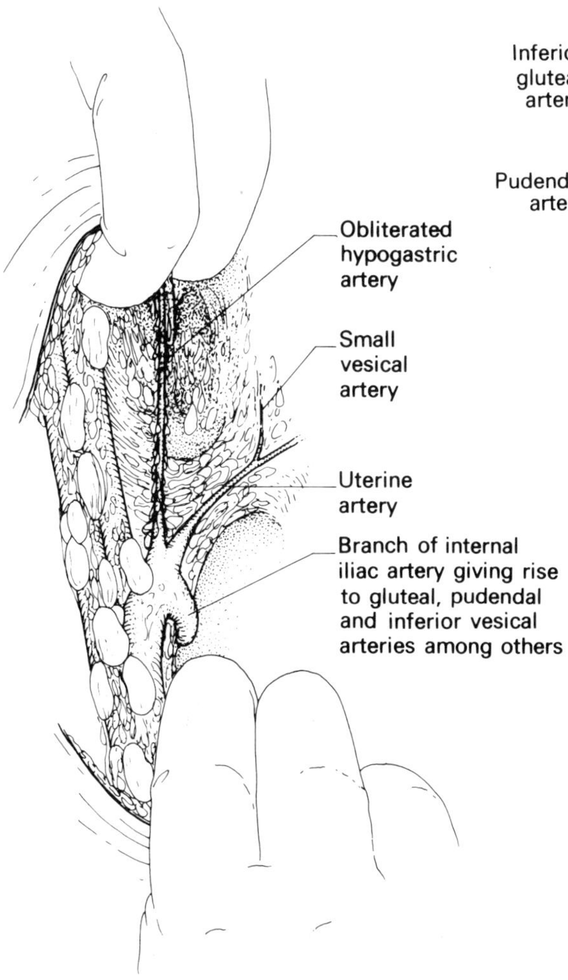

Fig. 10.7. Exposure of the branches of the internal iliac artery and the paravesical and pararectal dry spaces.

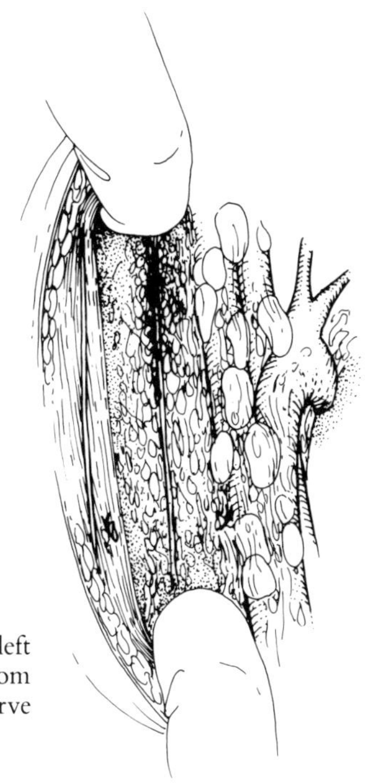

Fig. 10.8. Mobilization of the left common and external iliac arteries from the pelvic wall so that the obturator nerve comes into view.

often a little artery with accompanying vein which supplies the psoas muscle from the lateral side of the big vessels. This must both be ligated and divided, otherwise one can tear holes in the vessels. The common iliac vein is thin walled and has small tributaries which sometimes bleed when it is separated from its surrounding lymphatic tissue. This can usually be stopped by light pressure with a swab. If, however, this does not help because the hole is too big where the tributary has been torn from the main vein, it must be sutured using interrupted vascular sutures.

Step 5. Lymphadenectomy

The iliac lymph nodes are now removed by dividing the lymphatic bundle where the common iliac artery divides (Fig. 10.9). The upper end of the bundle of lymph vessels containing the common iliac nodes is then removed as far up as the aortic bifurcation (Fig. 10.10). This is facilitated if the assistant holds the caecum or sigmoid colon together with the ureter up out of harms way with a curved retractor. There is otherwise a danger that the ureter might be grabbed by the ring forceps. Removal of the lymph nodes is done as much as possible en bloc and, apart from the common iliac group, does not involve danger to the lower urinary tract (Figs 10.11, 10.12, 10.13).

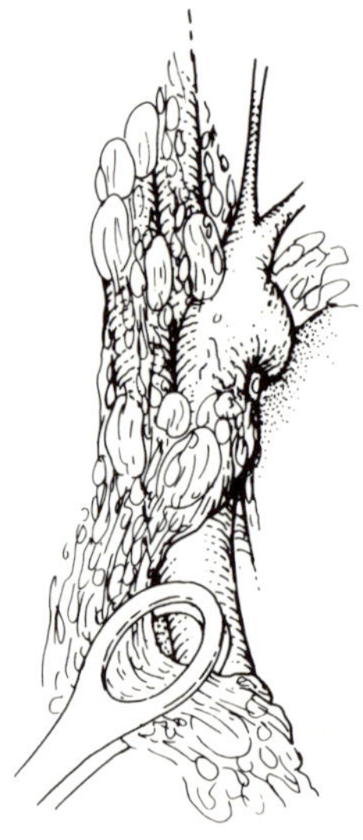

Fig. 10.9. The bundle of lymph vessels and nodes is picked up with ring forceps and divided at the level of the division of the common iliac artery.

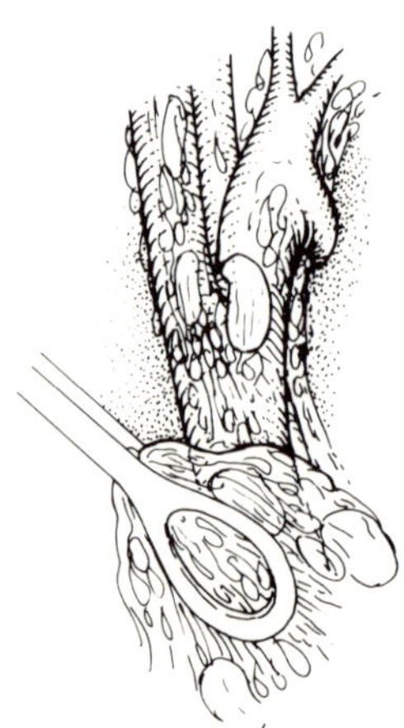

Fig. 10.10. The upper end is dissected in an upward direction. The ureter must be identified here, otherwise it may be grabbed by the ring forceps.

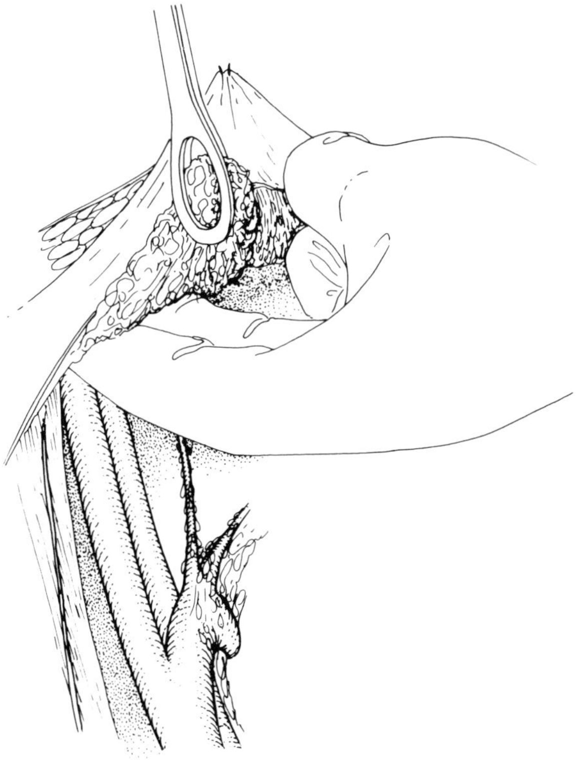

Fig. 10.11. The external iliac nodes are then removed as far as the inguinal ligament.

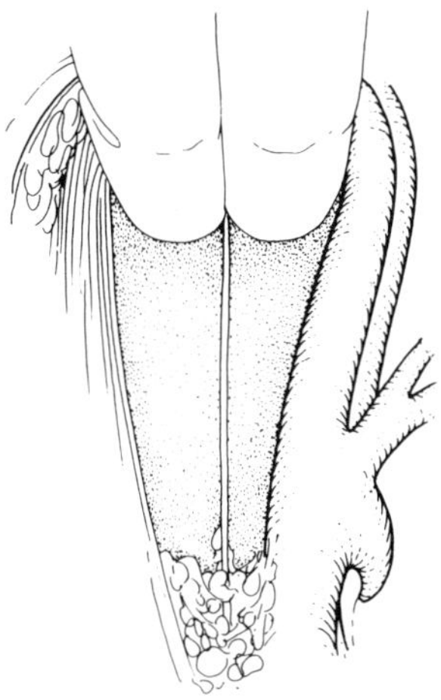

Fig. 10.12. Fat and lymphatic tissue is stripped from the obturator nerve.

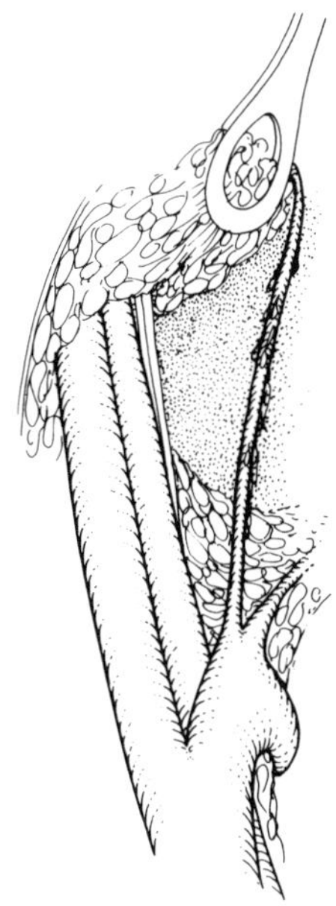

Fig. 10.13. The bundle is then pulled behind the iliac vessels and removed with the almond-shaped gland in the femoral canal.

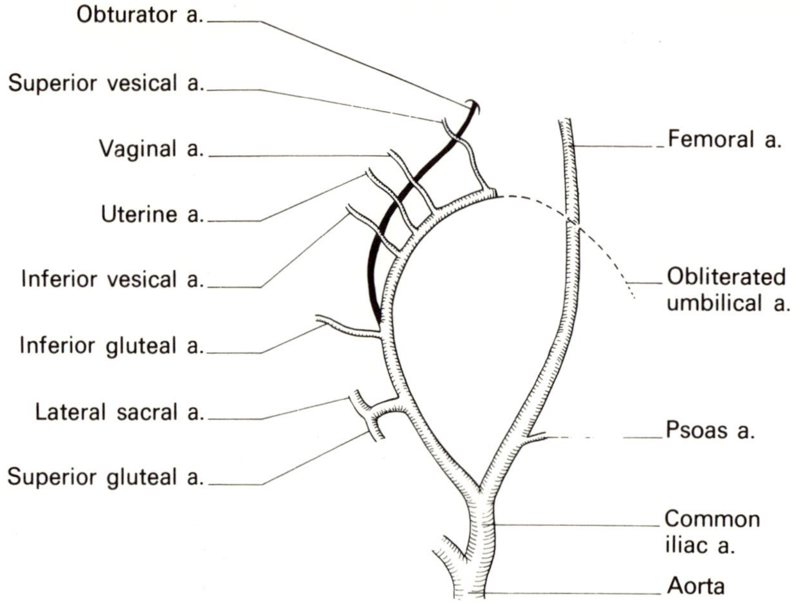

Figs 10.14, 10.15 and 10.16. Arterial distribution in the pelvis is very variable, particularly the origin of the obturator artery.

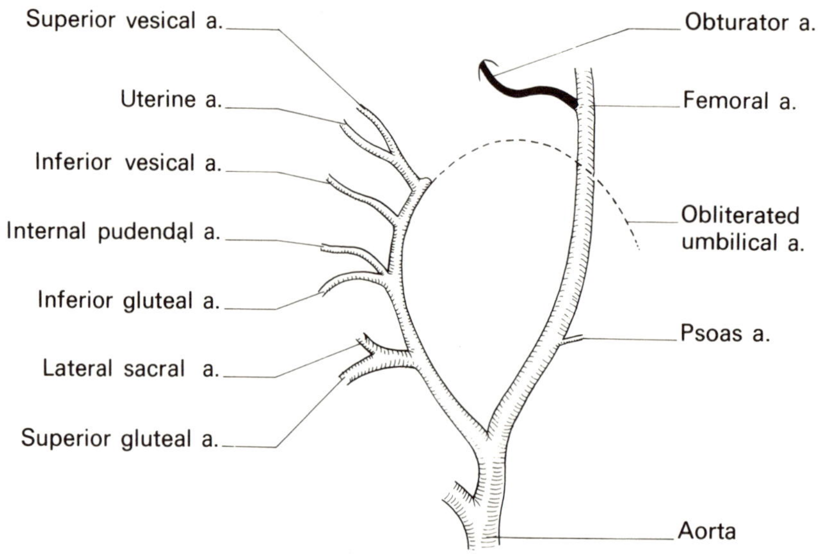

Fig. 10.15.

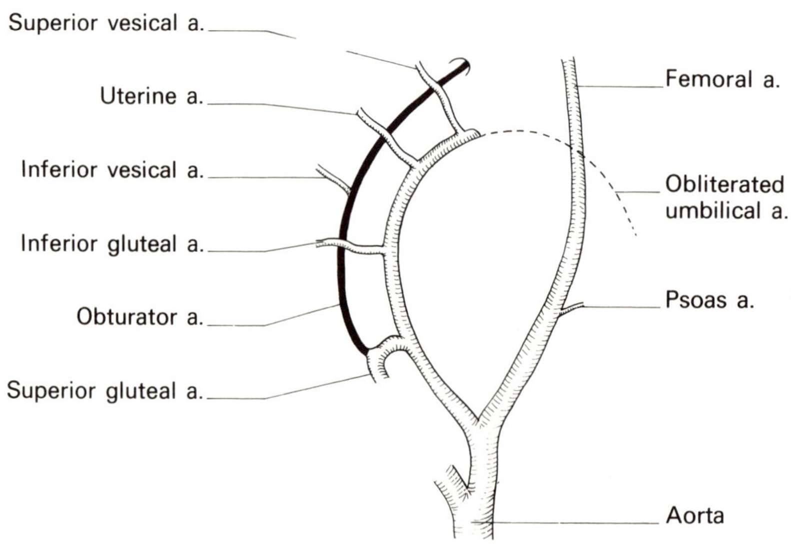

Fig. 10.16.

There is always a little bleeding, but this is readily controlled by light packing for a few moments. Any major bleeding is of course stopped by ligation. The en bloc technique may leave some smaller nodes behind. These are found and removed in the next step at the same time as dissection of the lateral retinaculum and removal of the perivesical and perirectal fat. The pre-sacral lymph nodes are removed at a later stage when the operation is nearly finished.

Step 6. Vascular ligation with dissection of the lateral retinaculum

There is great variation in the detailed vascular supply to the pelvic organs, but the following description will cover most situations. The greatest variation occurs in the obturator vessels but these can safely be doubly ligated and divided if they interfere with the dissection (Figs 10.14, 10.15 and 10.16).

The obliterated hypogastric and the uterine arteries have already been identified so they are now ligated and divided (Fig. 10.17). The superior vesical artery is therefore included in this and there is sometimes but not always a smaller branch which supplies the lower lateral wall of the bladder. This is also ligated because its preservation would interfere with an adequately radical dissection and its value as regards the lower end of the ureter is very doubtful. Ligation of the internal iliac (hypogastric) artery higher up is not recommended because this might interfere with the important blood supply to the bladder via the inferior vesical artery. This latter artery hugs the pelvic wall in its course and does not come in the way of the dissection. The same applies to other smaller arteries to the bladder and vagina

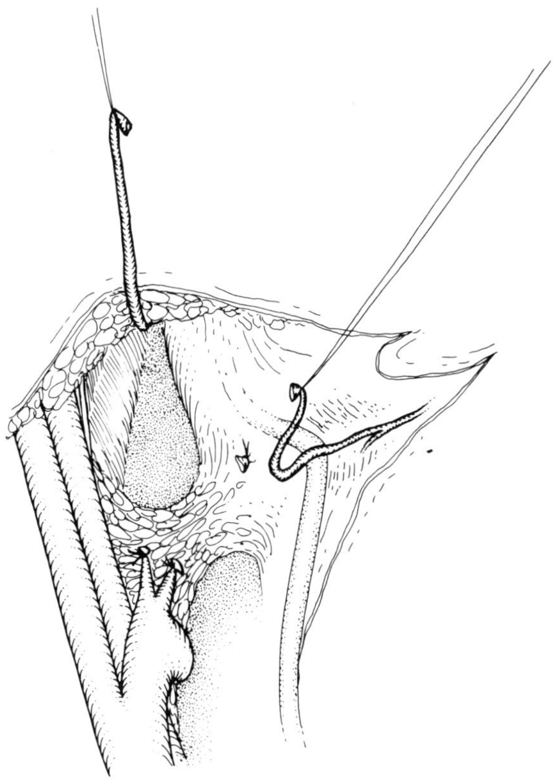

Fig. 10.17. The obliterated hypogastric and uterine arteries have been ligated and divided.

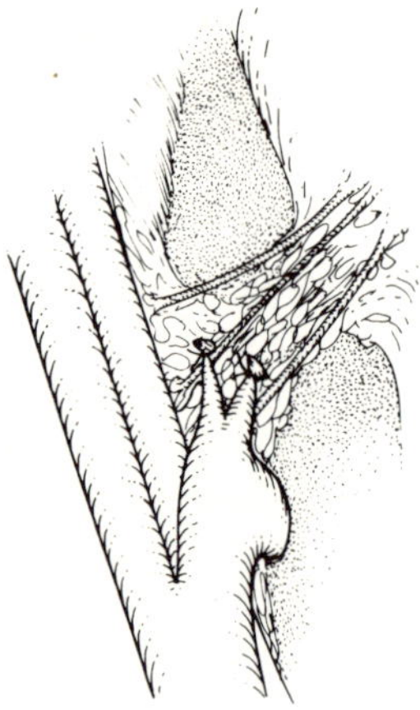

Fig. 10.18. Exposure of the veins in the anterior retinaculum. They are ligated individually.

which pass through the lowest part of the lateral retinaculum together with the main autonomic nerve supply to the bladder. Once the arterial ligation is completed all paravesical, paravaginal and pararectal fat is gently removed down to the levator ani muscles, leaving the rest of the lateral retinaculum a well-defined structure passing from the pelvic wall and floor to the uterus.

The next stage is meticulous dissection of all fat from this structure, gradually revealing the uterine veins and some veins which drain the bladder and vagina. These are usually 3 or 4 in number and sometimes large. We recommend ligation and division of these veins one by one (Fig. 10.18). The ligatures are placed as far laterally and medially as possible. This greatly facilitates later dissection of the ureter by avoiding unexpected venous bleeding in this region. This bleeding is a major problem for many surgeons and certainly one of the most frequent causes of ureteric damage. This can be avoided by patient and gentle removal of fat so that the veins are adequately displayed. This enables the ligatures to be placed right next to the organs from which the veins come—the uterus, vagina or bladder. The ureter is under vision and out of danger during this step. Some minutes spent over this manoeuvre will be saved many times over later on by the avoidance of troublesome bleeding in a region adjacent to the lower ureter.

During the dissection the surgeon may be able to discover and preserve additional arterial supply to the bladder if it exists.

Anatomical studies of the lateral retinaculum show that the middle part consists of veins, lymphatics and small arteries and a few lymph nodes (Fig. 10.19). The nodes are not visualized on foot lymphograms, either because they do not take up contrast or because they are so small. We still do not know if they drain the bladder or uterus or both, or what their significance is as regards

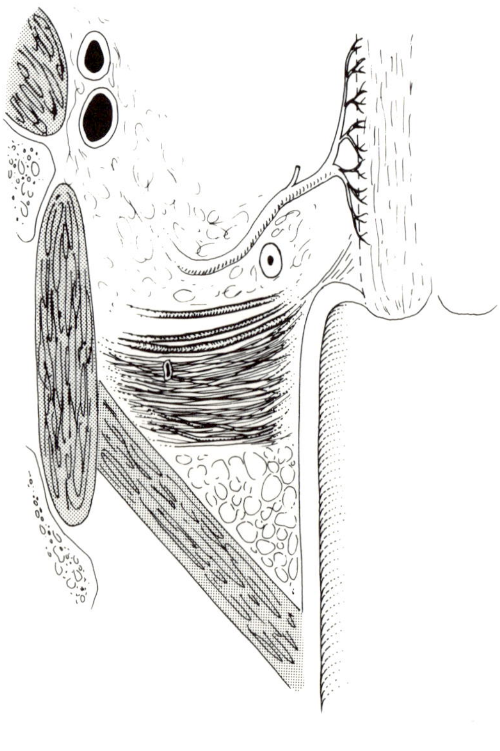

Fig. 10.19. Diagramatic cross-section of the lateral retinaculum showing the uterine artery in the upper part, the uterine and vaginal veins in the middle and the part of the hypogastric plexus which supplies the bladder and urethra in the lower part together with the inferior vesical artery.

carcinoma of the cervix. Patients can have metastases on the pelvic wall without these small nodes being involved. In any case they must be removed so that the excision can be satisfactorily completed.

While the lateral retinaculum is being dealt with, the hypogastric plexus gradually comes into view as a well-defined structure which must be treated with the utmost respect for it contains the main autonomic nerve supply to the bladder and urethra. It must be preserved as intact as possible because it supplies organs which are not going to be removed (Fig. 10.20). Figure 10.21 shows how the autonomic nerve supply divides into three parts, rectal, genital and a part to the lower urinary tract.

Damage to the whole hypogastric plexus is an unpleasant complication of radical hysterectomy due to clamping and cutting the whole retinaculum near the pelvic wall. This destroys most of the blood, and all the nerve supply to the bladder (Fig. 10.22). An atonic bladder with residual urine has been the commonest complication after the radical operation, but this can be avoided by preservation of the hypogastric plexus as described above. We do not believe that there is any other significant nerve supply to the bladder because bilateral excision of this plexus inevitably leads to a completely atonic bladder, lack of bladder sensation and retention with overflow incontinence. It is important also to realize that stretching and rough handling will seriously interfere with the subsequent function of the plexus.

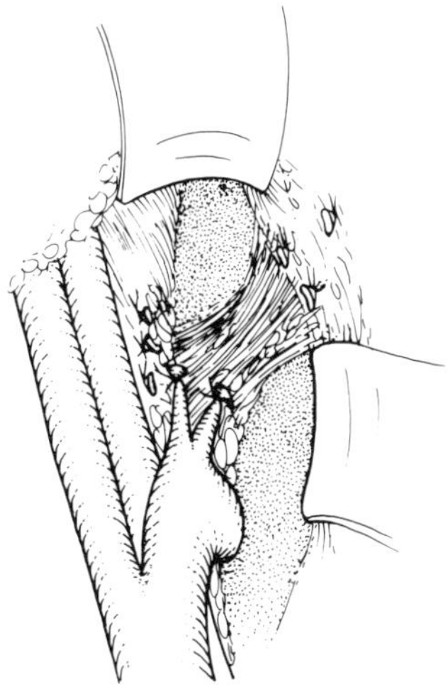

Fig. 10.20. After ligation of the veins as laterally and medially as possible, the part of the hypogastric plexus which supplies the lower urinary tract comes into view.

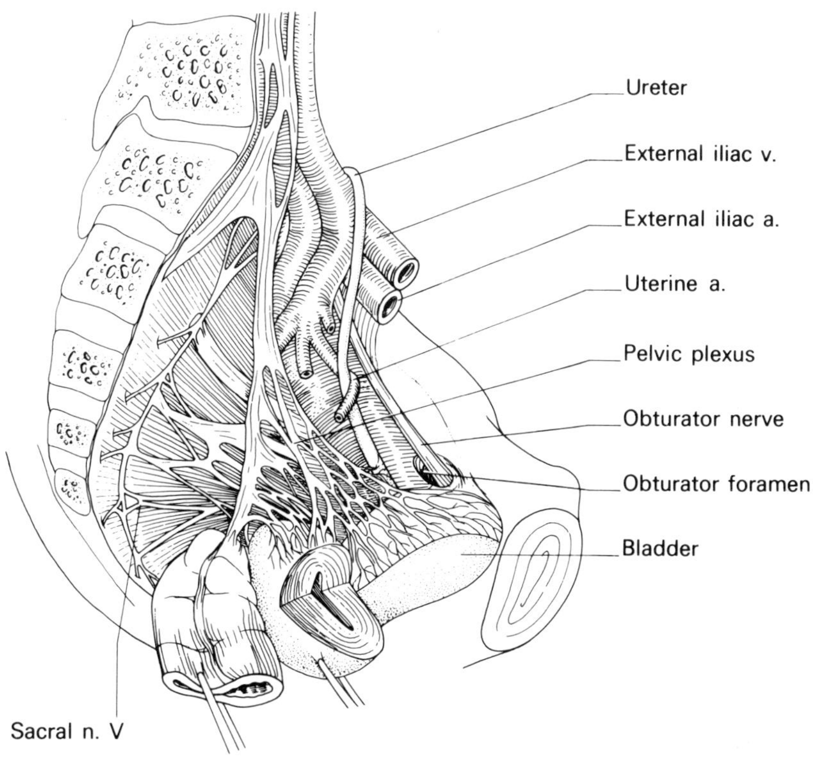

Fig. 10.21. Diagram of the autonomic nerve supply to the pelvic organs.

Step 7. Dissection of the bladder and ureter

The peritoneum over the bladder is now held up by 2 pairs of forceps and divided transversely where it is reflected from the uterus onto the bladder. The bladder is then lifted up and dissected free from the uterus and the upper 4–5 cm of the vagina in the region of the mid-line (Fig. 10.23). Blunt dissection is never used; the surgeon uses scissors all the time to divide bladder wall from the white fascia over the vagina. He must keep outside the thin perivesical fascia and thus avoid exposing bladder muscle. The bladder is freed as far as the upper part of the trigone. If any bladder muscle is left attached to the vagina, it is a sign that the surgeon is in the wrong layer. If he is in the right layer there is seldom any major bleeding so that this can, in fact, be termed the third 'dry space'. It is however, not quite so dry as the paravesical, the pararectal and the recto-vaginal spaces. This dissection of the bladder from the vagina can be extremely difficult in patients who have undergone conisation, Caesarian section or vaginal repair.

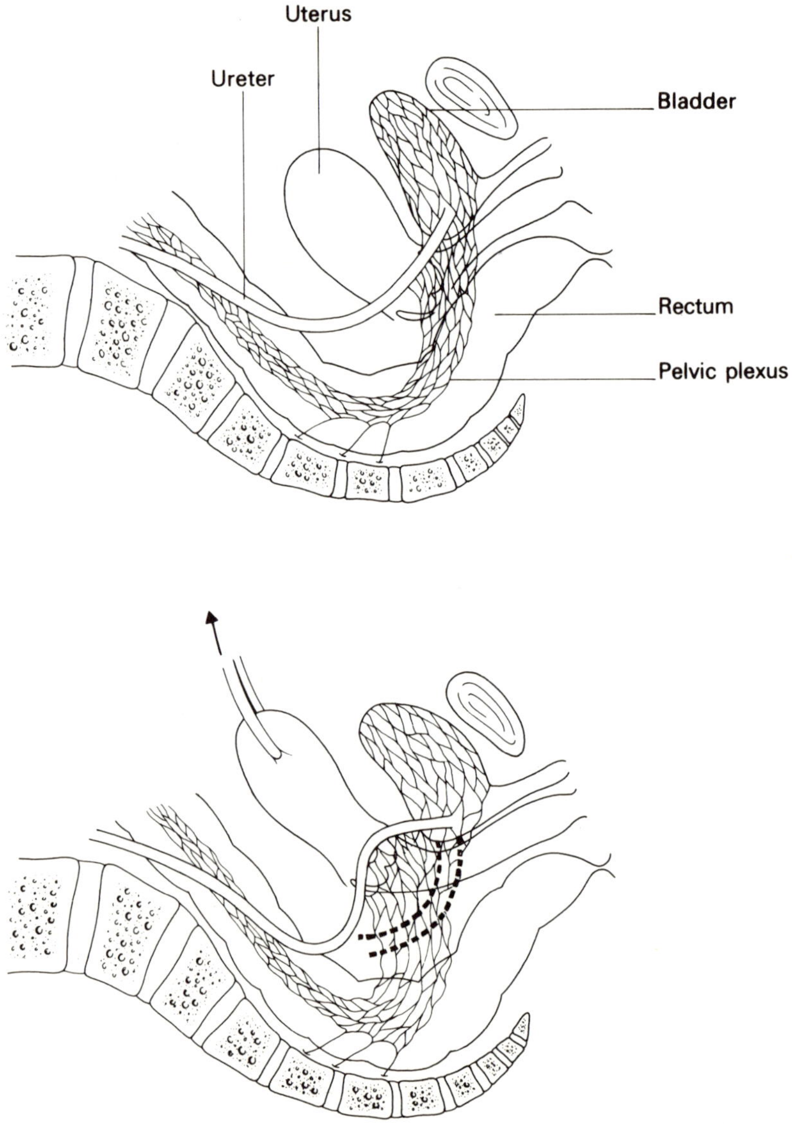

Fig. 10.22. Diagram of the nerve supply to the lower urinary tract showing how it is pulled upwards with the ureter when the uterus is lifted out of the pelvis. It can be severely damaged by clamping or by being stretched if it is not carefully dissected out.

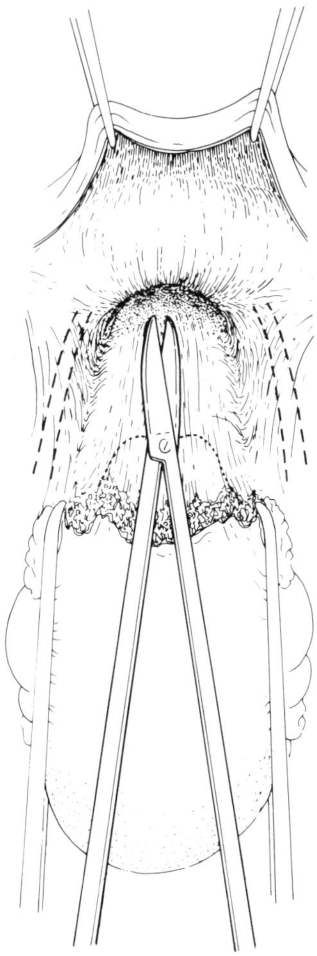

Fig. 10.23. Separation of bladder wall from uterus and vagina near the mid-line by sharp dissection. This opens the vesico-vaginal dry space and displays the anterior retinaculum containing the ureter on each side.

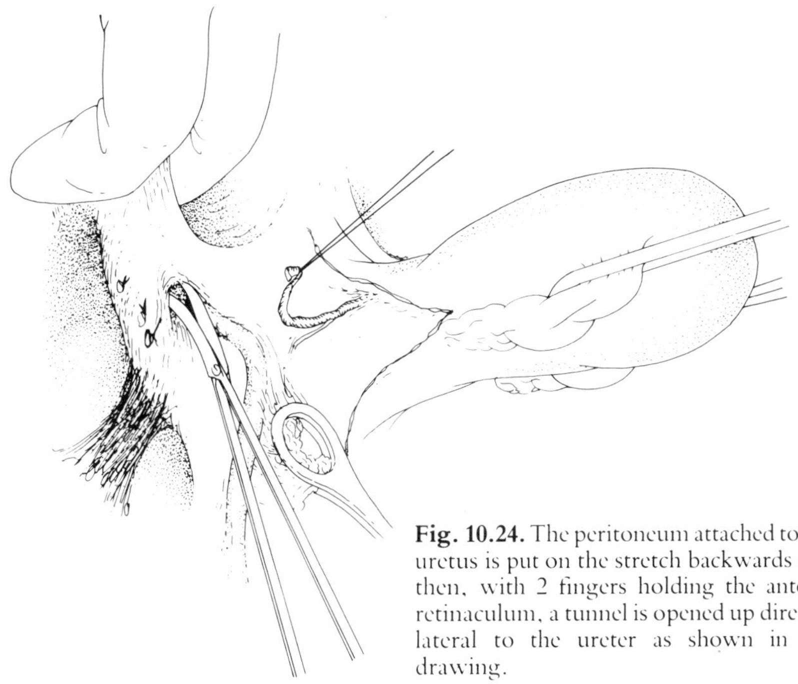

Fig. 10.24. The peritoneum attached to the uretus is put on the stretch backwards and then, with 2 fingers holding the anteior retinaculum, a tunnel is opened up directly lateral to the ureter as shown in the drawing.

When this mid-line dissection is completed the anterior retinaculum, also called 'the bladder pillar' or 'the vesico-uterine ligament', is beautifully demonstrated. It consists of fibro-muscular tissue and contains the ureter just before it reaches the bladder. The ureter cannot be seen here but it can be felt between the finger and thumb to divide the retinaculum into a superficial and a deeper part. During the next dissection, in which a tunnel is made alongside the ureter on its lateral side, the surgeon can always reassure himself about the safety of the ureter by feeling it. The ureter is put a little on the stretch by pulling the peritoneum to which it is attached, backwards (Fig. 10.24). Long curved forceps are then passed down on the lateral side of the ureter by opening and closing the blades and the tunnel so formed is opened by cutting down its lateral wall. This can be done with minimal arterial or venous bleeding because most of the vessels have already been ligated.

The anterior retinaculum is lifted up between two fingers so that a forceps can be passed through it just above the ureter into the vesico-vaginal space (Fig. 10.25). The forceps is left in position and the part of the retinaculum above it is divided.

This leaves a little tissue directly anterior to the lower end of the ureter just before it enters the bladder. This tissue is considered to be important because it seems to prevent kinking of the ureter after the operation and also may play some part in preserving its nutrition.

Next, the ureter is completely freed from the uterus and vagina on its medical aspect and from the deeper part of the retinaculum down to the bladder wall (Fig. 10.26). The bladder muscle should not be damaged and the ureter should not be stripped by traumatic blunt dissection. The periureteric fascia must be maintained intact. The hypogastric nerve plexus and the inferior vesical artery are under vision all the time and should not be damaged. Steps 2, 3, 4, 5, 6 and 7 are now performed on the other side.

Fig. 10.25. The anterior retinaculum is lifted up between two fingers and a forceps passed through just above the ureter into the vesico-vaginal space. The forceps is left in position. The smaller figure shows how the ureter divides the anterior retinaculum into a superficial and a deep part. It is divided along the dotted line.

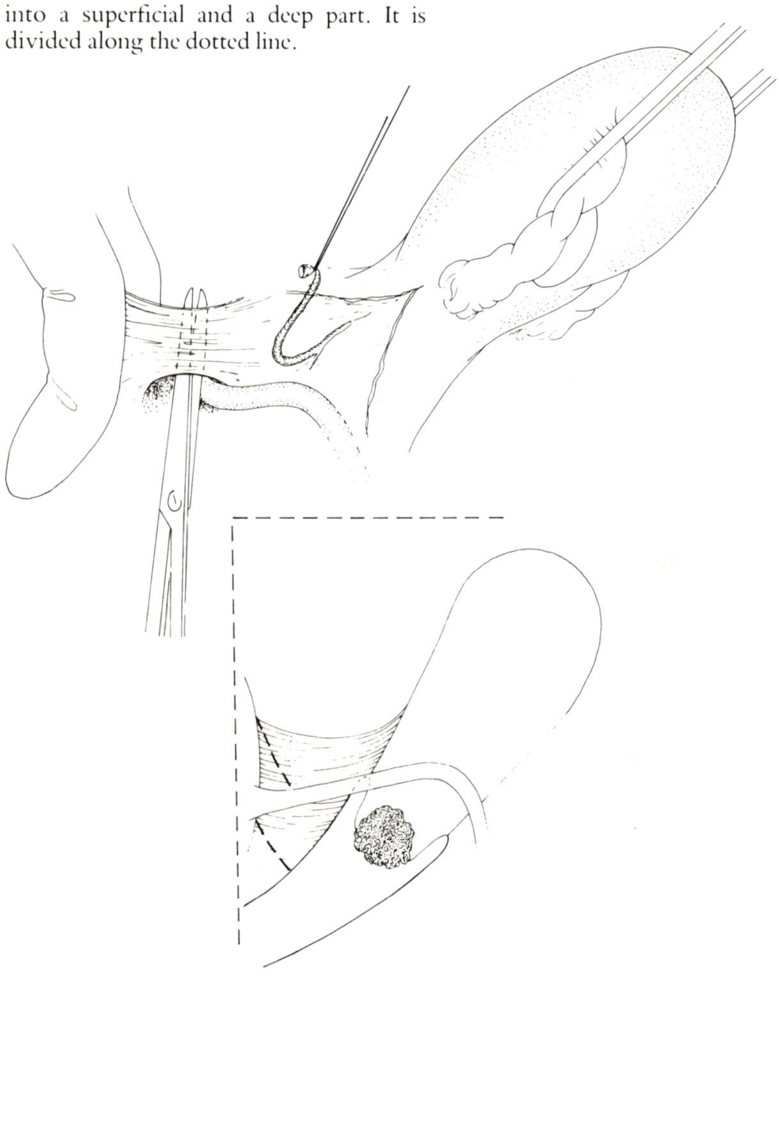

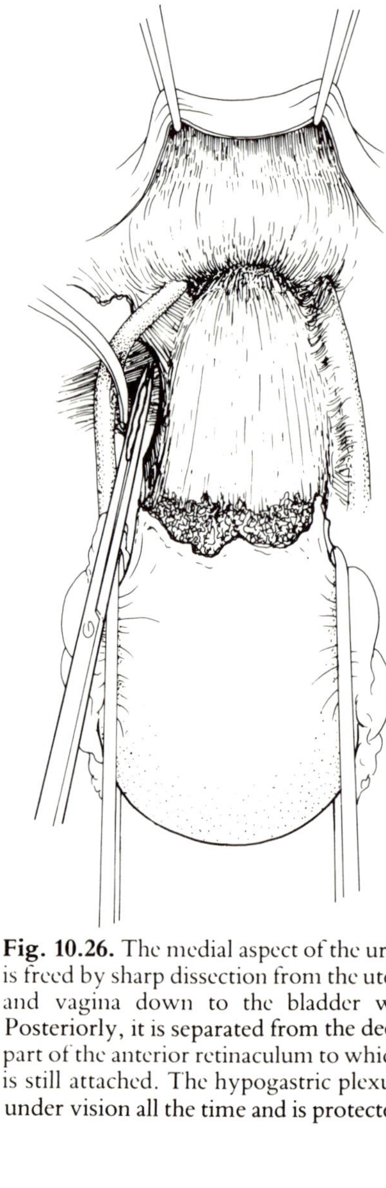

Fig. 10.26. The medial aspect of the ureter is freed by sharp dissection from the uterus and vagina down to the bladder wall. Posteriorly, it is separated from the deeper part of the anterior retinaculum to which it is still attached. The hypogastric plexus is under vision all the time and is protected.

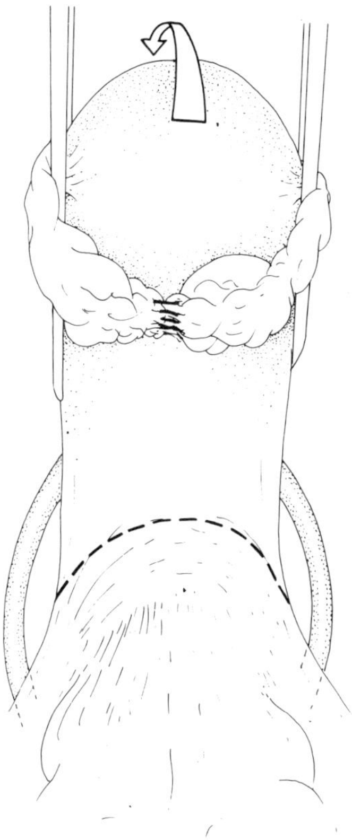

Fig. 10.27. The rectum is drawn upwards and the uterus forwards. The ureter is left attached to the peritoneum. The peritoneum is divided along the dotted line to open the recto-vaginal space.

Step 8. Mobilisation of rectum and division of the posterior retinaculum

The most hazardous parts of the operation as regards the lower urinary tract are now accomplished. The next step is to draw the rectum upwards with slight tension. This has the effect of putting the peritoneum on the stretch. The peritoneum is then divided along a line shown in Fig. 10.27, so that the ureter is left attached to the medial leaf as much as possible. It is only loosened from the peritoneum in about the last 10 cm of its course.

The posterior retinaculum is now gradually exposed by blunt dissection as the structure lying between the pararectal and recto-vaginal dry spaces and reaching down to the pelvic floor. It is also called 'the sacro-uterine ligament', and consists of fibro-muscular elements and the nerve supply to the uterus (mainly sympathetic fibres from the hypogastric nerves). The deeper part also consists of fibro-muscular elements and contains the autonomic nerve supply to the vagina together with some blood vessels. This deeper part is often called the paracolpos (Fig. 10.28). The more superficial part can be divided as far laterally as possible without ligation while the fingers of the other hand protect the rectum, ureter and

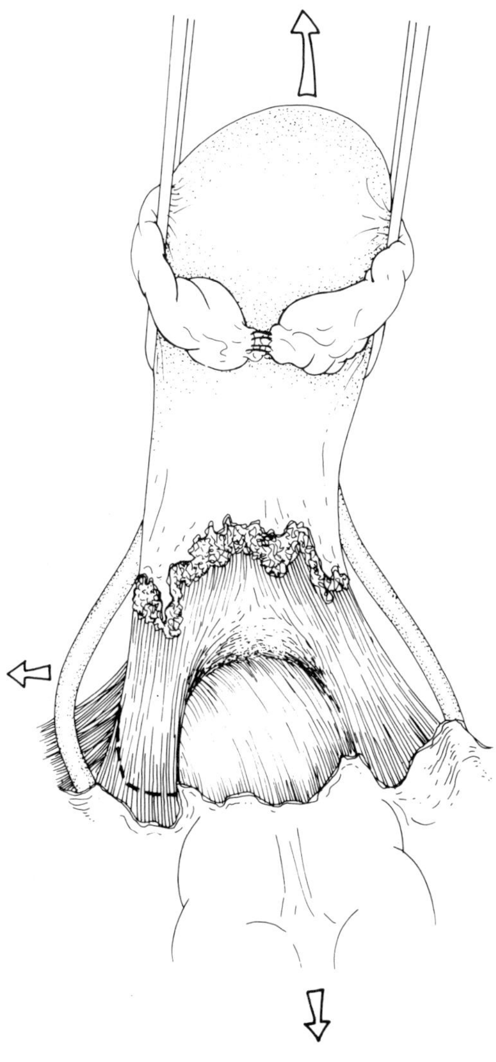

Fig. 10.28. The rectum is mobilised from the vagina in the region of the mid-line to display the posterior retinaculum on each side. The dotted line indicates where this is divided.

nerve supply to the lower urinary tract (Fig. 10.29). During this procedure the uterus and the rectum must be pulled upwards, the uterus somewhat forwards and the rectum backwards. The uterus will be found gradually to become more mobile so that it can be pulled further up out of the pelvis. This allows the rectum to be completely detached by blunt dissection from the posterior vaginal wall in the mid-line and on each side from the deep part of the posterior retinaculum. The rectum is now mobilised down to the pelvic floor without interference with its blood or nerve supply. This is in fact the fourth 'dry space' which must be made use of in this operation.

Up to this point the operation has been standardized. The surgeon must now decide how radical he will make the rest of the operation. The more lateral and the deeper he goes, the greater the danger of complications which involve the lower urinary tract. These include micturition dysfunction, bladder paresis and risk of fistula formation. It is possible to ligate an adequate amount of the deeper part of the posterior retinaculum (paracolpos) and remove up to 4 cm of the vagina without endangering the main part of the nerve and blood supply to the lower urinary tract. The deep portion (paracolpos) is now divided in one or more steps by using a strong curved forceps as shown in Fig. 10.30 and under vision as far

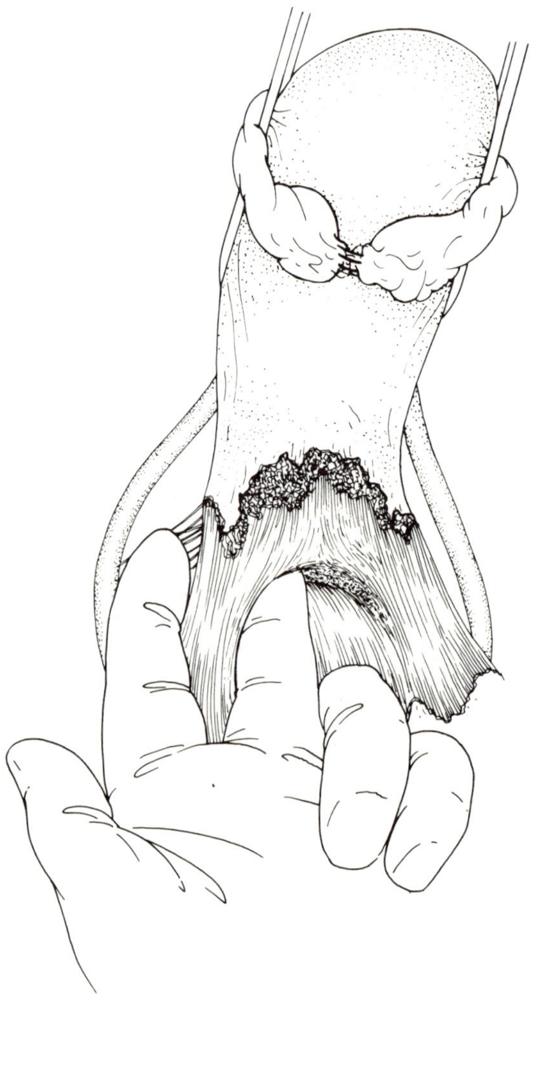

Fig. 10.29. Fingers on either side of the posterior retinaculum protect the nerve supply to the rectum and lower urinary tract.

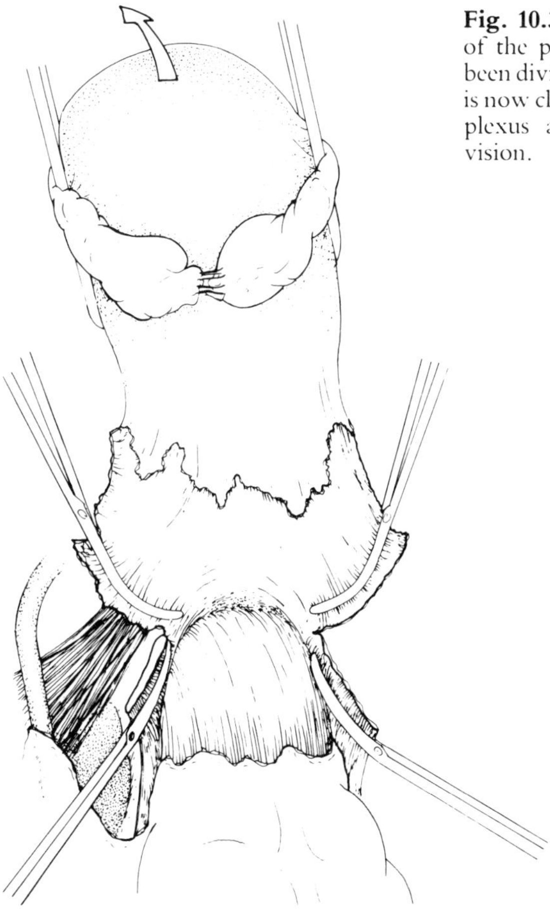

Fig. 10.30. The bloodless superficial part of the posterior retinaculum has already been divided with scissors. The deeper part is now clamped and divided with the nerve plexus and the ureter protected under vision.

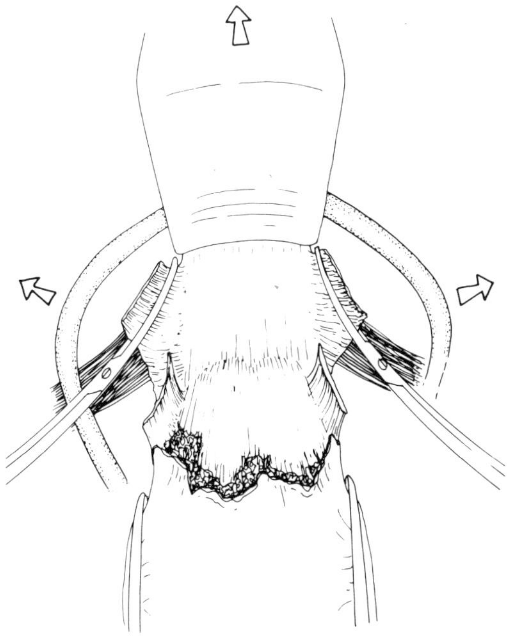

Fig. 10.31. Position just before the vagina is divided.

laterally as possible without endangering the plexus. The site of division is normally 3 to 4 cm from the cervix. These forceps should be strong and have longitudinal serrations on the blades so that they cannot slip off the tissue. The operator's and the assistant's hands protect the rectum, ureter and nerve plexus from damage. The procedure is facilitated by the assistant holding the uterus to the opposite side under a little tension.

Step 9. Removal of uterus, closure of vagina and revision of lymphadenectomy

The uterus is now removed by dividing the vagina at least 2 cm distal to the tumour. The anterior wall is incised with a knife while the assistant protects the bladder and ureters. The lateral and posterior vaginal walls are then divided symmetrically with scissors (Fig. 10.31). As soon as the vagina is opened, it is lightly packed from above to reduce risk of contamination. The cut edges of the vagina are then sutured with strong continuous sutures. The vagina should not be

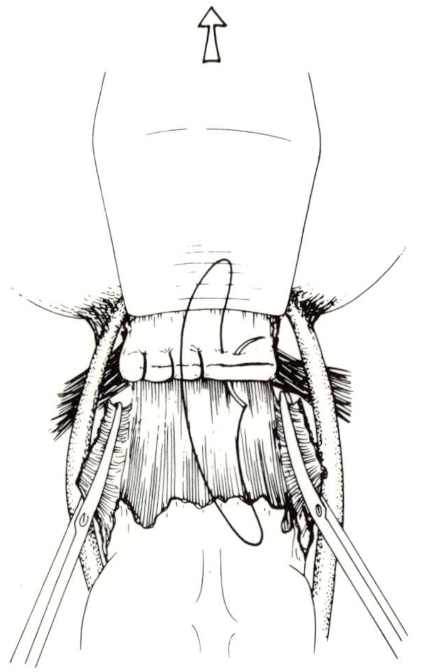

Fig. 10.32. The vagina is closed with a continuous suture.

left open because it can be the cause of later infection (Fig. 10.32). The deep part of the posterior retinaculum is attached by the vaginal suture to each corner of the vaginal stump to help to hold it up and reduce tension on the ureters.

If drainage via the vagina is used, a soft rubber T-drain avoids the risk of fistula formation due to damage by a stiff drain. This particular area should be left as undisturbed as possible because it has already been traumatized more than enough during the dissection. We prefer to close the vagina and rely on extraperitoneal suction drainage through the abdominal wall. This avoids haematoma and lymph cyst formation, thereby reducing the risk of compression and infection of the lower urinary tract. Compression and infection are causes of lower urinary tract complications in addition to surgical trauma. Pelvic cellulitis is a severe and possibly lethal complication.

At this stage it is confirmed that most lymph nodes have been removed and that there is no source of bleeding. There may be a little diffuse venous bleeding from the whole bare area in the pelvis. This stops when the abdominal pack is removed and any compression of the vena cava ceases. The pre-sacral glands, if they exist, are also removed. The lower urinary tract is not at risk here.

Step 10. Insertion of drain, peritonealization and wound closure

Suction drains are inserted through separate openings on each side of the lower abdomen. These should be extraperitoneal and reach down to the bottom of the obturator fossa. The drains should have multiple holes and must be soft enough to avoid compression of the external iliac arteries and veins. They should be at least 5 mm in diameter to assure good drainage. A drainage tube which is too small will become obstructed by clot which will lead to lymph cyst formation.

The peritoneum is sutured in such a way that tension is avoided and the ureters are supported. They are still attached throughout most of their pelvic course. If

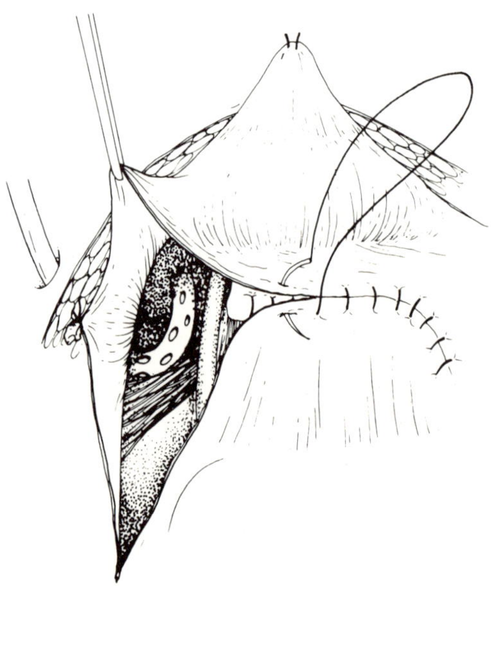

Fig. 10.33. Suture of peritoneum without tension and with ureters under vision.

they are left unsupported between the pelvic wall and the bladder, they tend to become kinked by fixation to the posterior wall. They must, of course, be kept in mind while the peritoneum is being closed because it is all too easy to pick a ureter up in a stitch as it lies just under the edge of the peritoneum (Fig. 10.33).

It is not usually possible to cover the whole bare area with peritoneum. This is of no consequence, as the re-growth of peritoneum is exceedingly rapid and the drains remove collections of fluid such as blood, serum and lymph. The abdominal wall is closed in the usual way.

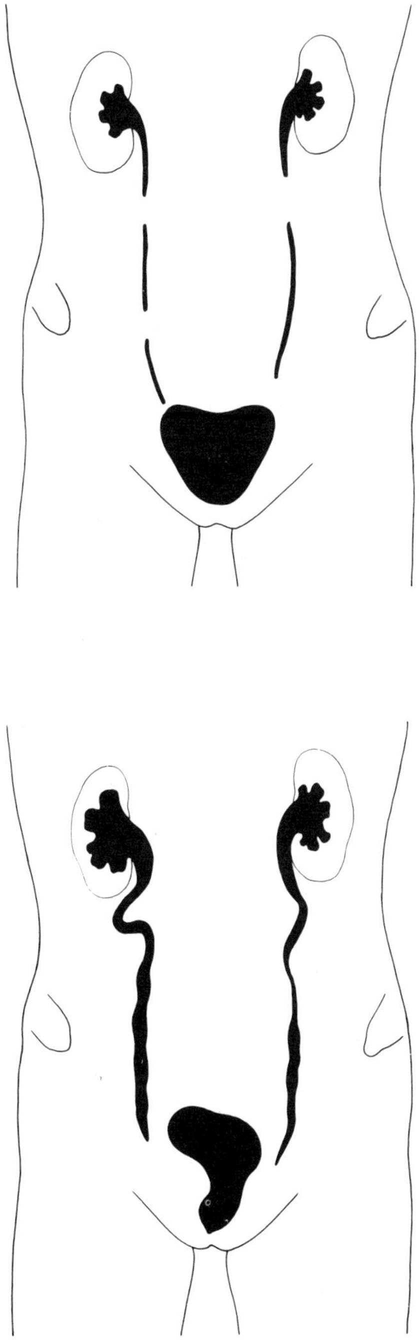

Fig. 10.34. Pre- and post-operative urography. The latter shows moderate hydrorephrosis and hydroureter with an impression in the bladder due to a lymph cyst on the right side of the pelvis.

POST-OPERATIVE CARE

Post-operative haematoma and lymph-cyst formation

We believe that haematoma and lymph-cyst formation can and should be prevented by efficient suction drainage which should be maintained until nothing more comes out. A considerable amount of lymph will drain out, simply because the lymphatic drainage system from the femoral and inguinal nodes has been removed.

If lymph is allowed to form a large collection in the pelvis, the danger of infection is great. Lymph cysts can even produce bilateral ureteric obstruction with uraemia whether they are infected or not. Good suction drainage will prevent collections forming by removing all the lymph and, in addition, lymph leakage ceases after 3 to 7 days. Bleeding in the form of oozing from the wound surfaces stops within a few hours, but can nevertheless amount to several hundred ml. This must be included in the total fluid loss. Infection, haematoma formation, lymph cyst formation with compression and kinking of the ureters are all serious complications which may result in hydronephrosis. They can lead to ureteric necrosis, stricture and fistula formation.

Noone can guarantee that these complications can always be avoided, but these rules of efficient drainage will go a long way towards preventing them. An isotope renography should be done one to two weeks after the operation and repeated later if it is pathological. It is surprising how many ureters are completely unaffected by this operation even though renogaphy is a very sensitive form of investigation. Post-operative urography is also recommended about the end of the second week, just before removal of the catheter (Fig. 10.34).

THE BLADDER

Either suprapubic or perurethral bladder drainage can be used after the operation.

An advantage of suprapubic drainage is that it can be continued until micturition is acceptable and the patient can attempt this simply by clipping the catheter. It also allows easy measurement of residual urine. The disadvantage is that it involves another drainage tube in the region of the suprapubic wound.

The urethra is intact and the bladder has not been opened, so a transurethral 14 F balloon catheter can be used in most cases.

Micturition can be attempted from about the 10th day. There is often temporary dysfunction of the hypogastric plexus due to dissection in the neighbourhood and oedema of the bladder wall and this leads to inadequate bladder function for some time. In our experience this is seldom more than about 4 weeks. The patient should be informed of this and encouraged to await eventual improvement.

'Bladder training' designed to preserve bladder capacity or assist bladder function does not appear to have much effect. As long as urinary infection is kept to a minimum, the bladder will look after itself and will regain a normal capacity. Evaluation of bladder and urethral function in a series of patients 2 weeks and one year after this operation showed that residual urine was at first very variable (0–300 ml on the same day) but had disappeared in all cases at one year.

First sensation, maximum bladder capacity and maximum urethral pressure were not significantly altered, and no patient became stress incontinent after the operation. An interesting thing was that about one third of the patients already had an almost normal micturition pattern at 14 days with insignificant residual urine. Very few showed an abnormal micturition pattern or assisted micturation by straining. This was in fact no more than in the pre-operative investigation, when the patient was nervous and in unfamiliar surroundings. The amount of residual urine at one year after operation was in fact less than that recorded pre-operatively. This interesting observation stresses the importance of psychological influences on bladder function and underlines the difficulties inherent in any investigation of micturition problems. We keep the catheter in place for 10–14 days, in order to avoid any chance of unnecessary distension of the bladder at this critical stage.

It has been found that the general post-operative abdominal discomfort interferes with bladder emptying if the catheter is removed too early. A bladder which has once been over-distended can take a long time to recover although the use of carbachol by mouth may be of assistance.

If the patient has residual urine after the catheter has been removed, we prefer intermittent catheterization 4 times a day after micturition has been attempted. The amount of residual urine very quickly falls to under 100 ml. Only one out of three patients had significant bacteriuria in the mid-stream specimen after the catheter was removed and this disappeared with treatment. None had any bacterial growth on examination of midstream urine or suprapubic puncture one year after operation. None of the patients had signs or symptoms of upper urinary tract infection.

If bacteriuria persists, and there is doubt about its origin, it is wise to take a suprapubic puncture specimen in the morning when the bladder is full. Patients with total bladder denervation with considerable residual urine can manage to keep the urine sterile. If there is hydronephrosis, the bacterial content of the urine should be watched very closely and treated according to the principles in Appendix B.

It has been postulated for a long time that the post-operative phase includes a period of bladder hypertonicity which appears after operation when the catheter is removed. This has been diagnosed as a result of simple cystometry and it has

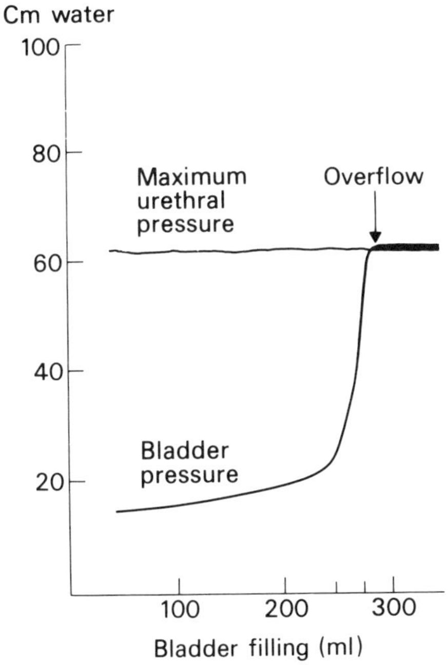

Fig. 10.35. Simultaneous pressure measurements in the bladder and urethra soon after radical hysterectomy showing overflow incontinence.

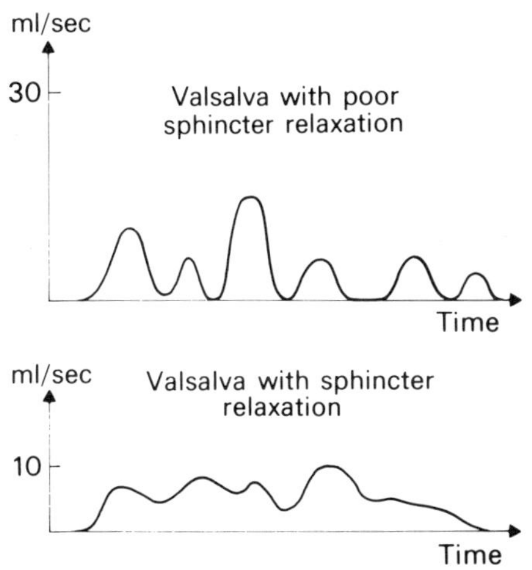

Fig. 10.36. Flow rate measurements after a radical hysterectomy which involved complete denervation of the bladder.

been suggested that the denervated or partially denervated detrusor muscle is responsible for this. There are indications, on the basis of simultaneous pressure measurements in the bladder and urethra, that this is an artifact. The situation in fact, is an overflow incontinence produced by the stiffness of the bladder wall resulting from post-operative oedema and temporary interference with nervous control. The main cause of this is interruption of the lymphatic drainage route from the bladder which is almost the same as that from the uterine cervix. If a cystoscopy is done at this stage, the whole bladder mucosa will be found to be grossly oedematous with the ureteric orifices buried in bulging epithelium. When it is filled to a certain volume, the bladder is mechanically incapable of further distension. A typical simultaneous pressure measurement is shown in Fig. 10.35 taken from a patient 2 weeks post-operatively before she was able to initiate micturition. She had no bladder sensation, no detrusor activity and no response in the urethra. The bladder was filled to 250 ml with little rise in intravesical pressure. When filling continued up to 275 ml, this small amount of fluid produced a marked and sudden rise in the intravesical pressure so that it rose above the maximum urethral pressure and a pure overflow incontinence occurred. It is easy to understand that simple cystometry with fast filling may lead to misinterpretation of this phenomenon. In fact, it is illogical to talk of hypertonicity of the bladder, for if this was the case a catheter would be unnecessary.

It is surprising to see how little the urethral pressure profile is affected in long term observation after radical hysterectomy where total bilateral resection of the hypogastric plexus has been performed, producing total denervation of the bladder. These patients do not become incontinent, although stress incontinence may occur when the bladder is full. After a while, they learn to empty their bladder satisfactorily by a combination of straining, pressure on the lower abdomen and simultaneous relaxation of the pelvic floor (Fig. 10.36). This latter has to be learnt as it is necessary in order to decrease urethral resistance. It is obvious that the micturition reflex arc is interrupted.

If the hypogastric plexus has been preserved intact, as described above, the detrusor muscle can contract and empty the bladder almost completely. The last few millilitres will remain, probably because of perivesical adhesions and rigidity in the bladder wall, and can be expressed by a Valsalva manoeuvre (Fig. 10.37).

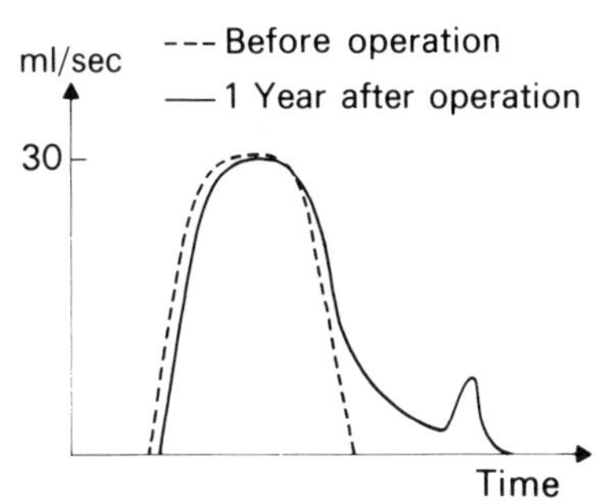

Fig. 10.37. Flow rate after radical hysterectomy. Micturition is nearly normal except that the last few ml are retained and then expelled by a valsalva manoeuvre.

THE URETERS

As mentioned before, the ureters and the periureteric fascia must not be damaged during operation either by compression, by forceps, incision of periureteric fascia or by stretching. As long as the ureters are kept intact throughout their length there need be no fear about compromising their blood supply with resulting necrosis or dysfunction. In practice the vessel which supplies the ureter from the common iliac artery just above the brim of the pelvis is always kept intact in a radical operation and this is a safeguard which ensures excellent blood supply to the lower half. There is no need to try to preserve any vessels below this which supply the ureter. Also, attempts to preserve the lowest vessel are illogical because they must make the operation less radical than is required. In addition, when the ureter is accidentally divided in the pelvis and reimplanted into the bladder, the results are satisfactory with good healing in spite of the fact that the lowest arterial branch must have been removed. Also, last but not least, this little vessel does not always exist.

It is wise to keep the ureter loosely attached to the medial leaf of the peritoneum over as long a distance as possible simply in order to avoid damaging it. There is then no danger of it being pulled on unnecessarily by retractors and at the end of the operation, when the peritoneum is being sutured, damage by stretching and kinking is prevented. Preserving the loose attachment to the peritoneum has nothing to do with preserving its blood supply. Hydroureter or hydronephrosis is commonly seen postoperatively but seldom lasts more than a few weeks after this method of operation.

Ureteric catheters

The use of ureteric catheters either placed pre-operatively or as a means of ureteric drainage post-operatively is not advocated. They are a possible source of infection and serve no practical purpose because the ureters are kept under vision during the whole operation.

Urinary leakage, immediately post-operative

If urine appears from a suction drain it indicates damage to the bladder or a ureter. The latter is more usual. The site of leakage should be determined without delay according to the principles described in Chapter 12. Immediate re-operation and repair is recommended as soon as the site of the fistula is determined. Urinary contamination of the large raw surfaces involved after this operation leads to a massive fibrous tissue reaction or 'frozen pelvis'. This makes later repair of the fistula difficult or impossible. A policy of immediate re-operation and repair is advocated up to about the fifth post-operative day.

Urinary leakage which appears after the drain is removed about the fifth day is seen either as a uretero-vaginal fistula or as an interstitial collection of urine in the iliac fossa and loin retro-peritoneally which is known as a urinary phlegmon. The diagnosis of this can be difficult and is often delayed some days or weeks. After a while it can become an enormous thick-walled fibrous cyst because of the tissue reaction to the urine. The best treatment of these cysts is direct retroperitoneal drainage to the surface or drainage to the vagina. This first step should be combined with adequate antibiotics. The next step, when the patient is over this stage, is consideration of how the fistula should be treated and what should be done with the damaged kidney. The most rational procedure in these particular cases can be nephrectomy if the other kidney is normal; it is suggested that the gynaecologist enlists the help of a urological colleague before making this decision. The condition is discussed in more detail in Chapter 12.

Uretero-vaginal fistula

This usually occurs 1–3 weeks after primary surgery, either because a cystic collection of urine in the pelvis finds its way out through the vaginal suture line or simply because there is a direct fistula from a ureteric injury which has produced necrosis. The principles of localization will be described in Chapter 12. The gynaecologist should avoid the use of a ureteric catheter as there is a great danger that he may make the fistulous opening bigger and ruin any chance of spontaneous healing. There is often displacement or a kink in the ureter at the site of the fistula and the ureteric wall is soft because of oedema and necrosis. The fistula should certainly be given a chance to heal spontaneously without being further damaged unnecessarily. First of all, one must be sure that drainage to the vagina is adequate. The opening in the vaginal wall should be gently enlarged to empty any cyst which has formed. This also avoids the risk of infection which is associated with fistula formation. Antibiotics should be used for a week or two in order to give the fistula a chance to heal spontaneously. If it does not heal or if hydronephrosis and/or hydroureter appear because of stricture formation, one should not hesitate to drain the kidney by percutaneous nephrostomy. The object is to avoid damage to the kidney by back pressure and to keep the region of the fistula free of urine. Keeping the fistula free of urine avoids to a great extent the massive fibrous tissue formation which always occurs around any interstitial collection of urine. Percutaneous nephrostomy also makes it possible at any stage to do antegrade ureterography, which delineates the fistula. Nephrostomy also acts as a 'safety-valve' drain after any repair operation which may have to be carried out. It offers, in fact, so many advantages and carries so little risk that it could well be used more often as soon as a fistula is discovered.

If a lymph cyst or a pelvic abscess is to be drained via the vagina, the surgeon should remember that the ureters now lie just above the top of the shortened vagina. We have seen damage to a ureter with fistula formation result from forced dilation of the apex of the vagina with forceps.

Ureteric stricture formation (without fistula)

The hydroureter and hydronephrosis which is seen immediately after the operation sometimes looks alarming on a urogram but usually disappears after a few weeks without any permanent damage to the kidney (Fig. 10.34). It must, however, be carefully followed up. There is no need to think of drainage of the ureter or kidney; an isotope renograph may still appear alarming even though a urogram looks almost normal. This is only because it is a much more sensitive test of ureteric function. The old saying, 'Treat the patient and not the X-ray picture' certainly applies here. The only reason for active treatment is the appearance on the renogram of signs of renal damage or of total obstruction. Ureteric catheterization is again not recommended owing to the danger of perforation. There are descriptions in the literature of gradual dilatation of a ureteric stricture by passing ureteric bougies. If there really is an intrinsic ureteric stricture, dilatation by bougie is not a real possibility. It is either impossible to pass instruments or there is a great risk of damage by perforation due to kinking. Such a ureter is no longer flexible and is fixed in an abnormal position, usually with angulation. Even if a bougie can be passed, the stricture contracts again because it is formed of fibrous tissue. We believe that where successful dilatation has been described, the stricture has not been intrinsic but a stenosis due to external compression, which might well have resolved by itself in time.

When the site of a stricture or stenosis which is producing significant obstruction has been determined by urography, percutaneous nephrostomy is an effective first step in treatment. This can be maintained for a month or more. Percutaneous nephrostomy has many advantages: the patient is mobile, the hazard of ureteric catheterization is avoided, any hydroureter or hydronephrosis disappears and potential back-pressure damage or infection of the kidney is avoided. Furthermore, a stenosis caused by external pressure on the ureter, for example by a haematoma, is given time to disappear. If the stricture becomes permanent (as shown by antegrade ureterography) the nephrostomy can be maintained until after operative correction of the stricture has been adequately carried out.

It is our definite opinion that the rational way of treating an intrinsic ureteric stricture is by direct surgical intervention involving reimplantation into the bladder. Permanent ureteric stricture with kidney damage occurs very infrequently and surgical treatment has a good chance of success.

About half of all patients who die of carcinoma of the cervix, whether they are treated or not and however they are treated, die of bilateral ureteric obstruction and uraemia caused by primary spread or recurrence of the tumour. Many of these have a severe superimposed renal infection. It is important that the same chain of events is not produced in cases that are potentially curable by causing bilateral ureteric obstruction with infection. Unilateral damage can also result in death of the patient but more usually results in loss of a kidney or chronic renal infection.

Vesico-vaginal fistula

This usually appears 1–2 weeks after operation when bladder drainage is removed and is due to known or unknown damage to the bladder wall or to an inadequate repair of an injury to the bladder. It is usually a small high fistula in the mid-line which should be repaired from the vaginal aspect as soon as possible. See Chapter 12. This is an additional operation, but it involves comparatively little inconvenience to the patient and at the same time has a good chance of success. Good post-operative bladder drainage and prevention of infection are essential. Any suprapubic operation on the bladder should be avoided for at least 3 months because of post-operative oedema, interstitial inflammatory reaction in the bladder wall and temporary impairment of the vesical vascular circulation. Suprapubic opening of the bladder may well lead to permanently reduced bladder capacity and interstitial fibrosis if it is done in the early stages after a radical pelvic operation.

Radical surgery and radiotherapy

See Chapters 11 and 12.

Later urinary complications after primary surgery

If the lower urinary tract has been shown to have returned to normal after operation and subsequently ureteric obstruction or reduced bladder capacity develops, the cause is in nearly all cases not an intrinsic lesion in the urinary tract but a recurrence of the tumour in the pelvis.

OTHER CANCER OPERATIONS

The following operations are also performed for radical treatment of various forms of cancer in the pelvis. If the surgeon understands the various steps of radical hysterectomy and lymph node dissection, he is well on the way to understanding how to protect the lower urinary tract in these other operations.

EXTENDED HYSTERECTOMY

This consists of removal of the cervix and uterus together with a cuff of vagina and may be used in the treatment of micro-invasive cancers of the cervix or carcinoma in situ of the cervix which involves the upper vagina. It is also useful if the surgeon has set out to do a radical hysterectomy and lymph node dissection and finds either metastases on the pelvic wall which are not removable or spread to the lymph nodes in the lumbar region. Both of these are considered to be contra-indications to the operation. An extended hysterectomy might then be a rational way of treating the primary tumour. This operation means that the ureter is in greater danger than in a simple hysterectomy. The only way to do this operation safely and at the same time to ensure sufficient removal of tissue is to expose and dissect the ureter free from where it crosses the uterine artery to its entry into the bladder. These patients have often had a diagnostic conisation performed previously, so it is very easy to get into trouble with the ureter if one does not dissect it out completely. For this reason the procedure cannot be completely standardized. The surgeon must not make the operation more extensive than necessary, and at the same time he must be certain of not damaging the ureter. This is most effectively done by exposing it so that it can be held out of the way under vision all the time.

The uterine artery should be identified at its origin as in step 6 of the radical hysterectomy. It can then be followed medially until it reaches the ureter which has already been identified on the medial leaf of peritoneum. During this manoeuvre, small vessels which go to the ureter or to the bladder will be found and need not be disturbed. The uterine artery is ligated and divided and the distal end held up as shown in Fig. 10.17. This exposes the beginning of the channel in which the ureter runs in the anterior retinaculum. Before dissecting further, it is wise to remove a little fat and so expose the uterine vein or veins which can be ligated and divided straight away to avoid unexpected bleeding later on. The channel can now be widened a little above the ureter by introducing and opening the blades of a pair of long curved forceps which are left in position. The bladder is then lifted and dissected free from the uterus and anterior vaginal fornix in the mid-line by sharp scissor dissection as described in Step 7.

The anterior retinaculum is held so that the forceps can be pushed through it in a antero-medial direction into the vesico-vaginal space which has just been opened up. The part of the retinaculum over the forceps is now divided as close to the uterus as possible while the ureter lies protected under the blades.

This is usually sufficient exposure of the ureter to avoid damage since it allows it to be pushed gently out of the operative field. It also allows sufficient exposure of the vaginal fornices to ensure an adequate cuff.

The recto-vaginal space is then opened as in Step 8 after pulling the uterus forwards and upwards and the rectum upwards and backwards so that the recto-uterine space can be opened up. It is not necessary to divide the deeper portion of the posterior retinaculum. The uterus with vaginal cuff can now be removed, while the ureter is protected as it lies loosely attached to the peritoneum.

The ureter is never dissected completely free from its attachments in any part of its course but it is nevertheless held under vision the whole time.

The operation is completed as in Step 10 of radical hysterectomy. We do not always advocate drainage.

The urethral catheter is kept in for 4 to 5 days. The urinary complication rate is much lower than after radical hysterectomy with lymphnode dissection.

PARTIAL OR TOTAL VAGINECTOMY

Excision of the upper part of the vagina is performed because of recurrence of ovarian or corpus uteri cancer in the vagina, or because of vaginal carcinoma in situ. After radical hysterectomy, it may occasionally be necessary to remove the rest of the vagina because of local recurrence.

Abdominal approach

In our opinion, it is impossible to remove the uterus and the whole vagina from above without destroying a significant amount of the blood and nerve supply to the lower urinary tract. If the uterus is intact, an extended hysterectomy can be done and more of the vagina removed. It must be realized that the more vagina is removed, the greater the chance of complications due to nerve and blood supply damage. Total vaginectomy has always been associated with a very high incidence of urinary fistula and also almost always results in complete denervation of the bladder. If lymph node dissection is not to be done, the operation can be summarized as follows.

Uterus intact

The ureters must be dissected out as in the extended or radical hysterectomy so that the operation is radical enough and to make sure that the ureters are preserved intact. The lateral approach is recommended which means that the pararectal and paravesical spaces are opened right down to the pelvic floor and all fat removed. The uterine artery and veins are ligated and the ureter treated in the same way as in radical hysterectomy (Step 6).

Uterus already removed

If the uterus has been removed, the same principles are employed but we advise the surgeon to pack the vagina first and not to start the operation by trying to expose the top of the vagina in the mid-line. This only endangers the ureters which can lie very near the vaginal remnant. The ureters should be identified from the lateral aspect and the rectum mobilized. The space between the bladder and the vagina is then identified and opened up in the mid-line. At this stage it is a good idea to remove the vaginal pack because it now takes up too much valuable space and then to decide how much of the retinacula and the vagina have to be removed. The surgeon must be ready to improvize here, but if he keeps to the principles described under radical hysterectomy, the ureters should be safe. It may be an advantage to start the operation by dividing the vaginal mucosa from below, for then the extent of the lesion can be identified more easily. This also applies if the uterus is intact.

Vaginectomy from below

Resection of recurrent or primary cancer in the vagina from below is of doubtful value because it is impossible to remove any infiltrative part of the tumour and the field of lymphatic spread cannot be examined.

We have no experience of *radical vaginal hysterectomy*. The indications for performing such an operation have now ceased to apply, therefore – although the operation classically performed was a masterpiece and gave less urinary complications than radical hysterectomy performed from above – we prefer the abdominal approach.

ANTERIOR EXENTERATION

This is, in fact, a radical hysterectomy with lymph node dissection together with removal of the bladder and urethra and the anterior vaginal wall. Urinary diversion in the form of an ileal bladder must be arranged at the end of the operation. The only indication for this is a cancer of the cervix with spread to the bladder and nowhere else. This is almost a theoretical state of affairs. If anterior exenteration is to be performed, the only practical detail which is worth noting is that it is useful to ligate the anterior division of the internal iliac arteries at the beginning of their course.

POSTERIOR OR TOTAL EXENTERATION

This is radical hysterectomy with lymph node dissection together with removal of the posterior vaginal wall including the rectum and anus. Some form of colostomy is provided. There is a great risk of infection and fistula formation, and the bladder and urethra are denervated. Mortality is much higher than in anterior resection and fistula formation very frequent.

Total exenteration involves the removal of rectum, uterus, bladder, urethra and vagina with lymphnode dissection with provision of ileal bladder and colostomy. This is an extensive operation which is seldom indicated.

REMOVAL OF CENTRAL RECURRENCE AFTER PRIMARY OPERATION

Operation on a central recurrence after primary operative treatment of cancer of the cervix or corpus uteri or after surgery combined with pre- or post-operative radiotherapy can occasionally be indicated.

The extent of the recurrent tumour must first be accurately mapped out by using all possible methods of investigation. There must be a reasonable chance of cure, bearing in mind that a second and more extensive surgical procedure is much more difficult than the first operation and carries a great and inevitable risk to the urinary tract. Radiotherapy is, of course, an alternative if it has not already been used but the results are disappointing. It is our view that if a ureter is involved in the recurrence, then any curative treatment is out of the question. It is better to use the most suitable form of palliation. It usually means that tissue in the pelvis which cannot be removed by any form of exenteration operation is involved by direct tumour infiltration. Anterior extenteration is only indicated when the recurrence is limited to the bladder wall.

Removal of central recurrence after full radiotherapy for carcinoma of the cervix

This is usually a hopeless situation because any operation involving the ureters and bladder carries a very high risk of fatal complications. Therefore some form of extended hysterectomy must be contemplated. Complete lymphadenectomy should never be attempted.

If there is infiltration into the bladder, excision together with that part of the bladder wall which is involved can be contemplated, but too often one or other of the ureters is involved. It is quite unnecessary to remove more of the bladder wall than is directly involved. These tumours do not spread in the bladder like a primary bladder cancer; they are limited to a local area and it is only necessary to remove this.

Attempts to reimplant an irradiated ureter into an irradiated bladder are doomed to failure in the great majority of cases. Poor healing with resultant fistula formation is almost inevitable. The only rational operation is therefore an extended hysterectomy combined with an ileal conduit. One should be careful not to use any part of the ureters which have been irradiated, to avoid the loop of small intestine which may have received a high dose because it was fixed by adhesions in the pelvis and to place the stoma in a part of the abdominal wall which was not included in an irradiation field. If the uterus and the rectum has to be removed after full radiotherapy there is a very high risk of urinary tract complication.

LARGE MALIGNANT PELVIC TUMOURS

The course of the ureters can never be predicted with certainty; they become infiltrated comparatively late and can be pushed in any direction by the expanding tumour. An intravenous urogram should be performed with additional lateral pictures. The surgeon should pass ureteric catheters pre-operatively in all cases and leave them in position during operation.

VULVECTOMY

In order to make sure that the operation is sufficiently radical it is often necessary to remove the distal part of the urethra. This does not need to lead to incontinence (*cf.* cancer of the urethra Chapter 13) but can lead to deformation of the remaining part of the urethra with stricture formation and micturition problems on account of the direction of the urinary stream. A later minor correction operation may be necessary.

REFERENCES

Asmussen M (1981) Radical hysterectomy without denervating the lower urinary tract. *Proc. I.U.G.A. Meeting, Stockholm.*

Asmussen M (1981) Bladder and urethral function after radical hysterectomy. *Proc. International Continence Society, Annual Meeting,* p. 99.

Asmussen M, Ulmsten U (1982) Immediate bladder dysfunction after radical hysterectomy (in press).

Bonney V (1974) in *Bonney's Gynecological Surgery, 9th edn,* ed. J Howkins & J Stallworthy. Baillière Tindall, London.

Curtis AH *et al.* (1952) Anatomy of the pelvic autonomic nerves in relation to gynecology. *Surg. Gynecol. Obstet.* **75,** 743.

Forney JP (1980) Effect of radical hysterectomy on bladder physiology. *Am. J. Obstet. Gynecol.* **138,** 374.

Glahn BE (1970) The neurogenic factor in vesical dysfunction following radical hysterectomy for carcinoma of cervix. *Scand. J. Urol. Nephrol.* **4,** 107.

Green TH, Meigs JV, Ulfelder H, Curtin RR (1962) Urologic complications of radical Wertheim hysterectomy. *Obstet. Gynecol.* **20,** 293.

Hohenfellner R (1965) *Die urologischen Komplikationen des Collum-Carcinoms.* Springer Verlag, Heidelberg.

Low JA, Mauger GM, Carmichael JA (1981) The effect of Wertheim hysterectomy upon bladder and urethral function. *Am. J. Obstet. Gynecol.* **139,** 826.

Mackenrodt A (1905) Ergebnisse der abdominalen Radikal-operation des Gebärmutter-scheiden-Krebses. *Z Geburtshilfe Gynäkologie.* **54,** 514.

Martius H (1971) *Die gynäkologischen Operationen.* Georg Thieme Verlag, Stuttgart.

Meigs JV (1954) *Surgical Treatment of Cancer of the Cervix.* Grune & Stratton, New York.

Nakano R (1981) The Okabayashi operation and its modifications. *Gynecol. Obstet. Invest.* **12,** 281.

Nelson JH Jr (1977) *Atlas of Radical Pelvic Surgery,* 2nd ed. Appleton, Century Crofts. New York.

Novak F (1956) Procedure for the reduction of the number of uretero-vaginal fistulas after Wertheim's operation. *Gynecol.* **72,** 506.

Palm L, Rønnike F (1977) Bladder function following either radiotherapy or radical operation ad modum Okabayashi for cervical cancer. *Dan. Med. Bull.* **17,** 113.

Seski JC, Dioko AC (1977) Bladder dysfunction after radical abdominal hysterectomy. *Am. J. Obstet. Gynecol.* **128,** 643.

Wertheim E (1911) *Die erweiterte Operation bei Carcinoma Colli Uteri.* Urban Schwarzenberg, Berlin.

Yagi H (1955) Extended abdominal hysterectomy with pelvic lymphadenectomy for carcinoma of the cervix – the Okabayashi operation. *Am. J. Obstet. Gynecol.* **69,** 33.

Chapter 11 Radiotherapy and the Lower Urinary Tract

Few gynaecologists are actually involved in the treatment of malignant disease by radiotherapy, but they see the patients who develop complications after the completion of irradiation. They must therefore know something about the biological changes involved in order to understand the mechanisms underlying these complications. They are then in a position to explain the situation adequately to the patient and to embark on the difficult problem of treatment.

Radiotherapy can be an effective form of treatment of pelvic cancer in the female, especially carcinoma of the cervix uteri. But, even when radiotherapy is properly applied, reactions in the lower urinary tract must be expected simply because of its proximity to the cervix. If the patient is to have an optimum chance of cure, the tumour-dose must be large and this means that normal tissue in the neighbourhood receives a dosage which is near the limit of tolerance. Reactions to this follow a known sequence of changes which can vary in intensity from what is tolerable to very serious damage. The critical dose for normal tissue varies from one patient to another. This is because that part of the irradiation dose which acts upon both normal tissue and tumour cells is influenced by age, obesity, vascularity and the extent of the tumour. The bigger the tumour, the higher the dosage needed to cure it. Certain other things tend to make the reaction in the lower urinary tract more severe, such as lower urinary tract infection and other pelvic infections. Previous operative interference with the bladder and ureters shortly before irradiation also increases the chance of complications. Irradiation lowers resistance to infection in the urothelium with the result that the chances of instrumental infection of residual urine in the bladder are greater than usual. This means that all kinds of infection in the pelvis must be effectively treated before radiotherapy begins.

CARCINOMA OF THE CERVIX TREATED BY LOCAL APPLICATION OF RADIUM, CAESIUM OR COBALT WITH OR WITHOUT EXTERNAL IRRADIATION

The former applies only to early cases and is an alternative to operative treatment. The aim of the radium insertion is to apply a very high central absorbed dose, about 60 Gy, to a block of tissue 2 cm on either side of the midline and 2 cm upwards from the tip of the cervix. This means that the ureters can sometimes receive almost as high a dose as they pass on each side of the cervix. The tissue dosage decreases according to the inverse square of the distance from the source.

The bladder base is kept as far away as possible by packing the anterior fornix with gauze. This moves the vesico-urethral junction and urethra out of harm's way but does nothing to move that part of the bladder base in the region of the mid-line just above the trigone where it is attached to the anterior wall of the uterus and cervix. This area of the bladder can therefore absorb about the same dose as the ureters. When the radium is applied (there are various systems) the total effective dose should be the same and therefore the complication rate should be about the same. There are, however, anatomical differences for no two women have exactly the same shape of bladder. These anatomical variations can produce major differences in dosage to normal bladder tissue. Previous surgery, such as conization of the cervix, and vaginal repair may possibly produce even larger variations.

Even though the dose fall-off in relation to distance from the radium source is very rapid, the lower ureters and the bladder base are so near that they cannot escape a high dosage, assuming that the radium source is inserted with optimum accuracy. Needless to say this is an ideal which is certainly not always reached, so it must also be taken into account as a possible source of overdosage to ureter, bladder base and especially the rectum which does not tolerate as much radiation as the bladder. In spite of these negative aspects, which may sound very formidable, it is quite certain that a large number of patients go through the radium insertion stage without serious complications.

THE BLADDER

The reaction in the bladder which can be expected may be roughly divided into the early and late phases of a continuous process. The patient begins to have symptoms of 'cystitis', that is to say urgency and a burning sensation on micturition, which usually begin 1–2 weeks after the first insertion. They may be aggravated by infection which results from the in-dwelling balloon catheter which is necessary during the few days the radium is in position. We prefer a small catheter, 14 F, with 2 ml saline in the balloon, as this is tolerated better than larger catheters. We prefer not to give the patients urinary antiseptics but rather to rely on a high diuresis. This is normally sufficient to hold infection in check and to clear it up within a short time after the removal of the catheter.

If a patient develops severe symptoms from either the bladder or rectum during the period of the radium insertion, this should never be ignored. It may well be a sign that the radium is not properly inserted. The patient should be re-examined at once because experience has shown that the worst complications occur in exactly these patients. Neglect of this precaution may be disastrous.

Biology and pathology

The effect of radiation, whether it consists of α, β or γ radiation or a combination of these, is to induce changes in cell nuclei which either inhibit reproduction or kill the cell. The exact mechanism is still not yet fully understood. Both normal cells and cancer cells are affected by radiation but the cancer cell, which divides more often and is more susceptible, is affected to a greater extent. The margin of difference may not be great because there is great variation between the various types of cancer cells and also between the different types of normal cells.

Radiation dosage is measured as energy absorbed in tissue and is expressed in Gray, which is the same as 1 joule per kg; formerly it was expressed in rad (radiation absorbed dose). One rad is equivlent to 100 erg per gram of tissue, which means that 1 Gray is the same as 100 rad.

The pathology of the reaction of normal bladder tissue consists of a phase showing cellular damage followed by a sort of repair process. This differs from the normal tissue response to injury because irradiated tissue gradually loses much of its ability to repair itself.

Early phase

To begin with, changes are seen in the submucosa where the capillaries become dilated and congested with intercellular oedema. Degeneration of the urothelium comes next, with the formation of vacuoles in the cytoplasm and destruction of the nuclei. Vacuole formation and hyaline changes are also seen in the smooth muscle, but they are less marked in comparison with the submucosa and the urothelium. The repair process begins within a few days with the appearance of a submucosal perivascular lymphocyte and polymorpho-nuclear infiltration. Desquamation of the superficial layers of the urothelium occurs, sometimes with disappearance of the whole thickness leading to ulceration. Submucosal haemorrhages are common. Fibrin and leucocytes cover these superficial desquamated areas.

At this stage the cystoscope will show increased vascularity and oedema of the mucosa on the lower posterior wall. The vascularity can vary from a moderate increase in the number of mucosal vessels to an appearance which resembles red velvet and looks like an acute haemorrhagic bladder infection except that it is limited to the bladder base. The tip of an in-dwelling catheter irritates the upper posterior wall and produces a red oedematous area known to urologists as a 'catheter tumour' which must not be confused with irradiation changes. This 'tumour' disappears a few days after the catheter is removed.

After removal of the radium, the changes regress—that is to say the visible vascular changes. However, the histological changes progress in the submucosa, the capillaries show narrowing of the lumen with endothelial proliferation and subendothelial fibrosis. Hyalinization of the connective tissue with generalized submucosal fibrosis progresses slowly and begins to involve the smooth muscle layers, replacing damaged muscle cells. So-called 'radiation fibroblasts', which look like malignant cells, can make histological differentiation of radiation damage from tumour cell infiltration exceedingly difficult. Fibrotic arteriolar changes gradually devascularize more and more of the bladder tissue. Cystoscopy at this stage may now reveal a reduced bladder capacity and a pale urothelium with capillary proliferation, petechial haemorrhages and superficial ulceration with flakes of necrotic epithelium. A superimposed infection (which is common because of catheters and the lowered resistance to infection) will cause alkalinization of the urine by breaking down the urea to form ammonia, which results in a white phosphatic deposit on all necrotic tissue. A diuresis should be maintained to discourage infection and remove necrotic products. Bacterial infection should also be kept to a minimum by drug treatment since it increases the damage produced by irradiation.

Late phase

The later changes in the bladder are largely the result of a generalized obliterative arteritis, often progressing to a complete arterial obstruction, combined with interstitial fibrosis. The process is slow but continuous and inexorable and it is this which accounts for the late development of ulcers and fistulae up to several years after irradiation.

This description applies, of course, to those cases which show the worst reactions. Most patients have considerably less reaction and show correspondingly less change on cystoscopy. Broadly speaking, the frequency of late complications increases for 3 to 4 years after irradiation and then diminishes, but radiation fistulae have been known to occur after 20 years.

If external irradiation is used after radium insertion, the whole bladder receives a considerable additional dose in spite of various methods of central shielding. This aggravates and prolongs the symptoms of the acute phase because a reaction is produced in the whole bladder. As part of the fibrous tissue reaction in the bladder wall, a significant ureteric obstruction may occasionally develop as a temporary phenomenon. Another complication at this stage is haemorrhage from the ulcerated bladder mucosa, which can become considerable. It can be difficult to control and, if it is accompanied by uraemia or acute pyelonephritis with septicaemia, it can herald a combination of complications which can threaten life. This situation usually indicates that the patient has received an irradiation dosage which was higher than she could tolerate.

In cases with large tumours where a high dose has been necessary and where there is invasion of the surrounding tissue very close to the bladder, such as the anterior vaginal wall, a vesico-vaginal fistula can develop because of necrosis in tumour tissue. As mentioned previously, reaction to irradiation depends not only on the total dose given but also on the dose fractions and the time-dose relationship. The reaction in the bladder increases considerably when more than 60 Gy are absorbed by the bladder wall as a total dose. Animal experiments have shown that this is especially so if a time-dose relationship of 10 Gy in less than 24 hours is reached. The risk of severe complications then becomes extremely high. This must be remembered if intracavitary cathetron after-loading techniques are planned because large doses up to 8 Gy can be given in a short period of time by this method. The standard dosage in external therapy is normally not more than 8 Gy in a week, given in 4 or 5 fractions.

REFERENCES

Buchsbaum HJ *et al.* (1978) Radiation cystitis, fistula and fibrosis. Chapter 18 in *Gynecologic and Obstetric Urology,* ed. Buchsbaum & Schmidt. WB Saunders, Philadelphia.

Dalrymple GV, Gaulden GM, Kollmorgen H, Vogel HH (1973) *Medical Radiation Biology.* WB Saunders, London.

Joslin CAF (1978 The biological effects of radiation therapy in gynaecological malignancy. Chapter 15 in *Scientific Basis of Obstetrics and Gynaecology,* 2nd edn, ed. RR Macdonald. Churchill Livingstone, London.

Meredith WJ, Massey JB (1970) *Fundamental Physics of Radiology,* 2nd edn. J. Wright & Sons, Bristol.

Rutledge F, Boronow RC, Wharton JT (1976) *Gynecologic Oncology.* J Wiley & Sons, New York.

Walter JB, Israel MS (1963) *General Pathology.* J & A Churchill, London.

Chapter 12 Urinary Fistula

The appearance of clear fluid from a post-operative drain or from the vagina during the first two weeks after a gynaecological operation is always a depressing event. At first it may only be a small amount and may even be intermittent; it is sometimes so little that it can encourage hope that it may be lymph or serum. After a while it becomes more profuse and, when the dressings are removed and the wound inspected, it reappears after drying with gauze with a characteristic inevitability which removes all doubt about its nature.

CLASSIFICATION

A fistula is defined as *a communication between two epithelial surfaces.* A urinary fistula is therefore a channel between an organ lined with urothelium and any other epithelium-covered surface, i.e. skin, vagina or intestine. We exclude congenital fistulae. As far as gynaecology is concerned, urinary fistulae can be divided into:

post-operative which in turn can be divided into immediate and late. Fistulae which occur after radical hysterectomy are somewhat different and are described in Chapter 10;

obstetric;

post-irradiation;

combined, which occur when operation is combined with irradiation, and

spontaneous and carcinomatous.

Gynaecological urinary fistulae are commonly uretero-vaginal and vesico-vaginal; other types are rare.

Repair of uretero-vaginal fistula is also discussed in Chapters 8 and 10.

POST-OPERATIVE FISTULAE

Immediate post-operative fistula

This is due to an injury which is not discovered at operation. If a ureter is involved, the fistula is usually uretero-vaginal, either unilateral or bilateral. It occasionally appears as a uretero-cutaneous fistula via the drain in the abdominal wound.

Fistula from the bladder is commonly vesico-vaginal but can appear as a leak from the suprapubic drain. The most frequent cause is a tear in the bladder wall due to too strenuous blunt dissection of the bladder from the anterior wall of the uterus during either an abdominal or a vaginal hysterectomy. Fistula between the urethra and the vagina can appear after any vaginal operation in which damage to the urethra has not been discovered or after urethral diverticulectomy if the sutures fail to hold.

Any of these fistulae can, of course, occur after inadequate repair of an injury which has been discovered at operation. In many cases the site of the fistula is obvious or is already suspected by the surgeon. If not, the methods described later in this chapter can be used to identify the exact site.

Later fistula

This develops one to two weeks after operation and is due to necrosis following direct damage, strangulation by a ligature, devascularization or as a result of inadequate repair of an injury. A vaginal suture which has inadvertently perforated the bladder wall can also lead to a fistula. All these accidents can occur with or without local or pelvic infection. If general pelvic infection is a part of the complication, good drainage is essential, both from the fistula and of any abscess that forms. A period of a few days with adequate drainage together with suitable antibiotics should be used to avoid any chance of a spreading infection when a repair operation on the fistula is contemplated.

A urinary phlegmon develops insidiously during the days after an operation or later as a result of injury to the ureteric wall with subsequent necrosis. Usually, any urinary leakage will find its way to the surface after a few hundred millilitres have collected extraperitoneally; occasionally this does not happen and the encysted collection of sterile urine builds up a massive fibrous reaction in connective tissue which effectively walls in the urine. The peritoneum, the common and internal iliac arteries and veins, the ureter itself and the psoas muscle are all involved in the fibrosis. Some days or weeks later, this mass is discovered in the flank or the pelvis. The patient has little in the way of symptoms and may, in fact, discover the mass herself. She may show a persistent pyrexia which may be the only clue. Infection in the cyst can spread rapidly with development of cellulitis, pyelonephritis and septicaemia. The diagnosis can be difficult, simply because it is an unexpected complication. Persistent pyrexia, otherwise unexplained, should always indicate a detailed clinical examination, preferably under anaesthesia. The discovery of a mass should lead to immediate suspicion of a phlegmon, chiefly because the mass was not there just before operation and, in the case of operation for malignant disease, it is too soon for recurrence of the tumour.

Puncture with a fine needle reveals urine and makes the diagnosis clear. The site of the lesion in the ureter can be found by intravenous urography and confirmed, if necessary, by ureteric catheterization.

Treatment consists of immediate drainage of the cystic collection to the surface. Theoretically if the diagnosis is made soon enough, one can re-operate and repair the damage, but in most cases it is the mass which has led to the discovery of the condition and it is then too late for repair because of the massive fibrosis. It is seldom that there is any choice other than nephrectomy but, before taking this step, a urologist should be consulted. A urinary phlegmon is a rare complication, but all gynaecologists, urologists and general surgeons should be aware of its existence. We have experience of a patient who developed a phlegmon 3 weeks after hysterectomy for a benign condition. The surgeon explored the mass and attempted to remove it – an operation which is technically impossible. The patient was then referred for treatment of an infiltrating abdominal tumour.

A vesico-vaginal fistula can appear many months or even years after combined surgery and irradiation for pelvic carcinoma. This is a rare complication of radiation necrosis. It is discussed in Chapter 11.

OBSTETRIC FISTULAE

These are rare in modern obstetric practice but, when they do occur, the injuries which produce them can be formidable. Forceps and vacuum deliveries, especially in combination with disproportion and possibly also with a full bladder, are the commonest causes. The injury occurs at the bladder base and may also involve the urethra. As soon as the injury is discovered an immediate repair should be performed.

A vesico-uterine fistula is an occasional complication of Caesarian section. The frequency increases with the number of sections which a patient must undergo because of scarring at the isthmus where the incision in the uterus must be made adjacent to the bladder wall. The diagnosis is never difficult and repair should be performed as soon as possible by separating the two organs, closing the openings and draining the bladder for 6–10 days.

Investigation of a fistula

If the diagnosis is in doubt, the fluid which leaks out can be collected and examined for urea in the laboratory. The presence of urea demonstrates that it is urine and not lymph or serum. The next step is to find out the exact location and size of the fistula by means of the following investigations.

Intravenous urography will often show contrast outside the urinary tract. There is almost always a hydroureter immediately above the site of leakage and this helps to decide which side is involved if there is any doubt. The leak can, however, be so small that the only indication on the X-rays is a collection of contrast in the vagina.

Clinical gynaecological examination and cystoscopy should follow. The normal ureteric orifice will show efflux of urine; but the ureteric orifice below the fistula will neither contract nor show efflux. Injection of methylene blue intravenously produces a blue efflux from the normal ureter and nothing from the damaged side. At the same time the blue colour appears from the fistula. After operations where the ureter has not been dissected free, very gentle ureteric catheterization is permissable (without a stilette). It will almost always be obstructed at the site of the fistula. Occasionally the catheter will pass the fistula site and can be passed up to the kidney. In this event it is well worth leaving it in-dwelling for 4–6 days.

Larger vesico-vaginal fistulae can, of course, be easily seen by vaginal examination; the smaller ones are best investigated by cystoscopy. With the instrument in the bladder and the water turned on, fluid will be seen to come into the vagina. The trigone and the bladder wall immediately behind the interureteric bar is inspected while a finger lifts it up from the vagina. All openings except minute ones will be obvious. Very small openings can be identified by using a thin curved metal sound or probe in the vagina and, at the same time, observing the bladder base through the cystoscope. These minute fistulae can also be demonstrated by putting methylene blue solution in the bladder and asking the patient to walk about with a tampon in the vagina.

As soon as the exact site of the fistula is recognized, no time should be lost in arranging for re-operation and repair. The sooner it is done, the easier it will be. Although the gynaecologist should be able to operate successfully on a simple fistula and possible also on a more complicated type, he will be well advised to refer post-irradiation and complicated or recurrent fistulae to departments which have experience of these operations.

In the treatment of urinary fistulae there is one rule that has proved true over and over again. This is that the first operation has the best chance of success. This implies that everything possible should be done to try to ensure this success.

Three operations will be described: the vaginal approach to a simple small fistula; the combined abdominal and vaginal approach to a larger, complicated fistula; and the treatment of a post-irradiation fistula using a vascular graft.

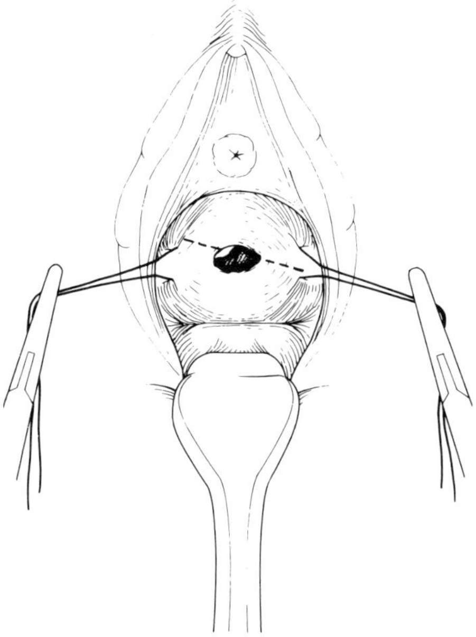

Fig. 12.1. Holding sutures used to draw fistula as far out as possible. Incision is made through fistulous opening in any convenient direction.

Operative surgery

The vaginal approach

The patient is placed in the modified lithotomy position. Holding sutures are placed on either side of the fistula so that the field of operation can be brought nearer the surface. They also demarcate the limits of the incision in the vaginal mucosa (Fig. 12.1). An incision is then made through the vaginal mucosa and fascia so that they can be dissected free from the bladder wall. This incision can be made in any convenient direction but it must pass through the fistulous opening and extend a sufficient distance on either side to permit exposure of about 2 cm of bladder wall in all directions around the fistula (Fig. 12.2).

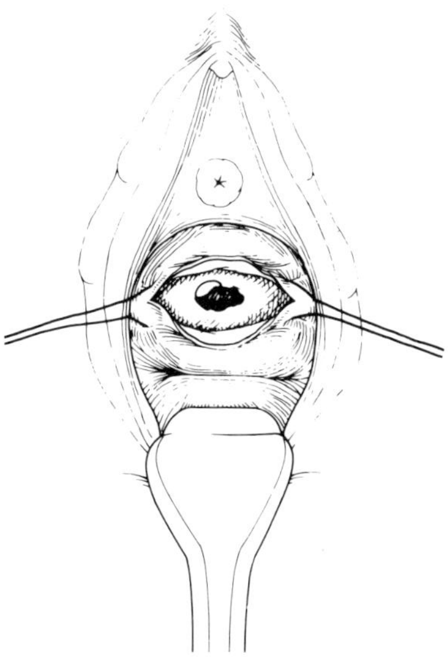

Fig. 12.2. Vaginal mucosa dissected free from bladder wall in all directions.

There is no need to trim the edges of the opening in the bladder wall if there is no necrosis. Fine absorbable ligatures on a thin, fully curved needle are used to close the edges of the opening. Interrupted sutures should be used and should only be tight enough to approximate the edges without tension. If it is necessary to pull the sutures tight, they will always cut out and the fistula will recur and become bigger. The sutures should pick up the whole thickness of the bladder wall including the mucosa (Fig. 12.3).

Any local bleeding should be stopped by pressure or by fine ligature in order to avoid any chance of haematoma formation between the bladder wall and the vagina. It is better not to use diathermy coagulation.

The vaginal wall is then closed using mattress sutures. The direction in which it is sewn up is immaterial, but again tension should be avoided.

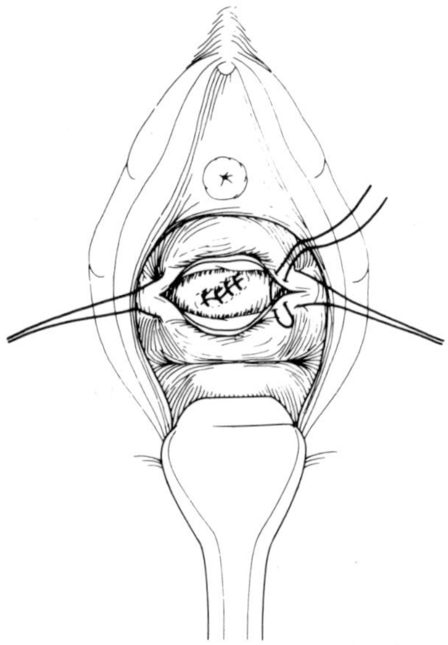

Fig. 12.3. Suture of opening in bladder wall with fine interrupted sutures without tension. Sutures go through all layers.

Bladder drainage can be perurethral or suprapubic. Perurethral drainage is quite adequate in most simple cases, using a 14–16 F balloon catheter. The object is to keep the bladder empty for about 10 days. It may be an advantage to use the stiffer, male type of balloon catheter and make a small hole on the distal side of the balloon so that there is no possibility of the collection of urine in the internal meatus region below the balloon. The patient should be ambulant from the first post-operative day. The use of bilateral ureteric catheter drainage to keep the bladder dry is not always effective. Urine can be passed alongside the catheters and there is an extra risk of infection.

When the catheter is removed, it is important to be sure that there is no residual urine after micturition. For the first day or two, therefore, a catheter should be passed immediately after micturition until it is quite certain that the bladder is being emptied. Any suspicion of urinary infection should be treated using drugs according to resistance determinations. The patient should drink sufficient extra fluid during the drainage period in order to produce a diuresis. This aids drainage and helps prevent infection.

The combined abdominal and vaginal approach to a more complicated vesico-vaginal fistula

We have taken as an example a fistula up to 2 cm in diameter which has been operated on before and where a ureteric orifice can be seen near the edge of the opening (Fig. 12.4).

A vaginal approach is often inadequate; the fistula cannot be brought near the surface because of post-operative fibrosis and for this reason, lighting and access are difficult. The prone or kneeling position can be a slight help in the simpler cases but its advantages are not great enough to make it worth using. It is

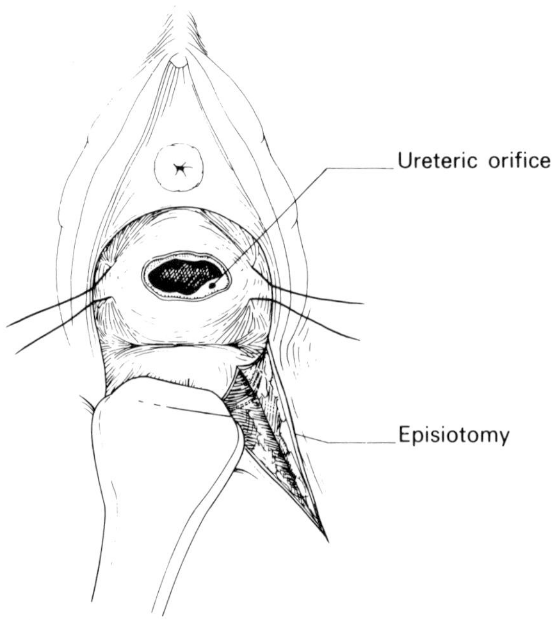

Fig. 12.4. A large high fistula near the left ureteric orifice. Holding sutures bring the opening nearer the surface. Episiotomy makes access easier.

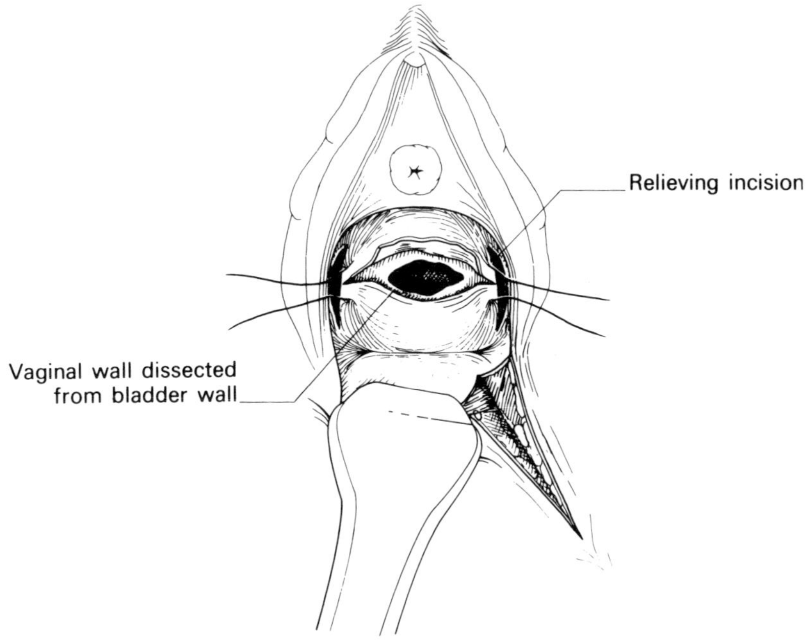

Fig. 12.5. Dissection of vaginal mucosa from bladder wall around fistula. Vertical incisions in the vaginal mucosa can be used to relieve tension.

a lot of bother for theatre staff and anaesthetist because it is something out of the ordinary and also—an important point—it automatically rules out the possibility of using a combined suprapubic approach if this found to be necessary. The modified lithotomy position should be used because this allows two surgeons to work together, one from above and one from below, each with necessary assistance.

The operation is started from the vagina. An episiotomy is recommended and, if necessary, the levator ani muscles can be divided for a short distance on either side to give better access. Holding sutures are placed well away from the opening on either side so that the fistula can be drawn down as much as possible towards the surface. Vaginal mucosa and fascia are dissected free from the region of the fistula as in the previous example. If necessary, vertical relieving sutures can

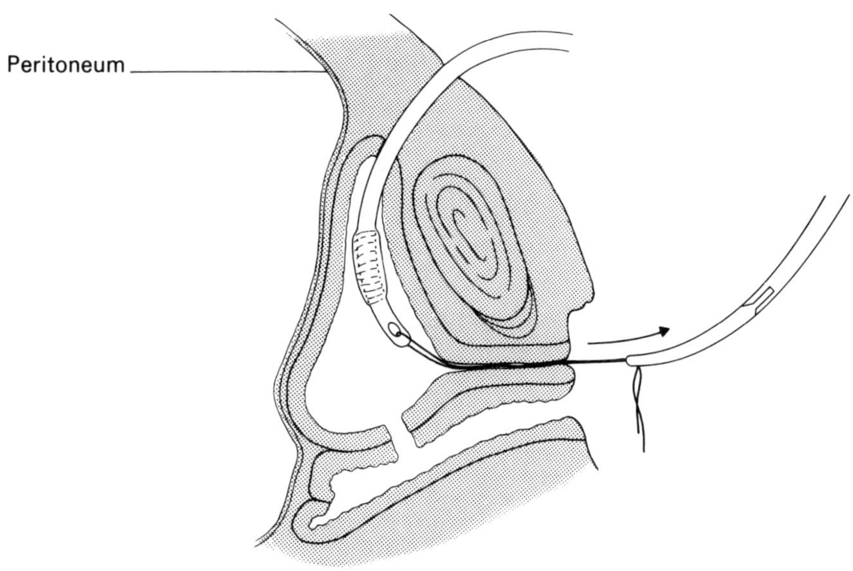

Fig. 12.6. Inserting a suprapubic balloon catheter when the bladder cannot be distended because of the fistula. A thin curved forceps is passed through the urethra so that its point can be felt suprapubically as near as possible to the upper border of the symphysis. The skin and underlying tissues are divided with a knife so that the forceps can draw the balloon catheter through the abdominal wall into the bladder.

be used at the junction of the anterior and lateral vaginal walls to allow mobilization up to 2 cm on either side (Fig. 12.5). If this dissection allows sufficient mobilization of the bladder wall around the fistula to enable it to be closed, then it is unnecessary to open the bladder suprapubically (Fig. 12.6). The indications for proceeding to the suprapubic approach are:

that the vaginal dissecton fails to give adequate access;
that one or both ureteric orifices are involved in the fistula or its repair and re-implantation is necessary;
that other organs such as the rectum or small intestine are involved in the fistula.

The abdominal approach through the open bladder gives excellent access with a good view of the fistula. It facilitates mobilization of the bladder base and makes re-implantation of a ureter feasible. It should, however, never be used by itself but always be combined with a vaginal approach. Urologists, who are accustomed to approach the bladder from above, should not neglect the combined method for it adds an extra and welcome dimension to the operation. It is an immense advantage to be able to see the fistula from both above and below and also it enables tension resulting from scarring in the vaginal wall to be relieved under vision, something which is impossible if the surgeon works only from above.

Ideally, perhaps, the operation should be performed by a urologist working from above and his gynaecological colleague working from below. One surgeon can, however, manage the whole operation but it takes much longer and becomes unnecessarily awkward.

REPAIR OF POST-IRRADIATION FISTULAE

The fistula which can be an almost insuperable problem is that which occurs after irradiation treatment of carcinoma of the cervix where the central dose has been so high that radio-necrosis results, either because of the local dose alone or because of its combination with external radiotherapy later. It may also be seen after combined surgery and irradiation. The lower urinary tract is so close to the cervix that, even when the radium insertions are correctly placed, the bladder base can receive a dangerously high dose. The most likely reason for fistula formation, however, is that the insertions are slightly out of position with the result that part of the bladder base receives a dose which is higher than normal tissue will tolerate. The result is a vesico-vaginal fistula. It occurs in 1–3% of cases in many published series and makes its appearance soon after the course of irradiation is finished. Sometimes it appears much later, even up to 20 years later. It is the more advanced cases that are affected. The frequency of fistula formation after irradiation is less than after surgical treatment but it is much more unpleasant for the patient and is more difficult to treat.

Investigation by palpation, colposcopy and cystoscopy must always be done carefully and gently under anaesthesia. The edges of the opening are necrotic and friable with little bleeding from the edge of the viable tissue. The bladder mucosa around the fistula is oedematous with a concentric area of radiation cystitis. It may be difficult to see the actual opening because of the necrotic tissue and the associated white phosphatic deposit. Rough instrumentation may very easily make the opening bigger. Intravenous urography must be done to determine to what extent the ureters are involved. The possible development of ureteric obstruction can be observed by isotope renography.

It has long been accepted by many gynaecologists that these irradiation fistulae should not be operated on for 1 to 2 years in order to allow for shedding of necrotic tissue and demarcation by clean fibrous tissue. This is not now, as a general rule, realistic advice because we have seen several examples of gradual extension of the area of devitalized tissue apparently resulting primarily from grossly infected urine with local cellulitis rather than irradiation. This produces an unnecessarily large area of necrotic tissue which can involve the ureters and imperil the function of one or both kidneys. It makes later repair extremely difficult or impossible. The period of waiting can be almost unbearably unpleasant, a life of urinary incontinence and social isolation for the patient.

We have learnt from experience that it is better to operate as soon as the infection can be brought under control. Very high doses of antibiotic are necessary to produce a high enough local concentration. Using a combined approach as described above, the necrotic and obviously non-viable tissue is removed until one reaches an edge of viable tissue that bleeds easily. If a ureteric orifice is involved, re-implantation of the ureter has only a small chance of success because of the devitalized ureteric wall. The irradiated lower end should be removed and the rest implanted as high as possible in the bladder wall. Early operation has about the same chance of success as operation many months later and is much preferable for the patient.

The surgeon must realize that to operate on irradiated tissue is not the same as to operate on normal tissue, even if it looks almost normal. Generally speaking, it is thinner, more fibrotic and less elastic and – most important of all – it is less vascular and therefore cannot generate a normal repair process. This means that healing after any form of suture or anastomosis is slow and may even not occur at

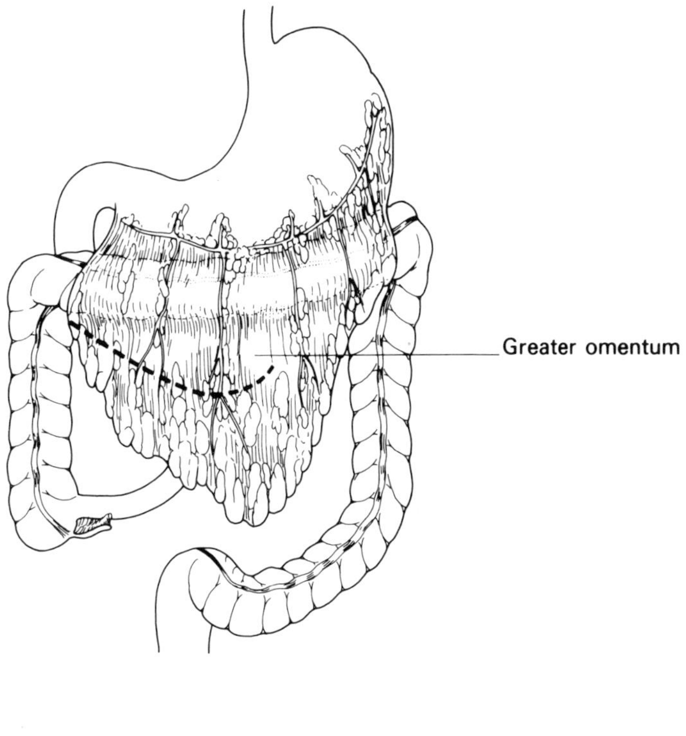

Fig. 12.7. The omentum can be used as a source of additional blood supply if it can be made to reach the base of the bladder. The dotted line shows a method of increasing its length a little.

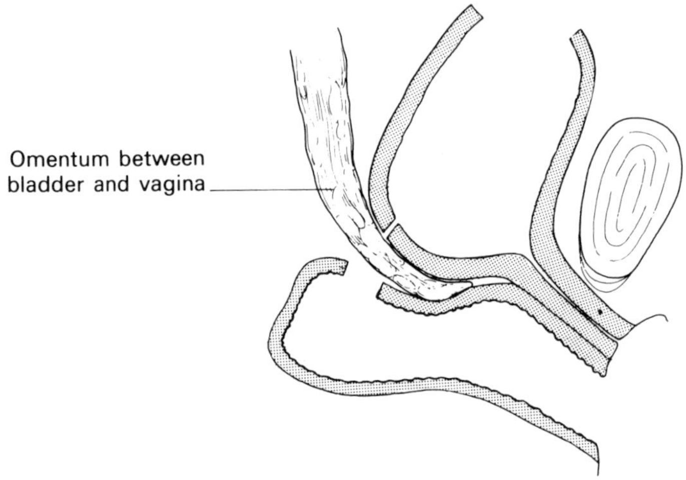

Fig. 12.8. The omentum is sutured between the bladder and vagina which have been separated from one another. It is best to close the fistulous opening in the bladder first from above and, after the omentum has been attached, close the vaginal opening from below.

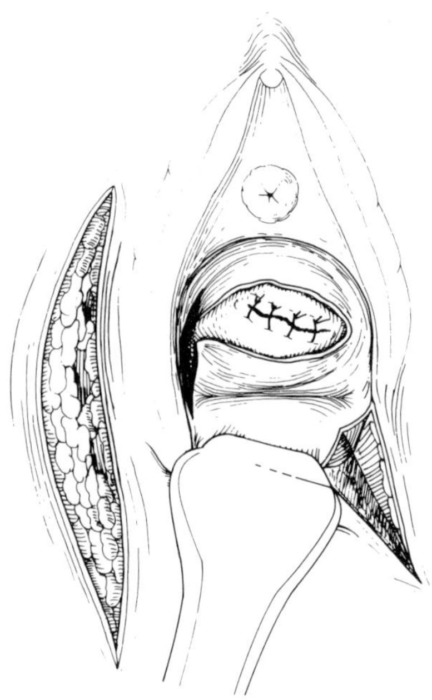

Fig. 12.9. The bulbo-cavernosus muscle with the adjacent fat can provide additional blood supply. It is approached through a separate incision in the vulva.

all. The consequence of this is that all non-viable tissue should be removed before suturing begins and that, when an anastomosis is contemplated, one of the tissues which are to be joined should have a normal blood supply. When the two edges of a fistulous opening have to be sutured together, they are of necessity both irradiated so some form of vascular graft must be prepared and brought to the suture line. Examples of this are omentum, gracilis muscle or the bulbo-cavernosus muscle. The details of the graft must vary according to the size and situation of the fistula so it is impossible to describe a standard procedure (Figs 12.7, 12.8, 12.9). The omental graft is the easiest to use but it is seldom that a long enough piece can be produced. The gracilis muscle is always long enough and is effective but has the disadvantage that its use involves an extra operation (Fig. 12.11). The bulbo-cavernosus muscles are readily available through the same surgical approach and are effective (Fig. 12.10). Whichever graft is chosen, tension must be avoided absolutely. It helps to do a total colpoclysis at the end of the operation.

Post-operative drainage should be by the suprapubic route rather than using balloon catheters in the urethra. Soft, thick-walled suprapubic drainage tubes with multiple holes can with advantage be used in combination with a diuresis and gentle suction. Drainage should be maintained longer than usual; 3 weeks is not too long. The patient can herself learn to work the suction apparatus. It is a great help to enlist her active support and participation in the treatment so that she can discover difficulties as soon as they occur. She should be ambulant from the first post-operative day so that she can use the toilet and attend to bowel function and perineal toilet herself. Efficient post-operative chest physiotherapy should be arranged to avoid coughing.

There are some vesico-vaginal fistulae, both irradiation and simple, that are so big and involve ureters and small and large intestine, and have such a degree of surrounding scarring, that repair is simply not possible. Fistula repair operations must have a real chance of success because repair involves a major operation with many possible complications which can be a danger to life. It is better to admit that permanent urinary diversion offers a better alternative in some cases. This decision should be taken in consultation with a urologist.

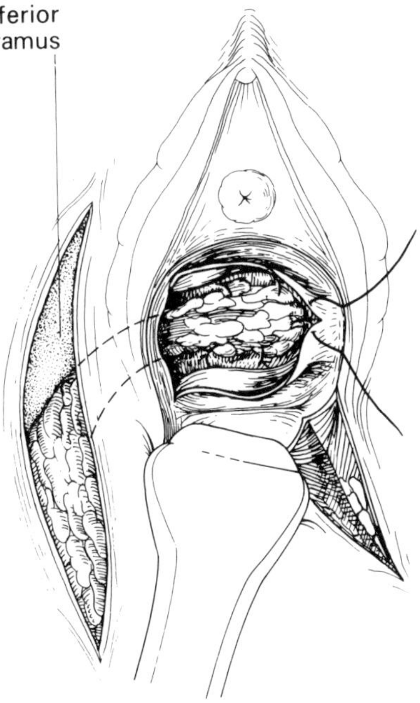

Fig. 12.10. The bulbo-cavernosus muscle with its surrounding fat is detached from the pubic ramus and passed through the lateral vaginal wall to provide additional blood supply to the fistula region. Episiotomy can with advantage be done on the other side.

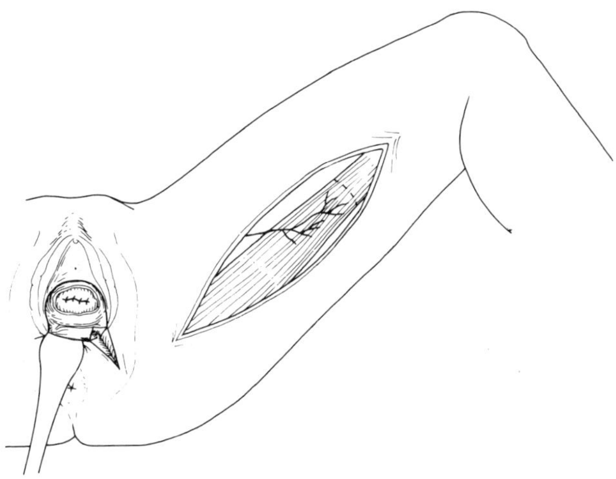

(a)

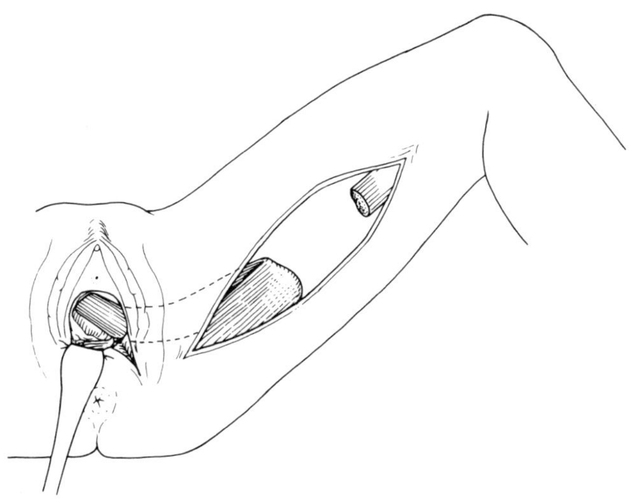

(b)

Fig. 12.11. Isolating the gracilis muscle in the thigh for vascular grafting.

(a) The muscle is divided below the point where its blood supply enters.

(b) The muscle is turned so that the cut end reaches the fistula area after passing through the lateral vaginal wall.

SPONTANEOUS AND CARCINOMATOUS FISTULAE

Vesico-intestinal fistulae occur as a complication of sigmoid diverticultitis or Crohn's disease and can also be seen after intra-cavitary irradiation for ovarian cancer or perforation of the uterus or cervix in the course of intra-cavitary radium implantation. In all these conditions there may be a considerable associated pelvic mass due to development of an abscess and it is this which is the reason for their appearance in a gynaecological department. The diagnosis is seldom difficult because of the presence of gas and faeces in the urine and because of the ease with which one can see the fistula in the bladder dome with the cystoscope. These cases can usually be very satisfactorily treated by removal of the local portion of intestine involved combined with closure of the fistula.

If the fistula involves the colon, a temporary colostomy is recommended. When irradiation has been used the situation is entirely different; resection of irradiated intestine as a primary operation is too often doomed to failure, so the surgeon must not do more as a first step than a proximal colostomy using normal bowel. After about 3 weeks it may be possible to think of a resection but adhesions and devascularization make the outcome so dubious that most cases get no further than the colostomy. This never has the effect of closing the vesico-colic fistula but it makes life more tolerable for the patient.

Malignant vesico-vaginal fistula can be seen in the patient with an untreated stage IV cancer of the cervix or advanced central recurrence after treatment of cancer of the cervix or after unsuccessful treatment of any other type of cancer in the pelvis. There is never any possibility of local treatment of the incontinence. Even though the patient has a short expectation of life, every effort should be made to help her by some kind of simple urinary diversion. Ureterostomy or percutaneous nephrostomy can be used. If the colon and rectum are intact a simple ureterocolic anastomosis may be an excellent solution, for it stops the leakage and avoids any form of external drainage.

SUMMARY OF MAIN POINTS CONCERNING VESICO-VAGINAL FISTULA OPERATIONS

Operate as soon as possible after the fistula is discovered.

Start all operations from the vagina because most can be repaired by this route.

Make use of episiotomy to improve access.

Get a good assistant and use instruments suitable for plastic surgery in a deep hole.

Make sure the lighting is as good as possible—a headlight can be a great help.

Avoid operating in the presence of active infection.

Remove all necrotic and doubtfully viable tissue.

Mobilize the bladder wall enough to avoid tension.

Avoid haematoma formation by careful haemotasis.

Insert sutures through all layers of the bladder wall.

Use partial or total colpocleisis when bigger fistulae are repaired.

Use suprapubic bladder drainage in all but smaller fistulae.

Give the patient sufficient fluid to ensure a diuresis during the whole period of bladder drainage.

Mobilize the patient as soon as possible and enlist her active cooperation in the treatment.

When micturition begins, make sure there is no residual urine.

REFERENCES

Keetel WC (1978) Vesico-vaginal and urethro-vaginal fistulae. In *Gynecologic and Obstetric Urology*, ed. Buchsbaum and Schmidt. WB Saunders, Philadelphia.

Kelly J (1979) Vesico-vaginal fistulae. *Br. J. Urol.* **51,** 208.

Lawson J (1978) The management of genito-urinary fistulae. *Clin. Obstet. & Gynecol.* **11,** 209.

Loughnane FMcG (1939) Transplantation of the gracilis muscle to cure stress incontinence in women. *Br. J. Urol.* **1,** 142.

Martius H (1956) *Gynecologic Operations*. Little Brown, Boston.

Moir JC (1967) *The Vesico-vaginal Fistula*. Baillière Tindall & Cassell, London.

Symmonds RE (1979) Prevention and management of genito-urinary fistula. *Clin. Obstet. Gynecol.* **21,** 13.

Williams JP (1976) Urinary fistulae. In *Urology*, ed. J Blandy. Blackwell Scientific Publications, Oxford.

Chapter 13

Benign and Malignant Conditions in the Urethra

The gynaecologist can be presented with any of the known abnormalities of the female urethra simply because of its proximity to the vagina. Women often find it difficult to be certain whether bleeding comes from the vagina or urethra, so it behoves the gynaecologist to regard the urethra as part of his territory.

Recently, the female urethra has been shown to be a much more complicated and delicate organ than was previously thought. It is an active muscular channel with a considerable nerve supply and a blood supply which is much greater than the needs of nutrition require. It deserves to be treated with great respect.

URETHRAL TRAUMA

Loss of almost the whole of the urethra has been described but is very rare. The reader is referred to Symmonds & Hill (1978) for guidance. Less severe injury of the female urethra is best treated by temporary suprapubic cystostomy. It is usually a complication of a fractured pelvis which itself may be one of multiple injuries. The urethra can be properly inspected and, if necessary, repaired after a day or two when the more serious injuries have been dealt with.

INFECTIONS

Acute urethritis usually occurs as part of a general infection of the lower urinary tract — a urethro-cystitis. This is a primary urethritis which spreads to the bladder and sometimes the upper urinary tract as an acute inflammatory process involving the urothelium.

Acute urethritis often occurs as part of an acute gonococcal infection in the female; oedema and inflammation of the mucosa is accompanied by a purulent yellow discharge from the external meatus. The urethra is tender on palpation and pus can be expressed from it. Smears will show intracellular gram negative diplococci. Micturition becomes difficult and painful with frequency and may occasionally become impossible because of the mucosal oedema. Catheterization may then be necessary. The infection extends upwards only to the trigone and internal meatus region; a generalized bladder infection does not occur unless there is a mixed infection. Further extension to the ureters and renal pelvis is very rare. Gonococcal urethritis never occurs as an isolated phenomenon, it is always an extension of a genital infection and responds to treatment at the same time as this. Whenever a gonococcal infection is found, simultaneous infection by syphilis should be borne in mind and excluded by serum tests. A primary chancre has been seen at the external urinary meatus and resembles the button-like ulcer seen in the male with oedema of the surrounding mucosa and inguinal adenitis.

Virus infection

Herpes simplex II or *herpes progenitalis* infection is sometimes seen at the external urinary meatus and produces marked dysuria, frequency and dyspareunia. Small vesicles appear which progress to painful ulcers 2 to 3 mm in diameter. The ulcers resemble those which commonly occur on the tongue and the inside of the cheek. If untreated they last one week to 10 days and then heal; another crop may then appear and so on for some weeks. There is often a mild inguinal adenitis. The urine is sterile. Treatment by antibiotics is seldom of any use; it is better to apply something locally which sterilizes the ulcers. A weak tincture of iodine is applied with a throat swab after having wiped away mucus and dried the ulcers. Creams containing local anaesthetic are of little help. Idoxuridine (IDU) can be tried in the form of an ointment. It should be applied as early as possible after onset.

Sterilization by a laser beam may prove to be the most effective method.

Intraurethral condylomata are best destroyed by diathermy through a urethroscope but can also be treated by local application of 5-Fluorouracil (5FU).

Low-grade urethritis

There is some evidence that symptoms can be produced by infection of the urethra by so-called 'fastidious' organisms such as Corynebacterium and Chlamydia which require special culture methods.

Non-bacterial urethritis

This type of urethritis can be seen as a form of chemical irritation which produces a burning sensation and a continuous desire to pass urine. Various cosmetic preparations, detergent soaps and bubble baths have been blamed for this, often rightly.

LESIONS AT THE EXTERNAL URINARY MEATUS

Urethral mucosal prolapse

This occurs in women after the menopause and is often symptomless and a chance finding (Fig. 13.1). It can become ulcerated and infected and then produces urethral bleeding with some dysuria. The cause is unknown. The urethral mucosa above the external meatus is normal. Treatment is only necessary when it causes symptoms. It should however always be carefully examined by taking a cytological smear and using the colposcope to exclude malignancy. It can be easily treated by excision of the prolapsed mucosa and suture of the cut edge to the surrounding mucosa of the introitus. This little operation can be done under local anaesthesia and no catheter is required afterwards.

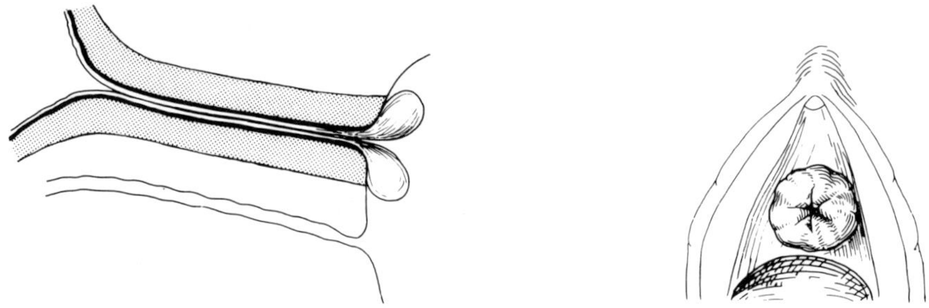

Fig. 13.1. Prolapse of urethral mucosa.

Urethral caruncle

Similar symptoms are produced by this haemangioma-like mass which is quite commonly found at the external meatus, usually on the posterior aspect. It consists of granulation tissue partly covered by epithelium; it bleeds easily when touched because of its rich vascularity but otherwise produces little in the way of symptoms. There is no special association with urethritis or urinary infection. The aetiology is unknown. Here also careful palpation, examination by cytological smear and colposcopy are necessary to exclude urethral carcinoma (Fig. 13.2).

The caruncle is best excised and the mucosal edges sutured with absorbable sutures. Histological examination is always essential.

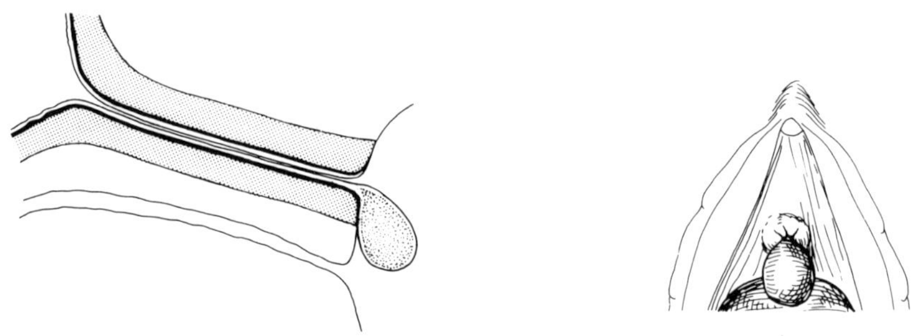

Fig. 13.2. Urethral caruncle.

Urethral stricture

Congenital stenosis is occasionally seen in adults. It takes the form of a short mucosal ring at the external urethral meatus which can be as small as 4 to 6 F. Dilatation simply splits the ring and produces a scar which may contract to form a real stricture. It is better to excise the narrow ring and suture the urethral mucosa to the mucosa of the introitus with fine sutures.

Acquired stricture also occurs at the external meatus in the form of a fibrous ring the lumen of which may be extremely small. It is sometimes a complication of the urethritis which follows the use of an in-dwelling catheter after gynaecological operations. The symptoms are usually prolonged micturition with a poor stream and recurrent infections. The Valsalva manoeuvre is often used to assist micturition. There is residual urine and flow studies show a slow stream, occasionally with fractionated micturition. The urethral pressure profile provides little help here.

A stricture is defined as a *constriction in the urethra which will not admit an instrument of size 20 F.* Gentle and patient dilatation under local interstitial anaesthesia (5–10 ml 0.5% lignocaine on each side of the urethra) is an effective method of treatment. A combined lubricant and antiseptic gel should be used in the urethra. Bleeding is a signal to stop for that day. After dilatation, the patient should maintain a diuresis. An indwelling catheter is not necessary. Some advocate sulphonamide for some days irrespective of whether the urine is infected or not. It is preferable to leave 50 ml 0.05% chlorhexidine in the bladder after instrumentation.

After treatment the flow-curve will become more normal and the residual urine disappears. Recurrence of the stricture, however, is common so periodic dilatation may be advisable. Oestrogen should be given to post-menopausal patients and can well be used in the form of a local application. A cytological smear should always be taken and, if possible, the vascular pattern examined with the colposcope to exclude carcinomatous change.

Strictures higher in the urethra are uncommon. They are occasionally seen in the mid-urethra after excision of a urethral diverticulum or urethrotomy and also after surgery for stress incontinence or anterior colporrhaphy. Forcible dilatation will simply split these strictures and make the scarring worse, so the surgeon must take his time and rely on repeated small dilatations up to 10 or 12 Hegar and not more.

Urethrotomy is not advisable; it can produce a worse stricture or even a 'rigid urethra' after some months. Gradual dilatation gives a better long-term result.

One must always remember, as mentioned above, that a stricture can be an early sign of malignant disease in the urethra so it is necessary to exclude this by cytology, urethroscopy and, if there is any further doubt, biopsy.

Bladder neck obstruction

This condition, which is common in the male, can occasionally be found in the female. The aetiology is unknown. It appears to restrict the normal opening mechanism of the vesico-urethral junction so that funnelling does not occur. This reveals itself as a poor stream and flow-rate, fractionated Valsalva-type micturition and considerable residual urine. Here also, the urethral pressure profile is no help. Cysto-urethroscopy shows a ring at the bladder neck which is rigid during a Valsalva manoeuvre and which can sometimes be felt by a finger per vaginam against the shaft of the instrument. The bladder is thick-walled and shows trabeculation on cystoscopy. High bladder pressures are produced during cystometry. The instrument can usually be introduced with no difficulty, but dilatation is of no lasting value — the neck contracts again shortly afterwards. The best treatment is transurethral resection by a urologist, or by an open Y – V plasty performed by the retropubic approach. The principles are shown in Fig. 13.3. Good results are usually obtained by these operations. Histology of the resected pieces shows fibro-muscular tissue without inflammatory reaction.

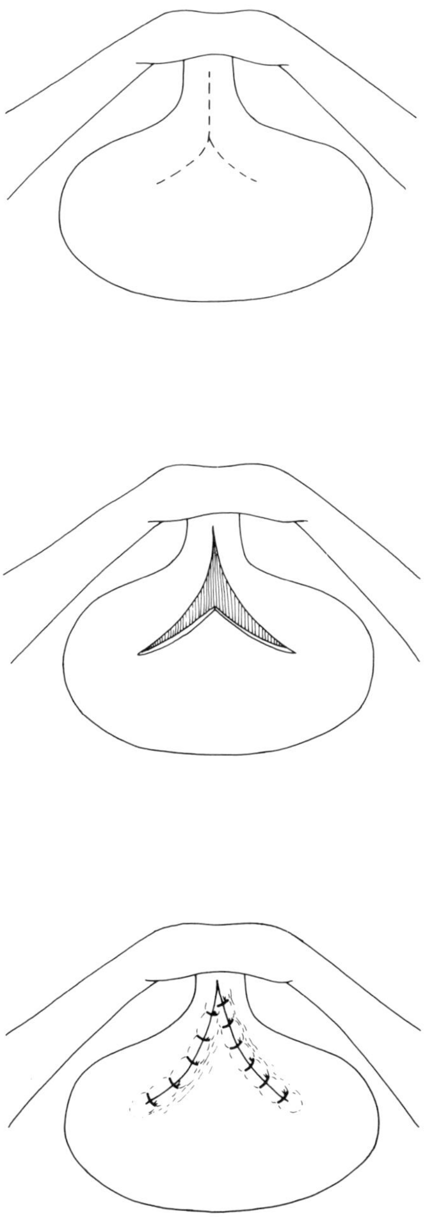

Fig. 13.3. Principles of V–Y plastic operation on vesico-urethral junction.

Urethral polyp

Small polyps are occasionally found in the urethra. They tend to develop a stalk and to prolapse out of the external meatus. They can be removed by division of the stalk or base using diathermy. Histological examination is also essential here. These tumours can be more or less fibromatous.

Urethral diverticulum

Some diverticula are congenital anomalies, possibly the result of migration of a ureteric bud or the development of an extra bud. These are found in childhood when investigating urinary leakage which occurs in addition to normal micturition.

A diverticulum is defined as a pouch formed in the wall of a larger cavity or tube. A diverticulum in the urethra differs from a diverticulum in the bladder in that its wall consists mostly of fibrous tissue and does not contain elements of the muscular layers as in the bladder.

The urethral diverticulum which gynaecologists and urologists have to treat in women appears to be acquired during adult life and is not a rarity. It can reach the size of a hen's egg. The opening from the urethra is found posteriorly or postero-laterally, usually more towards the upper end than near the external meatus and can be anything from 2 to 10 mm in diameter. The sac lies outside the muscular urethral wall, partially between the urethra and the vagina and partially alongside the urethra. In many cases it is composed of fibrous tissue without an epithelial lining and is adherent to everything in its neighbourhood including the vaginal wall. The aetiology is uncertain but the fibrous nature of the diverticular wall and its lack of an epithelial lining suggest that it is not basically a pouch of urethral mucosa. This however may simply be an impression which is due to the effects of long-standing infection. It may be the result of haematoma formation, perhaps from the submucosal venous plexus after a delivery. The haematoma ruptures into the urethral lumen and is then filled with urine. Distal obstruction in the urethra does not always occur and recurrent urethritis with infection of Skenes' glands is not necessarily an antecedent.

Symptoms

If the opening is below the point of maximum urethral pressure, the symptoms consist mainly of urinary leakage accompanied by a certain amount of dysuria. If the opening is higher up the urethra, there is little or no leakage but greater dysuria. There may also be local effects if infection is present, such as urethral pain and dyspareunia. The urinary leakage occurs for the most part after micturition and in connection with movement because the diverticulum fills during micturition and a little urine is squeezed out by pressure. Infection in the small amount of stagnant urine in the diverticulum can lead to stone formation, a phosphatic calculus being produced which can be a source of great discomfort. The risk of ascending infection is often the reason for operating on a diverticulum in the upper urethra.

The leakage can lead to a suspicion of stress incontinence because of the effect of straining and movement. Leakage, however, occurs soon after micturition, while in stress incontinence this is the one time when a patient can be almost certain that she will *not* leak, simply because the bladder is empty. After leakage has occurred from the diverticulum there is a tendency for the patient to be dry until after the next micturition. In stress incontinence the reverse is the case—she leaks more when the bladder is full.

Diagnosis

The most important step in making the diagnosis is to be aware of the existence of diverticulum. It is possible to overlook it entirely if one forgets to palpate the urethra from the vagina and does not examine the inside of the urethra with a cysto-urethroscope. A thickening is palpable through the anterior vaginal wall and pressure on this may sometimes cause urine or pus to appear at the external urinary meatus.

An abscess in one of Skenes' glands can be difficult to distinguish from an infected diverticulum. Here the urethra is normal on urethroscopy with the abscess adherent to one side of the urethral wall. It is important to recognize the difference, because the Skenes' gland abscess is best treated by marsupialization.

The surgeon can pass the cysto-urethroscope into the bladder to measure residual urine and then take the opportunity to feel the urethra from the vagina against the cystoscope. The diverticulum is felt as a somewhat soft ill-defined tumour attached to both the urethra and the vaginal wall. A stone can easily be felt. The cysto-urethroscope is then withdrawn so that the end is just inside the external meatus and the irrigating fluid is turned on. With the objective lens pointing backwards and a finger in the vagina as a guide, the inside of the urethra is inspected up to the bladder neck. The opening of the diverticulum will come into view. Occasionally, it is possible to pass the cystoscope tip or the end of a uterine sound into the diverticulum, again guided by the vaginal finger. If this can be done or if the opening is seen through the cysto-urethroscope, the diagnosis is made for certain and all that remains is to exclude other pathological conditions in the bladder. Histological examination after excision is always necessary because the development of a carcinoma in a diverticulum has been described.

A visual record can be obtained by injection urethrography. This is done by distending the urethra with contrast medium using a special type of catheter which has a balloon at each end of the urethra. The diverticulum should first be emptied by pressure from the vagina. X-ray pictures are then taken in antero-posterior and oblique planes. It can also be seen to fill on a video film (Fig. 13.4).

Treatment

Marsupialization should not be performed because this simply produces a urethro-vaginal fistula. Excision of the diverticulum with suture of the opening

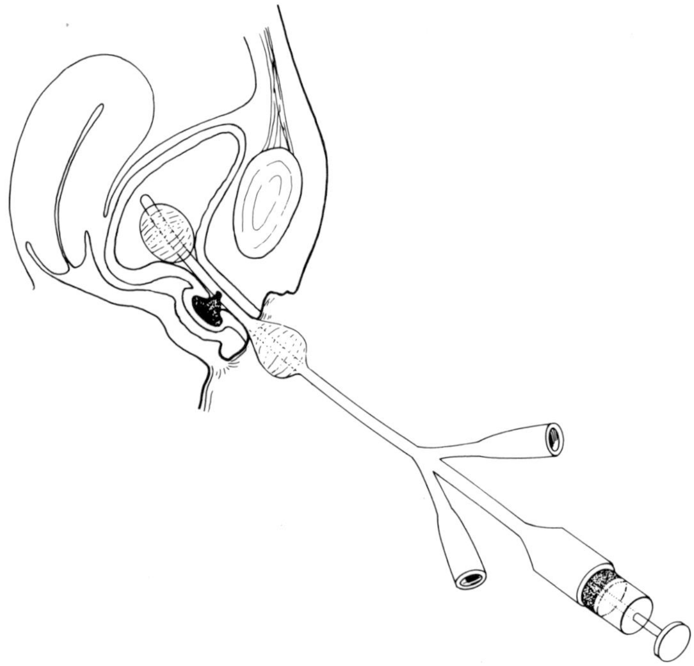

Fig. 13.4. Special catheter with two balloons used to demonstrate a urethral diverticulum by X-ray.

in the urethra is recommended. It is easier and safer to do this if the pouch is packed with ribbon gauze (using a pair of nasal forceps through the external urinary meatus and a guiding finger in the vagina). A catheter with a small balloon such as the Fogarty vascular catheter is preferable to gauze if it can be passed at the side of a cystoscope which is used to guide the catheter into the opening. A 24 F balloon catheter is then passed into the bladder and the balloon inflated; this allows accurate location of the urethral lumen and of the base of the bladder, and also prevents constriction of the lumen by the sutures.

The vaginal wall is dissected backwards, concentrating at first on dissecting it free on either side of the urethra (Fig. 13.5). This dissection can be made easier by holding a finger inside the vaginal wall especially where it is adherent to the diverticulum (Fig. 13.6). When the lower part of the diverticulum is exposed it is separated from the vagina by careful sharp dissection until it is possible to reach normal tissue above it. This may be the base of the bladder. The neck of the diverticulum is then exposed, doing as little damage to the urethra and its blood supply as possible (Fig. 13.7). At this stage it is an advantage to remove the packing or balloon from the diverticulum so that it can be grasped with a pair of artery forceps. By moving it from side to side one gets a better view of the neck and urethral wall, so that it can be removed by dividing the neck.

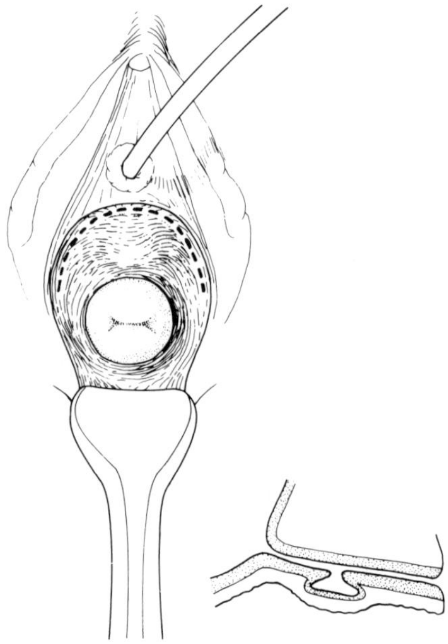

Fig. 13.5. Vaginal incision.

Removal of a diverticulum resembles in many ways the preliminary dissection of a cystocoele operation, especially a dissection after a patient has had a previous operation. The sac consists mostly of fibrous tissue and is adherent to everything with which it has come into contact, both urethral muscular wall and vaginal wall. This fact makes a serious injury to the urethra a possibility because the surgeon may believe he is removing the sac wall from its adherence to the urethra when in fact he is removing the whole thickness of the urethral wall in addition to the wall of the diverticulum. This results in the loss of a long and

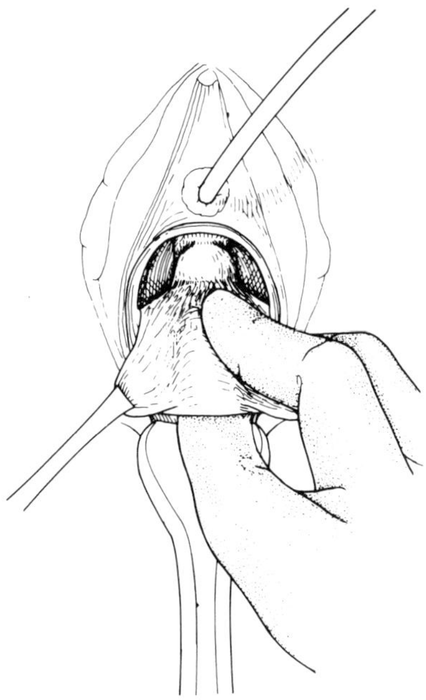

Fig. 13.6. Dissection of anterior vaginal wall from diverticulum.

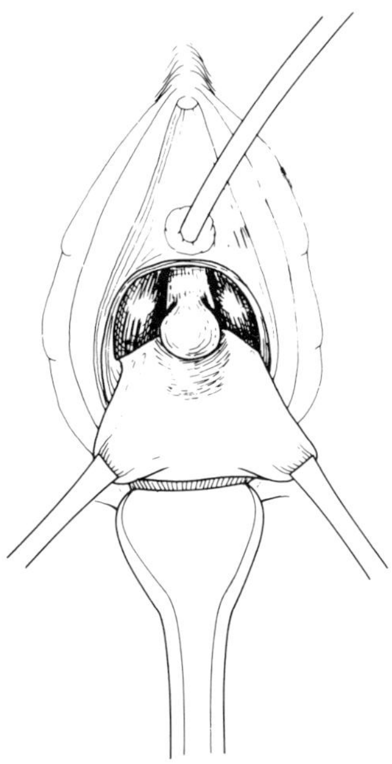

Fig. 13.7. Exposure of neck of diverticulum.

sometimes wide strip of the vaginal aspect of the urethral wall, which is an injury that is almost impossible to repair. At best one is left with an area of fibrous tissue which soon contracts to form a long and tough stricture. There may not even be enough urethral wall left to be closed around the catheter, so there is then also a danger of urethro-vaginal fistula formation.

The opening into the urethra should be carefully closed with small sutures. The original incision at the edge of the vaginal orifice is then loosely closed and the vagina lightly packed for 24 hours. If a catheter is put in it should be retained for a week to 10 days. Post-operative bladder drainage can be avoided altogether after smaller operations.

Gaertners cyst is seen in young women and must be differentiated from a urethral diverticulum by showing that the urethra is normal without any diverticular orifice. The cyst contains clear mucus without infection and should be treated by marsupialization which avoids the danger of damage to the urethra and bladder base, both of which may be in close direct relationship to the cyst.

PRIMARY CARCINOMA OF THE URETHRA

This tumour is a rarity compared with cancer in the bladder and cancer of the vulva. It occurs almost without exception in elderly women with a history of urethral bleeding or haematuria. Dysuria is less commonly a complaint. In many cases the history is surprisingly long. Histologically the tumour is a squamous cell or transitional cell carcinoma in the proportion of 3:1, and adeno-carcinoma is nearly as frequent as the transitional variety. Bizarre rarities are seen, such as sarcoma, mixed Müllerian tumour and mesonephroid tumour. Suburethral vaginal metastasis from endometrial uterine carcinoma is the most important differential diagnosis which must be remembered. Carcinoma of the urethra metastasises for the most part to lymph nodes, the tumours in the distal urethra to the superficial inguinal nodes and the tumours in the upper urethra to the external and internal iliac and obturator nodes. There is liable to be ulceration and secondary infection in the primary tumour which also tends to produce lymph node enlargement.

Diagnosis

Urethral prolapse with epithelial hypertrophy, urethral caruncle, carcinoma-in-situ and carcinoma can be difficult to distinguish from one another by simple clinical examination. It is therefore important that any urethral tumour, especially if near the external urinary meatus, should be investigated by cytological smear and by colposcopy. Both these examinations are very easy to do and often give conclusive results. If either of them reveal suspicion of carcinoma, a biopsy is necessary. At the same time as the biopsy, examination under anaesthesia should be performed, so that the tumour can be palpated from the vaginal aspect while the urethra is examined with the cysto-urethroscope. It is very important to identify the upper limit of the tumour by direct inspecton and to find out if there is any fixation of the urethra by bimanual examination under anaesthesia. This indicates spread to the paraurethral tissues above or below the urogenital diaphragm. If facilities are available, the urethral pressure profile will give an accurate picture of the effect of the tumour on urethral closure and helps to define the upper limit of resection. However, nearly as much information can be obtained by cysto-urethroscopy with simultaneous palpation of the urethra under anaesthesia.

Staging

There is as yet no accepted system of classification. Staging of these tumours is difficult because there are two types of epithelium involved, transitional in the upper part of the urethra and non-keratinizing squamous epithelium in the lower part. When a squamous tumour starts to invade adjacent tissue, there is no way of distinguishing it from a primary vaginal cancer. Direct invasion and lymphatic spread take place both inside the pelvis, to the obturator and internal iliac nodes and outside to the superficial inguinal group. There is no certain method of demonstrating intrapelvic lymphnode metastases from these tumours (Fig. 13.8).

The site in the urethra is important, both as regards the direction of spread and also as regards choice of treatment. The question of preservation of continence dwarfs almost all other considerations and has much to do with whether surgery is indicated or not.

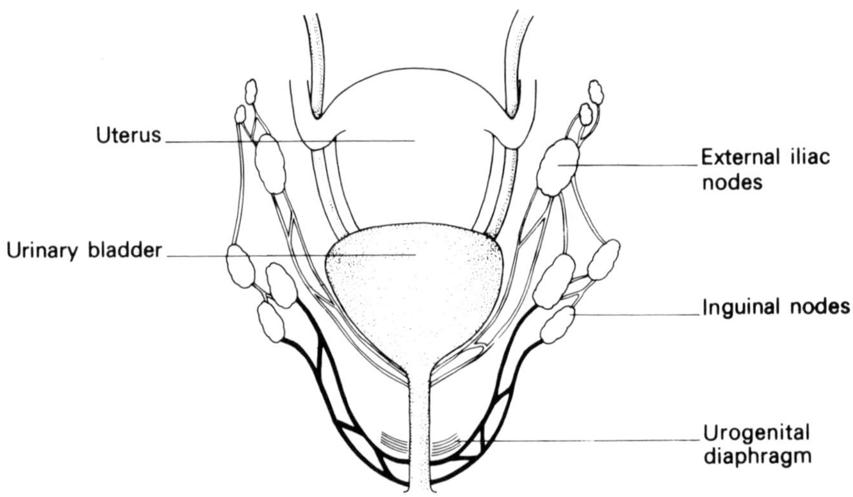

Fig. 13.8. Lymph drainage from urethra.

Treatment of the primary tumour

Carcinoma in situ is only discovered as an incidental finding at the external meatus as a result of the investigation of local changes such as leukoplakia, caruncle or polyp. The area involved can be removed just like a caruncle.

A urethral tumour which is limited to the distal centimetre and with no invasion outside the urethral wall can be effectively treated by surgical resection of the distal urethra. It is a safe rule that the distal half of the urethra can be removed without causing incontinence, so it is often possible to remove the tumour with an adequate margin of healthy mucosa (Fig. 13.9). The cut urethral mucosa must be accurately sewn with fine absorbable sutures to the introitus mucosa in order to avoid stricture formation at the junction. The urethral mucosa tends to retract upwards so every effort must be made to obtain an accurate adaptation. Even so, stricture formation can occur because it is difficult to avoid a scar in the form of a ring.

Since the urogenital diaphragm is located in the distal half of the urethra, removal of this part means that the patient may have difficulty in voluntarily interrupting the urinary stream during micturition. It does not lead to incontinence.

Sometimes a tumour in the distal centimetre can spread to the vulva without involving the deeper tissues. Surgical excision is still to be preferred and is, in fact, performed as if it were a vulval cancer which had involved the urethra.

Fixation of a malignant tumour anywhere in the urethra is a contra-indication to surgery. Radio-therapy is to be preferred.

If the tumour involves the upper half of the urethra the problem is not so simple. Any removal of the tumour will involve loss of continence. This suggests that removal of the whole urethra and bladder is therefore necessary together with lymph node removal in the groin or pelvis; and finally that anterior exenteration should be considered.

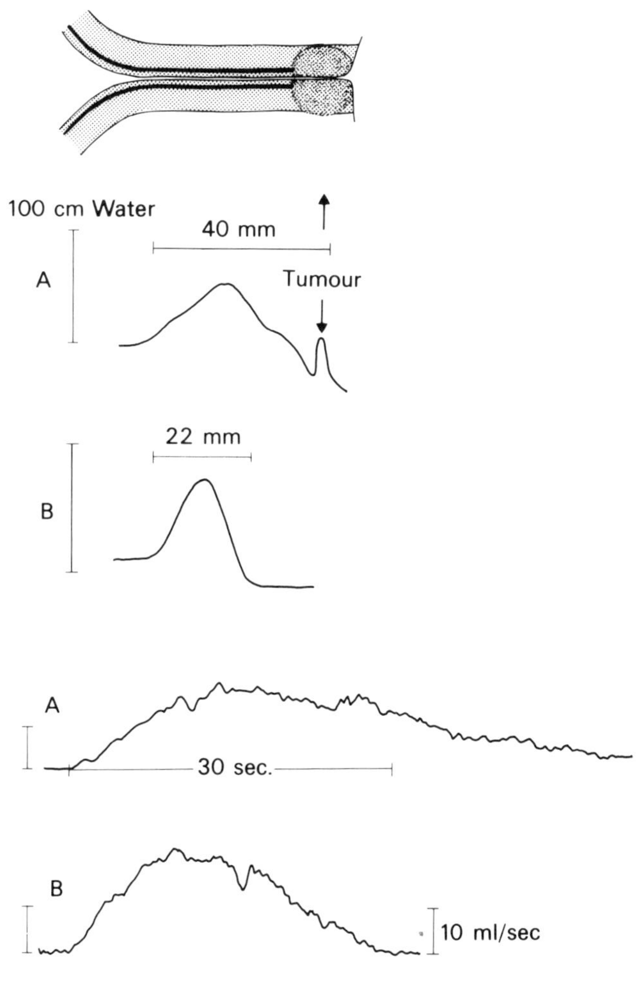

Fig. 13.9. Urethral pressure profile and flow measurement before (A) and after (B) partial resection of the urethra for carcinoma in the distal part. The tumour caused compression and obstruction.

These patients are often elderly women in the 70's, 80's and even 90's, with senile changes in cerebrum, heart, circulation and lungs. The prognosis, whatever the treatment, is poor due to the early spread of these tumours to lymph nodes within the pelvis. Urinary diversion, even if technically successful, is poorly tolerated in old age. The patients seldom manage to look after the ileostomy themselves and must be permanently hospitalized.

The rational treatment is radiotherapy, given as local tumour irradiation, using a tumour dose equivalent to about 70 Gy (7000 rads) either in the form of a local electron field or radium needle application. After-loading techniques can be used here with advantage, if available.

Treatment of lymphatic metastases

After local irradiation of a urethral tumour and if the patient is in good enough condition, the areas of secondary lymphatic spread can be irradiated. A low pelvic field can be used as long as the field of primary irradiation is shielded.

When the primary tumour is operable, the inguinal lymph nodes should always, if possible, be treated since more than half of the patients already have or will later develop inguinal metastases. Bilateral block dissection of the inguinal nodes can be considered in a younger woman, but an unshielded low pelvic irradiation field might be preferred. This includes the superficial inguinal nodes, the pelvic nodes and the primary tumour area.

Prognosis

The rarity of urethral carcinoma and the hitherto rather haphazard treatment has not contributed to the production of reliable survival figures. There is a general impression that it is a form of cancer with a poor prognosis. This is partly due to the age of the patients and partly due to the tendency to early dissemination. The mobile tumour in the distal urethra has undoubtedly the best prognosis.

Carcinoma of the urethra is a form of cancer where the main object of its management is not 5 or 10 years survival, but rather to make the patient's last year or two as comfortable as possible. Large operations involving radical changes in urine collection and disposal which are reasonable in younger women with considerable life expectancy are out of place. It is better to put more effort into treatment of symptoms and less into treatment of the cancer.

REFERENCES

Amussen M, Haveland H (1982) Primary malignant tumours of the female urethra. A report on 51 cases (in press).

Asmussen M, Ulmsten U (1982) The role of urethral pressure profile measurement-in female patients with urethral carcinoma. *Ann. Chir. Gynaecol.* (in press).

Bracken RB *et al.* (1976) Primary carcinoma of the female urethra. *J. Urol.* **116,** 188.

Chu AM (1973) Female urethral carcinoma – radiotherapy. *Radiology,* **107,** 627.

Grabstald H *et al.* (1966) Cancer of the female urethra. *J.A.M.A.,* **197,** 835.

Kolstad P, Stafl A (1977) *Atlas of Colposcopy.* University Park Press, Baltimore and Universitetsforlag, Oslo.

Packham DR (1971) Epithelial lining of the female urethra. *Brit. J. Urol.* **43,** 201.

Pointon R, Poole-Wilson D (1968) Primary carcinoma of the female urethra. *Brit. J. Urol.* **40,** 682.

Roberts M, Smith P (1968) Non-malignant obstruction of the female urethra. *Brit. J. Urol.* **40,** 694.

Robertson JR (1980) Urethral diverticula. In *Gynecologic Urology and Urodynamics,* ed. D Ostergard. Williams & Wilkins, Baltimore.

Spence H, Duckett J (1970) Diverticulum of the female urethra. *J. Urol.* **104,** 432.

Symmonds RE, Hill LM (1978) Loss of the urethra. *Am. J. Obstet. Gynecol.* **150,** 130.

Tanagho EA (1975) Anatomy and physiology of the urethra in urinary incontinence. In *Urinary Incontinence,* ed. KPS Caldwell. Sector Publishing Co, London.

Appendix A

Urine Specimens and their Examination

COLLECTION OF URINE SPECIMENS

All women harbour in the outer urethra several different types of organisms which are the same as those found in the introitus and on the perineum. Some of these are potentially pathological, such as the commonest—*E. coli,* which is of the same sero-type as the *E. coli* in the colon and rectum. It is therefore inevitable that urine which is sterile in the bladder will pick up organisms from the outer urethra on its way out and that secretions from the vagina, which also contain organisms, may be collected in the urine specimen. A sterile catheter can carry organisms from the outer urethra into the bladder and be a cause of infection of residual urine. Antiseptic solutions cleanse the introitus but have no effect on the bacterial content of the urethra and have the additional objection that they are liable to be mixed with the urine in the specimen jar so that bacteria are killed and cultures give false negative results.

Mid-stream urine specimen

The first part of the urinary stream functions as a kind of irrigation of the outer urethra and is discarded; the rest of the urine is then passed direct into a sterile container without contact with the labia. It is best to take the specimen when the patient first passes urine in the morning after sleep for this is the time when there are most cells and bacteria in the urine. In practice this is not always easy, but at any rate the patient should not have passed urine for 3 hours or more if this is possible. The whole introitus should be washed with a swab soaked in sterile normal saline. Antiseptic solutions should not be used. If there is a vaginal discharge or a menstrual period or other form of vaginal bleeding, a sterile swab or a tampon should be placed in the vagina. With adequate instruction, most patients can manage to provide a mid-stream specimen themselves in private and results show that these specimens are quite reliable.

Other methods of taking urine specimens

Obtaining a specimen of urine can sometimes be difficult because of mechanical obstruction of the urethra, obesity or severe infection in the introitus region or vagina. Urethral, vulval and vaginal tumours can make a mid-stream specimen impossible. Urine examination must not be neglected because of this; one needs to exclude the presence of sugar and protein and it is useful to know that the bladder urine is sterile. A urethral catheter can sometimes be used under these circumstances but is not recommended because it is often difficult to pass without contamination and the result as far as the bladder urine is concerned is therefore unreliable. It is preferable to use suprapubic puncture with a fine needle. This has the great advantage that the specimen is taken far from the contaminated area and that the result is definite and reliable. Suprapubic puncture can be done under all conditions of consulting room practice. Furthermore, it can be of great use in patients who have had or have complained of recurrent attacks of lower urinary tract infection. It allows a decision to be made as to whether the bladder or the urethra is the site of infection.

Technique of suprapubic bladder puncture

It should first be confirmed by palpation and percussion that the bladder is distended. The skin in the suprapubic area is cleansed with suitable antiseptic and wiped dry. A long needle (10 cm) about 1 mm in diameter with a 10 ml syringe attached is passed through the skin just above the upper border of the symphysis in the mid-line. The needle is then advanced backwards and a little downwards between the rectus muscles until it is felt to enter the bladder. Urine can then be aspirated into the syringe, after which the needle is removed. If there is any doubt about the direction in which the needle should be advanced after it has been passed through the abdominal wall a finger per vaginam can be used to palpate the trigone through the anterior vaginal wall and this gives the operator something to aim at.

Specimens from in-dwelling catheters

An in-dwelling plastic balloon catheter with an attached plastic drainage tube cannot be punctured with a needle without subsequent leakage. Disconnection of the drainage tube in order to obtain a specimen leads to infection in a high proportion of cases because the end of the catheter which has been outside the end of the drainage tube is not sterile owing to contact with the patient's thighs or bedclothes. Ideally, under these circumstances, a short piece of sterile rubber tubing should be inserted between the catheter and the drainage tube. This can then be punctured in exactly the same way as a specimen of blood is taken from a vein. Latex balloon catheters can be punctured without any subsequent trouble. It is recommended that the outside of the catheter or tube should be cleansed with spirit before puncturing. The spirit should be allowed time to dry.

LABORATORY EXAMINATION

The specimen can be examined in several different ways, as follows.

The cellular content

Normally, a mid-stream urine specimen contains epithelial cells, both transitional and squamous, a few white cells and the occasional red cell. Casts of epithelial cells from the renal tubules may be seen. This examination should always be done while the urine is still warm, that is to say before a sediment appears which contains mucus and phosphate crystals which obscure the cellular content and before the casts have disintegrated. A drop of urine is placed on a slide and a cover-glass placed on top. If desired the urine can be stained with methylene blue but this is not essential. If the specimen is macroscopically almost clear, the cell content is obviously small so it pays to let it stand 15 minutes on the bench and then take up a little from the deeper part with a pipette. The use of a centrifuge provides more cells and crystals on the slide but it can introduce artifacts because it makes all casts disintegrate and collects all the debris of dead epithelial cells. Using a fresh, uncentrifuged specimen may mean that there are very few cells in a normal specimen but this in fact means that recognition of a normal specimen is easy and quick. If there is an infection, cells will be very much more numerous and then centrifuging is unnecessary.

When infection has produced an inflammatory reaction with increased vascularity in the urothelium, there will be a manifest increase in the number of white (pus) cells sometimes up to about 100 per high power field, and red cells are increased to a lesser extent. There is also an increase in the number of desquamated epithelial cells. Bacteria can be seen singly or in clumps, especially if stained.

This microscopic examination is very easy to perform and requires only simple equipment. A high power microscope objective with ×400 magnification should be used. The approximate number of bacteria per high power field in the uncentrifuged specimen is related to the severity of the infection in that more than 1 per field represents a significant bacteriuria. The presence of pus cells without bacteria (sterile pyuria) is the classical sign of tuberculous infection, which must never be forgotten; pus cells can also commonly occur without bacteria after treatment of an acute infection and in various long-standing inflammatory conditions of the upper and lower urinary tracts. Radiation cystitis is an example of this, but here there are often also a number of red cells. Pus cells and red cells in sterile urine may also indicate urothelial cancer or a malignant tumour infiltrating the urinary tract from neighbouring organs.

In the great majority of cases, the clinical history of dysuria and frequency, the exclusion of other pathological conditions by clinical examination and the finding of pus cells and bacteria by direct examination of the urine is enough to prove that the patient has an acute bacterial infection of the lower urinary tract. This allows treatment to start at once without waiting for the result of urine culture.

Chemical examination

The pH must also be measured while the specimen is still fresh; it alters if the urine is allowed to stand a few hours. A clear, acid specimen makes a significant infection most unlikely. Albumin and sugar should also be excluded. This can all be done using commercially available dip sticks.

Quantitative bacterial culture

The mid-stream urine has the disadvantage that organisms can be grown from a normal specimen, which means that there is no definite dividing line between sterile and infected, all specimens are more or less infected. Where, therefore, do we draw the line? A general rule has been accepted by most laboratories and clinicians that 10,000 organisms per ml urine or less should be regarded as 'contamination'. One specimen with 100,000 organisms per ml means definite infection in the bladder urine in approximately 80% of cases. Any figure in between has no definite clinical meaning. This is a fairly good solution to the difficulty for it tells us what we want to know, whether there is an infection in the bladder or upper urinary tract. Isolated infection in the urethra needs to be examined by taking swabs and employing special culture methods. The cooperation of a bacteriologist should be sought before this is done. The results or urine culture are, of course, much more convincing if the same organisms are found in the same quantity in a second specimen taken a day or two later. The probability then reaches about 95%. Pathologists are naturally reluctant to commit themselves on the subject of infection in a urine specimen for it is obvious that the mid-stream urine is inherently liable to contamination and that laboratories have no control over this. It is not always possible for the patient to be sure that the urinary stream will pass directly into the specimen container without contact with the labia. Some printed instructions tell the patient to sit on the toilet while she collects the specimen, others recommend her to stand on the floor with one foot on the toilet seat. False positive results can also be due to the delay involved in sending the urine to the laboratory or to delay in the laboratory itself. Up to 1 hour at 20°C or up to 48 hours in a refrigerator is permissible, but not more. False negative results occur if the specimen is taken after a course of antibiotics has been started. The clinician is well advised to discuss all this with the pathologist concerned so that they can agree on how the reports shall be worded and whether the laboratory will report on the cellular content of the urine at the same time.

CULTURE METHODS IN THE CONSULTING ROOM, OFFICE OR OUT-PATIENT DEPARTMENT

It is not difficult for the gynaecologist to do a certain amount of bacterial culture himself and save a good deal of time. The simplest, most practical and inexpensive method which is at the same time reliable, is to use the dip-inoculum slide technique. This is an ordinary microscope slide (or something similar) which is coated with culture medium ready for use. It is removed from its sterile container and dipped into the fresh urine specimen; the surplus urine is then allowed to drip off and the slide is returned to its container and the top screwed on. It is incubated at 37°C overnight. If there is no incubator available, it can be left at room temperature (15 to 20°C) for 48 hours. About 0.01 ml of urine is reckoned to adhere to each side of the slide so the number of colonies can be counted and multiplied by 100 or compared with photographs of standard colony counts to obtain the number of bacteria per ml of urine. Recognition of the particular type of organism is a problem which can be solved to a certain extent by using a dip-slide coated with a special medium which allows only gram-negative organisms to grow. It is possible to identify *E. coli* on this medium by the characteristic metallic appearance of its colonies and the gynaecologist can learn to recognize others. However, if a gynaecologist wishes to go as far as this on his own, he will be well advised to use the same culture plates as the local laboratory uses, inoculating the urine with a loop onto blood agar and MacConkey media on the same plate and incubating overnight at 37°C. Final identification and resistance determination is then done in the laboratory if necessary. A second dip-slide can conveniently be sent for sub-culturing or a fresh specimen can be sent if the delay is not too great. It is here the dip-slide has its great advantage for it can be sent by post to the laboratory and read by the bacteriologist when it arrives. Another method uses boric acid in a small container. This prevents further bacterial multiplication during the transport period and has the advantage that the cellular content can be examined.

Why, then, bother to examine cultures at all when they can be so easily sent to the laboratory and examined more effectively there?

The answer is that many of the cultures which turn out to be negative can be identified in the consulting room and need not be sent to the laboratory at all. Furthermore a large number of the positive cultures are *E. coli* infections which the gynaecologist can learn to identify. They are from patients who have never been in hospital and who have therefore not yet acquired infection by drug-resistant bacteria. In this way, much time can be saved between examination and treatment and unnecessary treatment of the patient who has urinary symptoms with sterile urine can be avoided. In addition, after treatment is finished the urine can be shown to be sterile within 24 hours, which avoids waiting several days for a negative result from the laboratory. It is only in the case of infections which recur frequently or which do not respond to treatment that the help of the laboratory is needed.

Urine cytology

The cells in a mid-stream specimen can be fixed by mixing the specimen with an equal amount of 50% ethyl alcohol. It is then sent to a laboratory where the pathologist has experience of urine cytology. The examination can demonstrate malignant transitional epithelial cells where urothelial tumour formation is suspected—for example, because of haematuria in a patient where cystoscopy and urography are both negative. Urine cytology is however always a little uncertain, partly because the cellular debris can vary greatly in quantity and quality, and partly because the slight differences between benign and malignant transitional epithelial cells demand considerable experience on the part of the cytologist.

REFERENCES

Guttman D, Naylor GRE (1967) Dip-slide: an aid to quantitative urine culture in general practice. *Br. Med. J.* **3,** 343.

Hart EL, Magee MJ (1957) The mid-stream urine specimen. *Am. J. Nurs.* **57,** 1323.

Norden CW, Kass EH (1968) Bacteriuria of pregnancy. *Annu. Rev. Med.* **19,** 431.

Stamey T (1967) Office bacteriology. *J. Urol.* **97,** 926.

Appendix B The Clinical Interpretation of Urinary Infection

In theory, urinary infection in the female includes acute and chronic, symptomatic and asymptomatic inflammatory conditions due to growth of micro-organisms in the upper urinary tract (kidney parenchyma, calyces, renal pelvis and ureter) and the lower urinary tract (bladder and urethra) either individually or together.

In practice, there is no clearly defined line between acute and chronic or between symptomatic and asymptomatic. 'Inflammatory condition' can be used to mean pus cells in the urine specimen, the clinical picture found on examination or the histological appearance of urothelium. Micro-organisms in the urine are only what can be grown on standard culture media or seen with the microscope. Culture of anaerobic organisms or of viruses is not generally done. Bacteria can sometimes be found in significant quantities in the urine without histological evidence of inflammation. Conversely, histological evidence of inflammation can be seen in a patient with symptoms without growth of bacteria on culture. Many patients with, apparently, classical symptoms of a lower tract infection have repeatedly sterile urine specimens.

There is, however, in this complex situation one general rule regarding treatment. It must always be based on mid-stream specimens of urine which show a definite bacteriuria together with inflammatory cells.

Natural history of bacteriuria

The normal kidney does not excrete bacteria in the urine because they are not filtered through the glomerulus. The urine in the renal pelvis and bladder should therefore be sterile. The outer third of the female urethra is colonized by organisms which have a low pathogenicity as long as they remain there. But in many primary infections of the lower urinary tract there is a close correlation between the serotypes of the coliform organisms which can be cultured from the urine and those from swabs taken from the introitus and perineum.

Several epidemiological surveys have shown that 7% of women over 50 years of age, 4% of young women and 1% of schoolgirls have significant quantities of bacteria in a mid-stream urine specimen without any symptoms or demonstrable pathology. Seventy-five per cent of the bacteria are *E. coli*. It seems probable that women with bacteriuria rather than those with normal urine are the ones who develop attacks of acute infection, but this is not known for certain.

Attacks of lower urinary tract infection are not uncommon in young women when they start having sexual intercourse, so-called 'honeymoon cystitis'. These take the form of an acute inflammation of the urethral epithelium which spreads upwards to the trigone and bladder base. The inflammation tends to diminish spontaneously and reappear after subsequent intercourse. After a time the tendency to recurrence lessens for reasons which are not understood. It is probable that minor trauma to the external meatus facilitates the adherence of bacteria to the epithelial cell membranes so that pathological growth of bacteria which are already present becomes possible. Sometimes bacteriuria is a complication of a general disease such as diabetes, calculus disease or long-standing renal disease.

Hospital infections due to catheterization or instrumentation have for many years been a by-product of a woman's stay in a gynaecological department. They are caused by the patient's own organisms from the introitus and urethra which gain access to the bladder or to paraurethral tissues. These organisms are for the most part drug-sensitive but the hospital organisms which the patient acquires via an in-dwelling catheter by cross-infection are resistant to the commonly used urinary antiseptics.

Terminology

Many commonly used terms have never been acceptably defined. For example, 'pyelonephritis' means three different things according to whether it is used by a clinician, a radiologist or a pathologist. It can be seen in urograms in childhood as clubbing of calyces with scarring of the over-lying parenchyma, often in combination with ureteric reflux. These changes are found with and without bacteriuria, both in children and adults, but they have not been found in the adult after a typical attack of acute pyelonephritis. Histological renal scarring has been found as a congenital manifestation and is also seen as a result of the vascular changes found in diabetes and hypertension. Histological evidence of acute inflammation is most unusual in these kidneys unless there has been damage due to ureteric obstruction or to analgesic addiction.

Many now believe that vesico-ureteral reflux in infants (usually a transient phenomenon) can cause infected urine to be forced back into the renal parenchyma with resulting acute inflammation and development of fibrous tissue. The latest term—'reflux nephropathy'—reflects this explanation of the pathology.

The term 'cystitis' is used to describe a true inflammatory condition which is really a urethro-cystitis, but it also includes conditions with a similar symptomatology where the urine is sterile. An example of this is the so-called 'urethral syndrome'. It is better to speak of *upper urinary tract* and *lower urinary tract infections* and not to divide them into symptomatic and asymptomatic. Both are treated in the same way.

The importance of bacteriuria for the gynaecologist is twofold. It can flare up into an acute upper or lower tract infection after a pelvic operation and it can be the clue to the discovery of chronic renal disease. If a pathological, gynaecological condition has been found and the patient has infected urine, it is advisable to clear up the infection before any operation is considered. One course of a drug to which the organisms are known to be sensitive should be given, followed by examination of the urine. If this is unsuccessful, the reason should be found. Intravenous urography should be arranged, followed by cystoscopy. The objective is to pick out the small group of patients with chronic renal disease, that is—reflux nephropathy, hypertensive nephropathy, analgesic renal damage, urinary tract malformation, calculus, varieties of glomerulo-nephritis, a haemoglobinopathy, ureteric obstruction or diabetic renal complications. All these can lead to renal failure and therefore be a danger to life if major gynaecological surgery is unwittingly performed without knowledge of their existence.

Lower urinary tract infection

This tends to occur in attacks but the symptoms can vary from a most acute haemorrhagic cysto-urethritis to a mild inflammatory reaction which causes he patient little trouble. In young women who have not had previous attacks it can be treated after a mid-stream specimen has been taken and a recurrent attack can also be reasonably treated without further examination. The urine must always be re-examined to make sure that it has returned to normal. In women at or near the menopause who, for no obvious reason start to have attacks of lower urinary tract infection, great caution is necessary. It is often a signal that there is some underlying condition which may be found either in the urinary or the gynaecological tracts. Ovarian carcinoma, for example, can present by causing an apparently spontaneous onset of lower urinary tract infection.

About half the women who have symptoms of lower urinary tract infection have no pathological bacteria in the urine. A change from a predominantly vegetable diet to one rich in protein can produce dysuria and frequency owing to the highly acid urine. Certain drinks, such as coffee, tea, sherry and white wine have a similar effect in some women. Detergent soaps and bubble baths have an irritating effect on the urethra which can imitate infection. Hormonal changes, for example oestrogen deficiency in older women, are often associated with irritative symptoms, sometimes with true infection.

Upper urinary tract infection

The gynaecologist is most often confronted with this situation after a pelvic operation or even after catheterization or instrumentation of the lower urinary tract. Fever and loin pain associated with rigors occur in a patient with infected urine. A positive blood culture can be obtained soon after a rigor and will often show the same organisms as have been found in the urine. This is the classical 'catheter fever' which can proceed to a catastrophic fall in blood pressure and then becomes known as 'septic or bacteriaemic shock'. It can be rapidly fatal unless actively treated. The peculiar combination of high fever with the signs of shock is the clue to the condition.

Urinary antiseptic medication

There is no specific 'drug of choice' in the treatment of urinary infections. All drugs have their individual advantages and disadvantages. Choice is dictated by the urine specimens, by possible toxicity and by possible allergic reactions. Complicated medication which can be nephrotoxic should only be used in consultation with a nephrologist and/or a urologist.

Prophylaxis

Certain simple measures can be taken by the patient and her doctor to prevent urinary infection.

By the patient

Drink extra fluid throughout the 24 hours to produce a 'washout effect'.

Empty the bladder completely so as to avoid residual urine.

Empty the bladder in the night by drinking extra fluid in the evening or by using an alarm clock.

Empty the bladder after sexual intercourse.

Avoid exposure to cold.

Avoid antiseptic sprays, etc which alter the flora in the introitus.

By the gynaecologist

Discover and treat residual urine.

Take regular urine specimens from and, if necessary, operate on patients who are predisposed to infection because of prolapse, outflow obstruction, cystocele with residual urine, diverticula, etc.

Treat vulval and vaginal infections.

Treat oestrogen deficiency in elderly patients.

Follow up irradiated patients by taking regular specimens.

Follow up patients with neuropathic dysfunction after radical surgery.

Take catheterization seriously by adoption of a rigid antiseptic technique which is practised by all members of the team.

Arrange for all urethral instrumentation, cystoscopy, cystometry and urodynamics to be done with full antiseptic precautions.

Do all instrumentation as gently as possible.

In hospital, intermittent catheterization is preferable to an in-dwelling catheter.

If an in-dwelling catheter must be used, keep it attached to a closed drainage system and keep it closed when taking urine specimens.

Change in-dwelling catheters once a week.

Make sure that all drainage bags have a non-return valve.

Avoid long-term therapy unless it is given in consultation with a nephrologist or a urologist.

Avoid producing drug-resistance and rare bacterial strains by over-treatment.

REFERENCES

Asscher AW (1974) Asymptomatic infections of the urinary tract. *Trans. Assoc. Am. Physicians,* **69,** 56.

Brumfitt W, Percival A (1964) Pathogenesis and laboratory diagnosis of non-tuberculous urinary tract infection: a review. *J. Clin. Pathol.* **17,** 482.

Brumfitt W, Asscher AW (1973) *Urinary Tract Infections.* Oxford University Press, London.

Cox CE, Lacy SS, Hinman FJr (1968) The urethra and its relationship to urinary tract infection. *J. Urol.* **99,** 632.

Eykyn S, Newman CGH (1969) Suprapubic puncture. *Br. J. Hosp. Med.* **2,** 863.

Ferrie B, Glen E, Hunter B (1979) Long-term catheter drainage. *Br. Med. J.* **2,** 1046.

Freedman LR (1967) Chronic Pyelonephritis at autopsy. *Ann. Intern. Med.* **66,** 697.

Garrod LP, O'Grady F (1971) *Antibiotic and Chemotherapy.* E & S Livingstone, Edinburgh.

Gillespie WA, Linton KB, Miller A, Slade N (1960) Diagnosis, epidemiology & control of urinary infection in urology & gynaecology. *J. Clin. Pathol.* **13,** 168.

Kass EH (1956) Asymptomatic infections of the urinary tract. *Trans. Assoc. Am. Physicians,* **69,** 56.

Malek RS, Boyce WH, Wilkiemeyer RM (1973) Prophylactic systemic antimicrobial drugs and postoperative urinary infection. *J. Urol.* **109,** 84.

Miller A, Gillespie WA, Linton KB, Slade N, Mitchell JP (1958) Postoperative infection in urology. *Lancet,* **2,** 608.

O'Grady FW, Cattell WR (1966) Kinetics of urinary tract infection; 2, the bladder. *Br. J. Urol.* **38,** 156.

Slade N (1980) Postoperative urinary tract infections in urology and gynaecology: a review. *J. R. Soc. Med.* **73,** 739.

Wing AJ (1970) Infections of the urinary tract: 2, management. *Br. Med J.* **4,** 35.

Appendix C The Urinary Tract in Pregnancy

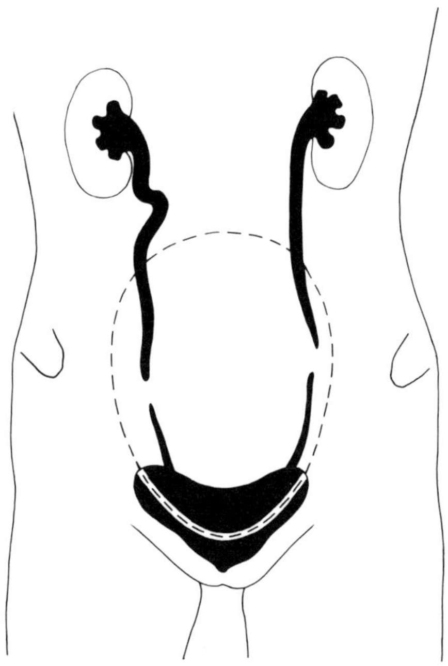

Fig. C1. Urogram in pregnancy.

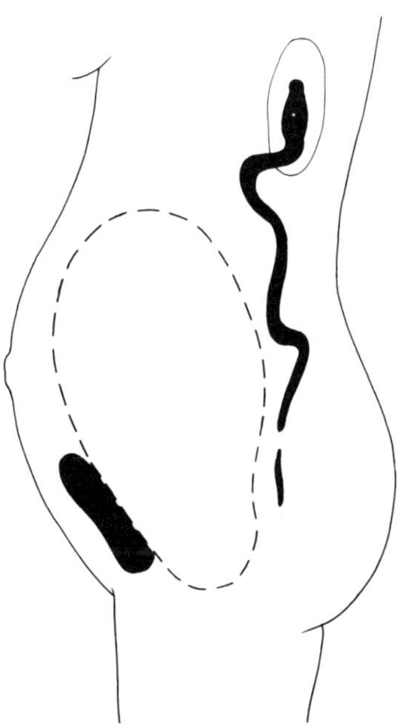

Fig. C2. Urogram in pregnancy: lateral view.

Early in pregnancy most women experience a certain frequency of micturition during the day, possibly because the enlarging uterus behind and above the bladder begins to have an effect on its capacity. This is apparently a simple mechanical effect which produces the desire to micturate when the bladder holds comparatively little urine. There is also a degree of polydipsia and polyuria which can contribute to the frequency. These symptoms begin about 6 weeks after conception and reach a maximum at 8–10 weeks. After this, when the enlarging uterus becomes an abdominal organ, the symptoms disappear and the bladder capacity increases until it holds more than is normal for the individual. It can commonly reach over 1000 ml in the later stages of pregnancy.

There is often dilatation of the ureters, which has been called 'the physiological hydroureter of pregnancy' in order to underline the fact that it is normally a harmless and temporary feature. There is moderate dilatation of the renal pelves and the ureters above the pelvic brim, while the ureters in the bony pelvis are not affected (Fig. C1 and C2). This is easily demonstrated in the renogram (Fig. C3) which shows normal kidney function with signs of intermittent obstruction. The condition reaches its maximum at about the 20th week and does not increase thereafter as pregnancy proceeds. It affects the right ureter more often than the left and the dilatation is greater on the right side. The capacity of the calyces, renal pelvis and ureter can be increased from 5–10 ml to 50 ml. The ureters are not only dilated but are also elongated so that their course can be altered and they appear on the urogram to be 'kinked'. However, if pictures are taken in two planes, these kinks will be found to be artifacts caused by the superimposition of two adjacent lengths.

After delivery, the ureteric dilatation quickly disappears. It takes from a few days to about 4 weeks for the ureters to return to normal. This physiological hydronephrosis has no adverse effect on kidney function even though it can look alarming on the isotope renogram. It is only when upper urinary tract infection occurs that permanent damage to the kidney becomes a possibility.

URINARY TRACT INFECTION

Asymptomatic bacteriuria

The mid-stream specimen of a woman in early pregnancy should be normal. About 4%, however, are found to have a definite bacteriuria without any

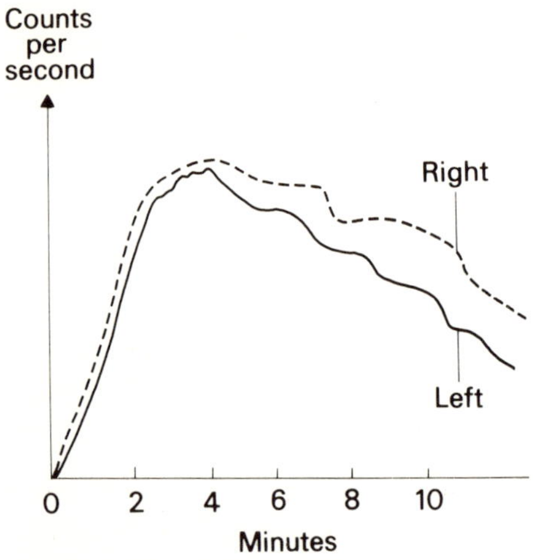

Fig. C3. Renogram in pregnancy showing delayed excretion in the third phase. This indicates hydroureter with intermittent emptying.

symptoms or signs of infection. This proportion is probably the same as in non-pregnant women and the bacterial strains are the same. It has been estimated that between a quarter and a third of pregnant women with bacteriuria will develop symptomatic upper and/or lower urinary tract infection if no precautions are taken. This is in contrast to non-pregnant women in whom only a very small proportion are at risk. Bacteriuria in pregnancy should therefore be regarded as potentially dangerous because it is impossible to pick out the patient who will develop severe infective complications. Moreover, the natural changes in the urinary tract which tend towards urinary stasis, together with the fact that the urine becomes an even better culture medium than usual because of the presence of sugar and protein, interfere with the normal self-cleaning mechanism of the urinary tract and make a urinary infection a danger to mother and child. Anomalies in the urinary tract, renal damage resulting from the prolonged use of analgesics, reflux nephropathy, renal calculi, diabetes mellitus and various types of anaemia which are all known to predispose to severe infective episodes in the non-pregnant woman, take on an added significance in pregnancy. They are not only a risk to the pregnancy in themselves but also can lead to repeated severe urinary tract infections. Infection which does not clear up with treatment is said to be associated with low birth weight of the foetus and with premature labour. There is also a suspected relationship between persistent urinary infection and the development of hypertension during pregnancy.

The precise meaning of simple bacteriuria in pregnancy in the absence of demonstrable pathology in the urinary tract or elsewhere is undecided. In the majority of cases it seems to do little harm but all must be thoroughly investigated and treated because of those who develop serious infections.

The practical consequence of this is that all pregnant women should have a mid-stream specimen of urine examined in each of the first, second and third trimesters. Patients with diabetes or the other predisposing factors mentioned above should have specimens examined more frequently.

It should be possible to culture the same pathological organism from two mid-stream urine specimens taken at a few days' interval to be sure that it is not a contamination or a chance organism picked up from the urethra. Catheter specimens are not necessary and should be avoided. Any special recommendations concerning the use of individual drugs during pregnancy should be looked for and followed.

After treatment, regular bacterial examination of the urine every two weeks should ideally be continued throughout the remainder of pregnancy. In practice, however, two successive negative specimens at a fortnight's interval is sufficient.

Prophylactic long-term medication should be avoided. It is better to watch frequent urine specimens for infection and then treat it if it appears. If the bacteriuria cannot be cleared up by drug treatment then there is almost certainly some abnormality in the urinary tract which should be localized and treated if possible.

After delivery, the same frequent examination of the urine should continue for three months, by which time the urinary tract should have returned to normal. Those with asymptomatic bacteriuria in whom the urine becomes and remains sterile need no further treatment or investigation. If bacteriuria is still present or recurs after treatment, a second course of treatment using a different drug which has been proved to be effective against the particular bacteria can be tried. If further recurrences cannot be prevented by courses of urinary antiseptic, it is best to avoid continuous medication and hold the patient under close observation with simple prophylactic precautions. Those women who have developed and been treated for a more serious urinary infection in pregnancy should later have a general clinical and urinary tract examination which should include urography in order to rule out reflux nephropathy and other abnormalities. Iodine sensitivity can be a problem which makes it impossible or at least inadvisable to do urography, but here isotope renography can be a great help. The object of this examination is to check the blood pressure (especially when there has been a rise during the pregnancy), to look for evidence of renal failure and to make sure that the urine remains normal. It is seldom that anything new is discovered and it has little relevance for the gynaecologist except during a subsequent pregnancy.

Symptomatic bacteriuria

UPPER TRACT INFECTIONS

Acute or subacute upper urinary tract infection usually occurs in the second trimester and can vary from an indefinite malaise without any of the classical symptoms to a severe illness with high temperature, rigors, vomiting, pain in one or both loins and frequency and pain on micturition. The urine is in all cases the clue to the diagnosis; it is true that in certain exceptional cases an acute attack can begin with a rise in temperature and general symptoms before there is evidence of infection in the urine and that, in unilateral cases, the affected ureter may become blocked by oedema so that only clear urine from the unaffected kidney comes into the bladder. This stage, if it happens at all, is short-lived and a urine specimen will become obviously infected. Microscopic examination shows masses of cellular debris mixed with pus cells and red cells, with groups of bacteria here and there. Culture shows *E. coli* in most cases, but other organisms may occur in patients with longstanding infection that have already been investigated or in cases with complications such as calculi.

Clinical examination in acute cases shows a high temperature, often over 40°C, associated with dehydration. Cases limited to the right side can at first sight look like acute appendicitis, but the higher temperature, absence of definite signs in the right side of the abdomen, together with the evidence of infection in the urine should lead to the right diagnosis. Vomiting may be a prominent symptom in acute pyelonephritis in early pregnancy, so much so that it suggests hyperemesis gravidarum, but here again the main clues are the high temperature and the infected urine.

Treatment should start as soon as the diagnosis is clear and be based on bed-rest, increased fluid intake and antibiotics. One must, of course, not forget to take a urine specimen for culture and resistance determination before the antibiotic is started.

The course of the disease under effective antibiotic treatment is about 4–6 days until all signs of infection have vanished. Not all cases, however, behave so well because, although the general condition may have improved, pain and tenderness may persist in one loin, the kidney becomes palpably enlarged and is clearly the cause of persistent trouble. This means that the ureter from this kidney has become obstructed and a pyonephrosis is developing. Some of these patients may indeed have had a hydronephrosis before the pregnancy with a partial stenosis at the junction of the renal pelvis and ureter. The diagnosis can be safely confirmed by isotope renography. In this situation the most effective treatment is drainage of the renal pelvis by catheterization of the ureter. It is very important to use a catheter without its stilette because the ureteric wall is thinner than before the pregnancy and may well have become softer because of the inflammatory reaction, all of which makes the chance of a perforation more likely. In the vast majority of cases a size 8 ureteric catheter can be passed into the oedematous orifice without difficulty, and thereafter it passes onwards to the junction of the renal pelvis and ureter where there may again be difficulty. Rotation of the catheter, combined with retraction a few centimetres followed by re-insertion, will usually achieve the desired result, which is obvious by the appearance of infected urine from the end of the catheter. It is sometimes necessary to irrigate the catheter with 2–4 ml sterile saline which is injected by using a small syringe and an intravenous needle (size 16) which is passed into the catheter. The cystoscope is then withdrawn from the bladder causing the catheter to drain into a sterile vessel.

The basic rule about leaving an in-dwelling ureteric catheter is that it should be removed as soon as possible, preferably within 24 hours. One must remember that the renal pelvis will not only drain itself *through* the catheter but also *around* it into the bladder; probably increasing amounts of urine come down this way as time goes on. The catheter under these circumstances has fulfilled its function of acting as a drain and may become a foreign body which does more harm than good. In addition, it is difficult to keep the outer end of the catheter sterile, so there are several good reasons for not retaining it more than a few hours.

If it is impossible to pass the catheter into the renal pelvis, there is a danger that the condition will progress to a pyonephrosis and if the pyonephrosis persists then operation cannot be long delayed. There is no doubt that a nephrectomy is an unnecessarily formidable operation when it is possible to achieve the necessary result with something easier and shorter. It is better to drain the kidney in the simplest manner and then re-consider the situation after the pregnancy is over. The operation of choice is either percutaneous or open nephrostomy.

ACUTE LOWER URINARY TRACT INFECTIONS

Acute infection of the lower urinary tract in pregnancy does not differ essentially from the same condition in the non-pregnant patient either in symptoms or treatment. There is neither the high pyrexia nor the profound general illness associated with upper tract infection. After-treatment and follow-up are the same as described above.

URINARY CALCULI

Development of calculi is very uncommon in pregnancy, probably because the altered physiology of the kidneys tends to produce conditions in the collecting tubules and calyces which reduce the chance of crystal formation. However, attacks of renal colic do occasionally occur, possibly due to a stone which had formed before the pregnancy began.

Clinical examination may reveal a stone which can be felt in the lower end of the ureter by rectal or vaginal examination. If a calculus can be felt there, it saves a great deal of time and trouble in coming to the correct diagnosis.

The patient should be admitted to hospital as an emergency for observation. The next step will be a straight X-ray of the abdomen to include the kidneys, ureters and bladder. This may be sufficient to confirm the presence of a calculus, but if there is still doubt, it is permissible to do a limited urography. The preliminary film will have already been taken, so one more film is taken 20 minutes after injection of contrast intravenously. The irradiation dosage must be kept to a minimum. Isotope renography can also be of help.

Relief of pain is the first necessity, preferably using intramuscular analgesics. The great majority of stones pass spontaneously if the patient is given extra fluid to increase urine production. Analgesics should be given and she should be encouraged to be active rather than at rest in bed. The intravenous urogram will indicate whether there is any haste about relieving the obstruction by removing the calculus. Renal concentration sufficient to give a fairly dense picture at 20 minutes after contrast injection means that there is no cause for immediate alarm, especially if the other kidney is normal. On the other hand, if the urogram shows a gross hydronephrosis with little concentration of contrast, this is an indication that there is a threat of permanent renal damage if the obstruction is not relieved. Obstruction by calculus at the upper end of the ureter is more likely to need treatment than impaction at the lower end. If a calculus has reached the lower ureter then it is practically certain that it will come out into the bladder. There is always time for the gynaecologist to get advice from a urologist, who should be consulted as soon as the diagnosis is made. There is no essential difference between the principles of treatment of a calculus in pregnancy and in the absence of pregnancy.

Renal colic can occur very late in pregnancy, just before labour begins and then presents a difficult problem. The best solution is to give analgesics and make every effort to put off doing anything to the calculus until after labour is completed. It is, perhaps, comforting to remember that a normal kidney will tolerate almost complete obstruction of its ureter for three weeks and then make a good recovery. A solitary kidney will survive even longer.

Operative surgery

If there is any question at all of surgical removal of a calculus in pregnancy, a urologist should be consulted. Every effort should be made to postpone uretero-lithotomy until after the pregnancy is over. This is possible in most cases. Even apparently urgent situations such as sudden calculus obstruction at the pelvi-ureteric junction in a solitary kidney near term, can be dealt with without recourse to surgery by close supervision of the electrolyte and serum creatinine changes and close and continual cooperation between the gynaecologist and the urologist. The gynaecologist is ready to induce labour or to do a Caesarian section, the urologist is ready to drain the kidney by the quickest and safest route. The only situation which might make surgical treatment of the obstruction take preference over all other considerations is the deadly combination of sudden obstruction and acute pyelonephritis in a solitary kidney at the end of pregnancy. This must be an extremely rare, almost theoretical situation.

REFERENCES

Brod J (1956) Chronic pyelonephritis. *Lancet,* **1,** 603.

Brown ADG (1978) The effect of pregnancy on the lower urinary tract. *Clin. Obstet. Gynecol.* **5,** 151.

Buchsbaum HJ, Schmidt JD (1973) The genito-urinary tract in pregnancy. In *Cynecologic and Obstetric Urology*. WB Saunders, Philadelphia.

Kincaid-Smith P, Bullen M (1965) Bacteriuria in pregnancy. *Lancet,* **1,** 395.

Leigh DA, Grunberg RN, Brumfitt W (1968) Long-term follow-up of bacteriuria in pregnancy. *Lancet,* **1,** 603.

Little P (1966) The incidence of urinary infection in 5000 pregnant women. *Lancet* **2,** 925.

Meares EMJr (1978) Urologic surgery during pregnancy. *Clin. Obstet. Gynecol.* **21,** 907.

Norden CW, Kass EH (1968) Bacteriuria of pregnancy: a critical appraisal. *Annu. Rev. Med.* **19,** 431.

Waltzer WC (1981) The urinary tract in pregnancy. *J. Urol.* **125,** 271.

Whalley PJ (1967) Bacteriuria of pregnancy. *Am. J. Obstet. Gynecol.* **97,** 723.

Appendix D Practical Help for the Woman with Urinary Incontinence

Urinary incontinence is an absolute bar to normal social intercourse. In many countries women with urinary fistulae are treated as unclean, like lepers. In the western world we like to think we are more enlightened, but, in practice, we treat urinary incontinence in exactly the same way. There is every reason, therefore, to help these people to live a more normal existence. Simple practical advice can be very effective and the equipment which is necessary is cheap and available in most countries. It is after all almost the same as has been developed for baby-care.

MANAGEMENT OF INCONTINENCE

For a variety of reasons, a number of gynaecological patients must live with incontinence of urine. In the great majority this is a temporary state of affairs, in the unlucky few it may be a permanent problem. Those with incontinence need help from the gynaecologist who has treated them and from their general practitioners if they are going to manage successfully at home. Some departments still demand a waiting period of many weeks or months to get rid of the necrotic tissue around a fistula. This is a tremendous burden on the patient and those who live with her. It is in many cases unneccessary but, as it has been an almost traditional method of treatment, there are still many patients who have to go through this waiting period.

More and more surgical and gynaecological departments have nursing sisters on their staff who are specialists who can advise and supervise incontinent patients before and after discharge from hospital. Local authorities have District Nurses and Health Visitors who are specially trained and can visit the patient in her home. These nursing sisters acquire so much practical experience that their advice to individual patients is of enormous value. They have seen all the problems associated with home life and have a solution to most of them. Above all they are optimistic and encouraging and able to lighten the heavy psychological burdens which inevitably worry incontinent patients. Help from one of these sisters is essential for the patient in whom leakage is a permanent problem, for example—the woman who has undergone several unsuccessful operations for stress incontinence. Under these conditions the help can sometimes be so effective that the patient prefers to continue in this way rather than embark on another operative attempt at cure or go over to a permanent urinary diversion. Practical guidance on the same lines is also needed for the woman with neurogenic bladder dysfunction.

Many countries have associations which can be of assistance; these are either publicly or privately supported and have branches in most of the bigger towns. They can give information on various types of absorbent material, special clothing and mechanical aids and can also tell the patient where and how to get them. They perform another useful function in that they allow the patient to meet others in a similar situation; this can be of great practical help in many cases. They are often the same associations who are so helpful with ileostomy and colostomy patients.

There is no completely satisfactory appliance for incontinent women to wear. Intravaginal tampons and similar devices which are primarily designed for use during menstruation have a limited power of absorbing urine and for this reason are inadequate except for very short periods where the leakage is minimal. They can be used with some success where there is a fistula from one ureter because the volume of urine is less, but are on the whole unsatisfactory and must always be worn with an external absorbent pad in case movement squeezes urine out from a soaked intravaginal tampon. Intravaginal devices which mechanically compress the urethra, such as rings, pessaries and inflatable balloons, can be tried and are sometimes successful in severe stress incontinence.

Most patients therefore rely on external absorbent pads without any intravaginal tampon and choose one of the many varieties which are combined with a pair of plastic pants designed to protect the clothing. Newer materials have been used with success such as duralite, which is a specially treated nylon, and the fabric which has been developed primarily for the use of cross-country skiers. This is non-absorbent, it allows the passage through it of sweat or urine which is absorbed by a layer of material on the outside. This is very comfortable to wear and avoids irritation of the skin by direct contact with urine and the chilling effect of contact with a soaked pad or garment. This principle is used in the pants where the absorbent pad is worn in a pouch on the outside of a tight-fitting garment (Fig. D1). The pad is changed without removing the pants. Daily washing is

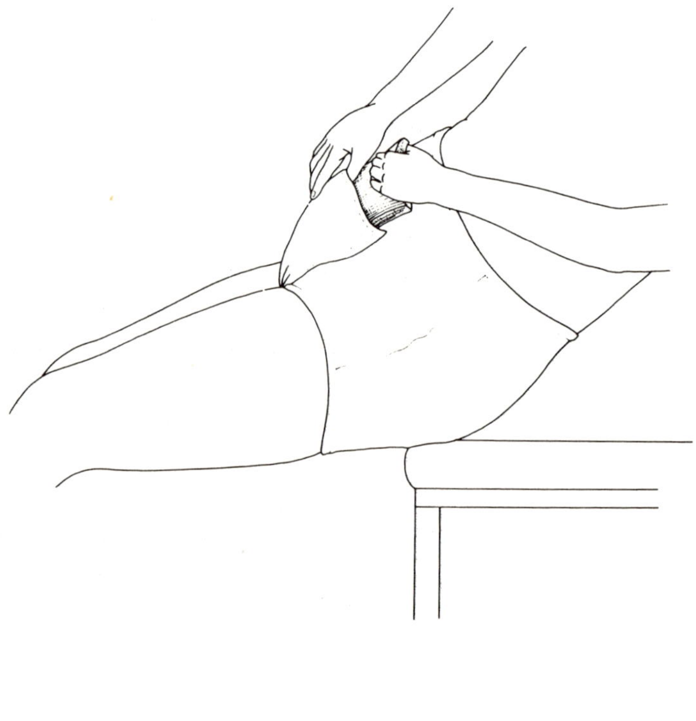

Fig. D1. Absorbent pad placed in pocket in tight-fitting pants of special material.

necessary otherwise the pants cease to function correctly. They should not be used at night, for alterations of position during sleep will cause leakage around the sides of the pad. They can be very effective while the patient is active during the day. Several types of stretch fabric have been used to make pants which simply keep a pad in position and disposable pants are, of course, on the market made of thin plastic material shaped like a bikini which retains the pad in position.

The pads themselves can be obtained washable or disposable and in various sizes or thicknesses. The patient can also make them herself from items obtained on prescription from her doctor if she lives in either Britain or Scandinavia or in several other countries (Fig. D2). The absorbent cotton wool is worn next to the skin, the gauze serves to retain the layers in position.

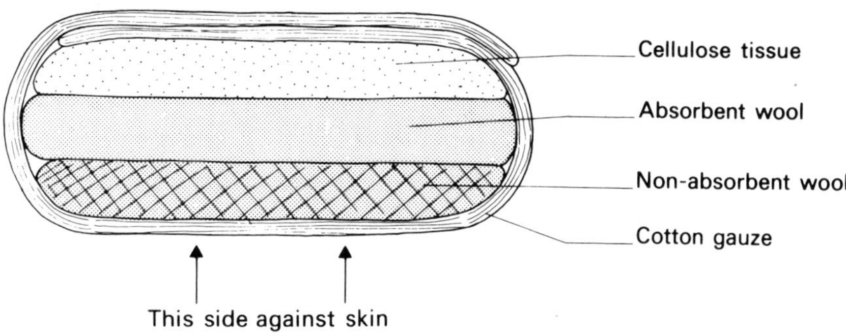

Fig. D2. Method of making up absorbent pad from layers of material.

A pad of this type can absorb up to about 250 ml over a period of several hours, but in practice is reliable up to 150–200 ml. This means changing 4 to 6 times a day. Special deodorants are available and should be used to avoid the ammoniacal smell of decomposing urine.

The areas of skin which come into more or less continuous contact with urine should be treated carefully by frequent washing with baby soap. Antiseptics and antiseptic soaps should not be used because they may irritate the skin and produce a mild inflammatory reaction. The skin should in fact be treated in exactly the same way as a baby's skin in the napkin area. The patient may well know more about this than her doctor.

During the night protective pants are unsatisfactory except where the urine leakage is very slight. It is often better to sleep on absorbent material which is laid across the bed on top of a plastic sheet which protects the ordinary sheet and mattress; these absorbent pads measure 75×60 cms and can absorb up to 500 ml of urine without discomfort. Advice on suitable clothing should be obtained as this helps the patient to lead a more normal social life.

In many countries there are special shops where experts give advice and can help by providing equipment. Information can usually be obtained through urological and gynaecological departments of hospitals, who are well informed about the various possibilities for help in their locality.

REFERENCES

Mandelstam, Dorothy (1977) *Incontinence*. Heinemann Health Books, London.

Stanton SL (1977) *Female Urinary Incontinence*. Lloyd-Luke, London.

Shepherd AM, Blannin JP (1980) A clinical trial of pants and pads used for urinary incontinence. *Nursing Times*, **76**, 1015.

Index